Evidence-Based Practices and Treatments for Children with Autism

D1264814

Evidence-Based Practices and Treatments for Children with Autism

Brian Reichow

YALE CHILD STUDY CENTER, NEW HAVEN, CT, USA

Peter Doehring

CHILDREN'S HOSPITAL OF PHILADELPHIA, PHILADELPHIA, PA, USA

Domenic V. Cicchetti

YALE CHILD STUDY CENTER, NEW HAVEN, CT, USA

FRED R. VOLKMAR

YALE CHILD STUDY CENTER, NEW HAVEN, CT, USA

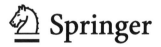

Editors
Brian Reichow
Yale Child Study Center
New Haven, CT
USA
brian.reichow@yale.edu

Domenic V. Cicchetti
Yale Child Study Center
New Haven, CT
USA
dom.cicchetti@yale.edu

Peter Doehring
The Children's Hospital
of Philadelphia
Philadelphia, PA
USA
doehringp@email.chop.edu

Fred R. Volkmar
Yale Child Study Center
New Haven, CT
USA
fred.volkmar@yale.edu

ISBN 978-1-4419-6973-6 (hardcover)   e-ISBN 978-1-4419-6975-0
ISBN 978-1-4419-6974-3 (softcover)
DOI 10.1007/978-1-4419-6975-0
Springer New York Dordrecht Heidelberg London

Springer is part of Springer Science+Business Media (www.springer.com)

CONTENTS

PART I
INTRODUCTION

Chapter 1
Evidence-Based Practices in Autism: Where We Started 3
Brian Reichow and Fred R. Volkmar

Chapter 2
Development, Procedures, and Application of the Evaluative Method for Determining Evidence-Based Practices in Autism 25
Brian Reichow

Chapter 3
On the Reliability and Accuracy of the Evaluative Method for Identifying Evidence-Based Practices in Autism 41

Domenic V. Cicchetti

PART II
TREATMENT REVIEWS

Chapter 4
Evidence-Based Treatment of Behavioral Excesses and Deficits for Individuals with Autism Spectrum Disorders 55

*Michael D. Powers, Mark J. Palmieri, Kristen S. D'Eramo,
and Kristen M. Powers*

Chapter 5
Evidence-Based Treatments in Communication for Children with Autism Spectrum Disorders 93

Patricia A. Prelock, Rhea Paul, and Elizabeth M. Allen

Chapter 6
Treatments to Increase Social Awareness and Social Skills 171

Suzannah J. Ferraioli and Sandra L. Harris

Chapter 7
Cognitive Behavioral Therapy in High-Functioning Autism: Review and Recommendations for Treatment Development 197

Jeffrey J. Wood, Cori Fujii, and Patricia Renno

Chapter 8
Psychopharmacology in Children with PDD: Review of Current Evidence 231

Lawrence Scahill and Susan Griebell Boorin

PART III
RESEARCH TO PRACTICE

Chapter 12
Practicing Evidence-Based Practices 309
Ruth Blennerhassett Eren and Pamela Owen Brucker

Chapter 13
The Implementation of Evidence-Based Practices in Public Schools 343
Peter Doehring and Vincent Winterling

Chapter 14
Evidence-Based Practices in Autism: Where We Are Now and Where We Need to Go 365
Fred R. Volkmar, Brian Reichow, and Peter Doehring

FOREWORD

In the past decade, we have witnessed increased public and media attention on autism and its spectrum disorders. Public attention also has brought to the fore the enormous impact the diagnosis of autism can have on parents and families. These parents embark on a path with many questions and a search for answers. Among the most critical of questions is, "what can be done to help my child now?" The urgency that families experience in seeking alternative courses of action is met with a vast array of programs, fixes, and seemingly definitive answers, many of which have no basis in fact and can even distract from very promising options. The urgent question of individual families is embraced by the science community as well – both seek to identify whether there are interventions, treatments, programs, or regimens that genuinely help. We need a resource that can tell us what we know based on the most recent and rigorous evidence and what seems very promising that is in the process of development. We finally have that resource and are indebted to the editors and contributors of this book in bringing it to fruition. The book covers a broad array of interventions – psychosocial, educational, biological, and alternative therapies – and sifts through a vast amount of research to draw informed conclusions.

Evaluation of treatments for autism spectrum disorders is challenging to say the least. Autism encompasses several domains of functioning that are appropriate targets for intervention. Communication and language, social skills, repetitive and self-stimulatory behaviors, limits in play and self-care, and hyperactivity, anxiety, and other areas of functioning may or may not be involved in the symptom presentation and in varying degrees and combinations. Evaluation of treatment outcome is complex because there is no single critical outcome that is a common metric for all approaches or for all children. Contrast this with interventions directed toward more circumscribed goals (e.g., reducing blood pressure or eliminating an infection) and the challenge becomes clear. Thus, evaluation of treatment requires a tempered view that eschews simple answers and verdicts about one or two treatments having "the" answer. Autism's many facets preclude a single answer, at least at present.

Treatments for autism vary in their focus and comprehensiveness. A very successful program in relation to social behavior or communication may leave untouched other domains of functioning that also are in need of intervention. Even within a given domain (e.g., social behavior), the goals (e.g., interpreting social cues, listening to others, or interacting) may vary for different interventions and for youths of different ages (e.g., preschool, teens). We want to satisfy the query of which treatment is better, but more often than not the treatments have not been compared and, because of varied goals, are not directly comparable.

The task of presenting treatments that have evidence is not all that straightforward. The quality and quantity of evidence represent as much of a spectrum as does autism. Controlled research is difficult to conduct and sacrifices often need to be made along the way in deciding whom to include, what will be evaluated after treatment, whether and how long follow-up will be conducted, and more. Thus, one does not merely tally the studies in support of an intervention and convey the count. As accomplished in this book, it is critical to elaborate the nuances of the evidence and how they will be addressed to reach meaningful conclusions.

The success of this book stems from how these and other complexities are handled. It would have been understandable if the editors and contributors conveyed that the topic is too complex or that we do not know enough to reach any conclusions at this time. When it comes to clinically relevant topics and the lives of individuals, this would be academia gone awry. The important problems in science (and life) invariably are complex and action is required without knowing all that we would like or even need to know. The editors and contributors were keenly aware of this, acknowledge the complexities, and still give us meaningful and helpful conclusions. The book brings together a remarkable set of chapters that embrace complexity, convey what we know that can be useful now, and identify what the next steps ought to be to ensure further progress.

There is a natural tension in science that encompasses hope and frustration. Hope stems from advances in our understanding and breakthrough findings (e.g., a new diagnostic method, very early identification of a clinical problem, a genetic or neurological underpinning). These advances are pregnant with implications that something useful is close at hand and will make a difference. Frustration stems from the fact that, as with any pregnancy, there is a gestation period and implications may not be delivered quickly enough to those in need of help right now. The book bridges the gap between hope and frustration by conveying that there are interventions that make a difference now. Progress in research is still needed but much has been made. As work continues, an equally daunting challenge is to ensure that our best interventions at present reach the public and those who provide services to them. The editors of this book have made remarkable contributions to understanding autism already and we are indebted to them for yet another such contribution on the key topic – what do we know that will help – based on our best science, presented by a stellar list of contributors.

Alan E. Kazdin
Yale University
2010

Brian Reichow, Ph.D., is currently an Associate Research Scientist at the Yale Child Study Center and Coordinator of Action-Based Research for the Autism Center of Excellence at Southern Connecticut State University. He began his training in autism at the University of North Carolina at Chapel Hill, where he earned undergraduate degrees in Psychology and Elementary Education and completed his graduate training in Special Education at Vanderbilt University. Before returning for his graduate degrees, he was a teacher of children with autism in the public schools of North Carolina. He has used his experience and knowledge from being a teacher to help guide his research, which focuses on increasing the effectiveness and efficiency of instruction for children with autism, identifying evidence-based practices for individuals with autism, and increasing the use of evidence-based practices in classrooms.

Peter Doehring, Ph.D., is currently Director of Regional Programs at the Center for Autism Research, at The Children's Hospital of Philadelphia and The University of Pennsylvania. He works to describe, implement, and research programs for training and intervention related to autism spectrum disorders (ASDs). He is particularly interested in how we might build capacity for evidence-based assessment, education, and treatment in community-based settings that are accessible to a broad and diverse population. He was originally trained in Canada as a clinical-research psychologist, where he worked to develop research and early intervention programs for children with ASD at the local and regional level. From 1999 until 2008, he served as statewide Director for the Delaware Autism Program (DAP), one of the largest and most comprehensive public school programs specializing in ASD in the USA.

Domenic V. Cicchetti, Ph.D., is a Yale psychologist and statistician with a longstanding interest in analyses of rating scales and reliability data. As the author of numerous articles and a textbook, he has published extensively in the area of autism including work on the reliability of rating scales, of diagnostic criteria, innovative approaches to diagnosis, screening tests, and assessment of agreement on treatment effects and rating scales. Corecipient (with Dr. Sara Sparrow) of the first Connecticut Psychological Association's "Award for Distinguished Effort by a Connecticut Psychologist, Utilizing Psychological Knowledge and Skills, Which Has Made A Material Contribution to the Welfare of the Public" at Fairfield Connecticut, on December 7, 1984. The award was for the development and publication of the Vineland Adaptive Behavior Scales (Sparrow, Balla, and Cicchetti, 1984). He is also a Fellow in the American Statistical Association, the highest award the organization can bestow upon its members.

The award was given "For contributions in behavioral and biomedical statistics, particularly assessment of psychometric properties of clinical diagnostic instruments, and for innovative methodologies for interexaminer reliability assessments."

Fred R. Volkmar, M.D., is the Irving B. Harris Professor of Child Psychiatry, Pediatrics, and Psychology and Director of the Yale Child Study Center, Yale University School of Medicine. An international authority on Asperger's disorder and autism, Dr. Volkmar was the primary author of the DSM-IV autism and pervasive developmental disorders section. He has authored several hundred scientific papers and has coedited numerous books, including *Asperger Syndrome, A Practical Guide to Autism*, and the third edition of *The Handbook of Autism and Pervasive Developmental Disorders*. He has served as associate editor of the *Journal of Autism*, the *Journal of Child Psychology and Psychiatry*, and the *American Journal of Psychiatry*. He has also served as co-chairperson of the autism/MR committee of the American Academy of Child and Adolescent Psychiatry. Starting in March 2007, he became editor of the *Journal of Autism and Developmental Disorders*.

CONTRIBUTORS

Elizabeth M. Allen
Department of Communication
Sciences and Disorders,
University of Vermont, Burlington,
VT, USA

Susan Griebell Boorin
Yale Child Study Center,
Yale School of Medicine,
New Haven, CT, USA

Pamela Owen Brucker
Department of Special Education
and Reading, Southern Connecticut
State University, New Haven, CT, USA

Domenic V. Cicchetti
Yale Child Study Center,
Yale School of Medicine,
New Haven, CT, USA

Peter Doehring
The Children's Hospital of Philadelphia,
The University of Pennsylvania,
Philadelphia, PA, USA

Kristen S. D'Eramo
The Center for Children with
Special Needs, Glastonbury, CT,
USA

Ruth Blennerhassett Eren
Department of Special Education
and Reading, Southern Connecticut
State University, New Haven, CT, USA

Suzannah J. Ferraioli
Douglas Developmental
Disabilities Center, Rutgers,
The State University of New Jersey,
New Brunswick, NJ, USA

Cori Fujii
UCLA Department of Education,
University of California at Los Angeles,
Los Angeles, CA, USA

Sandra L. Harris
Douglas Developmental Disabilities
Center, Rutgers, The State University
of New Jersey, New Brunswick,
NJ, USA

Susan L. Hyman
Golisano Children's Hospital at Strong,
University of Rochester, Rochester, NY,
USA

Alan E. Kazdin
Department of Psychology,
Yale University, New Haven, CT, USA

Susan E. Levy
The Children's Hospital of Philadelphia,
The University of Pennsylvania,
Philadelphia, PA, USA

Mark J. Palmieri
The Center for Children with Special
Needs, Glastonbury, CT, USA

Rhea Paul
Yale Child Study Center,
Yale School of Medicine,
New Haven, CT, USA

Kristen M. Powers
The Center for Children with Special
Needs, Glastonbury, CT, USA

Michael D. Powers
The Center for Children with Special
Needs, Glastonbury, CT, USA
Yale Child Study Center,
Yale School of Medicine,
New Haven, CT, USA

Patricia A. Prelock
Department of Communication Sciences
and Disorders, University of Vermont,
Burlington, VT, USA

Brian Reichow
Yale Child Study Center,
Yale School of Medicine,
New Haven, CT, USA

Patricia Renno
UCLA Department of Education,
University of California at Los Angeles,
Los Angeles, CA, USA

Celine Saulnier
Yale Child Study Center,
Yale School of Medicine,
New Haven, CT, USA

Lawrence Scahill
Yale Child Study Center,
Yale School of Medicine,
New Haven, CT, USA

Roseann C. Schaaf
Department of Occupational Therapy,
Thomas Jefferson University,
Philadelphia, PA, USA

Sara S. Sparrow
Yale Child Study Center,
Yale School of Medicine,
New Haven, CT, USA

Katherine D. Tsatsanis
Yale Child Study Center,
Yale School of Medicine,
New Haven, CT, USA

Fred R. Volkmar
Yale Child Study Center, Yale School
of Medicine, New Haven CT, USA

Vincent Winterling
Delaware Autism Program,
Wilmington, DE, USA

Jeffrey J. Wood
UCLA Department of Education,
University of California at
Los Angeles, Los Angeles, CA, USA

PART I

Introduction

CHAPTER 1

Evidence-Based Practices in Autism: Where We Started

Brian Reichow and Fred R. Volkmar

ABBREVIATIONS

ABA	Applied behavior analysis
APA	American Psychological Association
ASDs	Autism spectrum disorders
ASHA	American Speech–Language–Hearing Association
DSM-III	Diagnostic and Statistical Manual of Mental Disorders 3rd edition
DSM-IV	Diagnostic and Statistical Manual of Mental Disorders 4th edition
EBM	Evidence-based medicine
EBP	Evidence-based practice*
EBT	Evidence-based treatment
EIBI	Early intensive behavioral intervention
EST	Empirically supported treatment
FAPE	Free and appropriate public education
FDA	Food and Drug Administration
ICD-10	International Classification of Diseases and Related Health Problems 10th edition
IDEA	Individuals with Disabilities Education Act
IEP	Individualized education program
ISP	Individualized support program
LEAP	Learning experiences and alternative programs for preschoolers and their parents
LRE	Least restrictive environment
NRC	National Research Council
PECOT	Patient exposure to intervention, control group, outcome, and time course

*In the social sciences the conceptualization of evidence-based medicine assumed multiple names (e.g., evidence-based treatments, empirically supported treatments, evidence-based practice). Although some researchers point out intricate differences between the terminologies (see Drake et al. 2004; Kazdin 2008; Hamilton 2007) the term "evidence-based practice (EBP)" is used for the remainder of this book (unless otherwise noted) to represent the process of using empirical evidence, clinical judgment, and client values to make treatment decisions.

B. Reichow et al. (eds.), *Evidence-Based Practices and Treatments for Children with Autism*, DOI 10.1007/978-1-4419-6975-0_1, © Springer Science+Business Media, LLC 2011

PICO   Problem intervention,
            comparison, outcome
PRT   Pivotal response treatment
RCT   Randomized control trial
SIGN   Scottish Intercollegiate
            Guidelines Network
SSED   Single subject experimental
            design
TEACCH   Treatment and Education of
            Autistic and Communication
            related handicapped Children
UCLA   University of California at
            Los Angeles

WHERE WE STARTED

Sadly, the early history of intervention research in autism (1943–1980) can be relatively briefly summarized. In his initial description of autism, Kanner (1943) provided some follow-up information on the cases he had seen. Apart from one child "dumped in a school for the feeble minded" (Kanner 1943: 249), the other children (then between 9 and 11) had shown some development of social skills although fundamental social difficulties remained. Kanner's original paper was not particularly concerned with intervention and, over the years, the varying conceptualizations of autism have led to marked changes in intervention. The emphasis on parental success and some social oddity (which was also noted by Kanner, who emphasized it because he believed the disorder to be congenital and hence not likely entirely attributable to psychopathology in the parents) led various clinicians in the 1950s to postulate a strong role for experience in the pathogenesis of autism (Bettelheim 1950; Despert 1971) and to mistaken attempts to "fix" the child through psychotherapy. Such attempts persist in some countries, particularly France, to the present day even though prominent analysts, such as Anna Freud, cautioned against such notions (see

the review by Riddle in 1987). Diagnostic controversy (e.g., whether autism was the earliest form of "childhood schizophrenia") also contributed to confusion about best treatment practices. However, the growing recognition that autism was a biologically based condition (Rimland 1964) coupled with evidence that it was not the earliest manifestation of schizophrenia (Kolvin 1971; Rutter 1972) and had a strong genetic basis (Folstein and Rutter 1977) and a strong brain basis (Cohen and Young 1977) led to a major shift in thinking and stimulated a large, and ever expanding, body of research on these conditions (Volkmar, in press). It became clear that efforts to remediate autism via intensive psychotherapy were also misguided (Riddle 1987) and that structured educational (Bartak and Rutter 1973; Schopler et al. 1971) and behavioral (Ferster 1961; Lovaas et al. 1966a, b, 1971) interventions were associated with positive behavior change.

Educational interventions in the 1950s and 1960s were, at best (and when available), spotty. Schools could, and did, decline to serve students whose behavior was more challenging. Children with autism were frequently turned away from schools and their parents were advised to place them in residential institutions. Fortunately, some parents did not heed this advice and either found schools willing to work with their child or started programs of their own. These programs, many of which continue to exist today, were some of the first to implement behavioral and drug treatments for autism (Greden and Groden 1997; Lettick 1981; Simonson et al. 1990; Sullivan 2005). A host of interventions was tried including a vast array of medications, reinforcement schedules and paradigms, and aversive conditioning techniques. Much of this early work remains difficult to interpret given the small sample studies, lack of controls, and often lack of clarity about what was actually being studied. Several factors led to improved research on treatments for autism.

During the 1970s, several lines of evidence began to suggest that autism was a distinctive disorder, apart from other conditions, childhood schizophrenia in particular. The recognition of autism as an official diagnostic category in the landmark *Diagnostic and Statistical Manual*, 3rd edition (DSM-III; American Psychiatric Association 1980) facilitated both research and public awareness of the condition. Well before DSM-III appeared, the founding, in 1971, of the *Journal of Autism and Developmental Disorders* (originally called the *Journal of Autism and Childhood Schizophrenia*) provided an important forum for research to be disseminated. Intervention programs began to be more closely allied with universities and research programs. These programs took various forms. For example, the Treatment and Education of Autistic and Communication related handicapped Children (TEACCH) program was founded by Eric Schopler in 1972 as a statewide program for children in North Carolina (Mesibov et al. 2005; Schopler 1997). The TEACCH model was eclectic, drawing from structured teaching, work with parents, and specific curricular materials. Programs based in technologies derived from the field of applied behavior analysis (ABA), such as the UCLA Young Autism Project directed by Lovaas (Lovaas 1987; Lovaas and Smith 1988) became increasingly sophisticated with expansion into new areas of behavioral intervention including pivotal response treatment (PRT) approaches (Koegel and Koegel 2006; Schreibman and Koegel 1996; Schreibman and Ingersoll 2005) and incidental teaching (McGee et al. 1999). Other programs emphasized more developmental principles, e.g., the Denver model began in 1981 as a demonstration day treatment project (Rogers et al. 2000). Sometimes programs were originally based at a center, e.g., the Douglas Developmental Center at Rutgers University (Harris et al. 2005), and were designed to serve older children; often, as was true at Douglas, the focus expanded to include preschool children and an emphasis on treatment in more integrated settings. Some models, such as the individualized support program (ISP) at the University of South Florida (Dunlap and Fox 1999), were concerned with parent training while others, such as those developed by Strain and colleagues as the Learning Experiences and Alternative Programs (LEAP) for preschoolers and their parents (Strain 2001; Strain and Hoyson 2000) were concerned with facilitating peer-mediated social interactions.

Much of the early research in autism suffered from serious limitations. Although behavioral studies frequently used rigorous single subject experimental designs (SSEDs), there were relatively few studies and they typically contained small samples. Given the disparate research traditions of the various disciplines involved in studying autism there were often basic failures in integrating research findings with clinical work. Further complicating the picture were the multiple lines of research that proceeded quite independently from each other, with few attempts to look at treatments in combination. Even within the area of psychopharmacology, which has a long tradition of large-sample controlled studies, randomized control trials (RCTs) were relatively few.

Legislation and judicial decisions had an important impact on treatment and, indirectly, on models of treatment and research on service and service delivery. Before 1975, probably a minority of children with serious disabilities (of all kinds) received an education within public school settings. Schools could, and often would, turn away students who they felt could not be appropriately provided for within the public school setting. In many schools, parents would be turned away and were often told to put their children in institutional settings where there was little proactive programming or education and limited opportunities for the child to acquire relevant, adaptive, "real-life" skills (Volkmar and Wiesner 2009). As a result, many individuals with autism were placed in these institutions; probably unsurprisingly, the major function of such placements was that it helped them learn to live in (i.e., remain in) institutions and outcomes were often poor (Howlin 2005). Some parents, particularly of more able children, were able to provide an educational program or start their own specialized treatment programs.

Passage of the Education for All Handicapped Children Act (Public Law 94–142) in 1975 by the United States Congress marked a sea change for children with autism, their parents, and public schools because it established the child's right to access a free and appropriate public education (FAPE) within mainstream settings – the "least restrictive" environment (LRE). The Individuals with Disabilities Education Act (IDEA; Public Law 108–446, § 118 Stat 2647) applies to early education as well as school based and transitional services. It and a related law, the Americans with Disabilities Act (Public Law 101–336, § 12101 Stat. 327 1990) provide specifically for support to enable children with autism and other developmental and psychiatric disabilities to attend public school. The law mandated a "free and appropriate public education" with disability determination and needs based on assessment of the child and with a number of safeguards in place to protect the rights of the child to such an education. The development of a data-based individualized educational plan (IEP) was a further stimulus to the use of data in monitoring the effectiveness of school-based services. Similar legislation in the United Kingdom mandated special services with major changes in educational practice (see the discussion by Farrell 2009). As we discuss later, mandates for providing services below the usual age of school entry, i.e., to infants and toddlers, had important implications, particularly for young children with autism.

Several other factors also impacted intervention programs and research on treatment during this period. In addition to Public Law 94–142, a series of court decisions began to change patterns of care for more severely disabled children and adults; these included entitlements to truly rehabilitative, as opposed to custodial, programming and community-based, as opposed to institutional, services; a number of long-standing institutions were forced to close (Berkman 1997; Mandlawitz 2005). As legal mandates for school-based services came into place, they converged with several lines of research findings that underscored the importance of exposure to peers as a source of learning and teaching (Charlop et al. 1983; Harris and Handleman 1997) and of the special importance, given the learning style in autism, of including an explicit focus on generalization (Koegel and Koegel 1995; Schreibman and Koegel 2005), communication (Paul and Sutherland 2005), and acquisition of adaptive "real-life" skills both in more cognitively impaired (Fenton et al. 2003) and higher functioning individuals (Klin et al. 2007).

These factors led to several major changes in programs providing service to children with autism. There was an increased focus on the use of schools as the major locus of intervention. Although models varied somewhat from state to state, the emphasis was on supporting children with autism, as much as possible, in general education classroom settings or, when this was not possible, including them in activities to the extent that this was appropriate (Koegel et al. 1999; Wolery et al. 1995). Similarly, the emphasis on generalization of skills led to greater inclusion of parents and family members, and community settings for teaching even for more cognitively and behaviorally challenged youngsters (Carr and Carlson 1993). These converging trends led many programs to consider changes in their format, e.g., with a move away from center-based to school-based and in-home services (through parent training) as well as to greater use of community teaching.

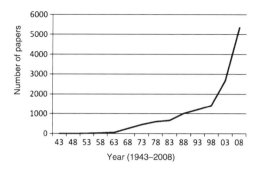

FIGURE 1.1

Number of Research Papers on "autism" Published between 1943 and 2008 Presented in 5 Year Blocks that were Located in the Medline Database

During the 1980s and 1990s, several factors led to major changes in how programs were provided. Research began to increase in both quality and quantity during this period (Volkmar, in press). Figure 1.1 shows rates of publication, in blocks of 5 years, from the first description of autism by Kanner in 1943 up to 2008.

Research began to increase in the late 1970s as a consensus on the validity and neurobiological basis of autism began to emerge. The publication of DSM-III in 1980 and the official recognition of autism was also a stimulus to this effort, as were the developments of various rating scales or checklists and other measures that facilitated subject characterization and research comparability. Similarly, the consensus in the (DSM-IV; American Psychiatric Association 1994) and its convergence with the *International Classification of Diseases and Related Health Problems*, 10th edition (ICD-10, World Health Organization 1992; Volkmar et al. 2009) together with increased federal support for research (particularly multi-site research) has resulted in a veritable explosion of work since 2000, with an average of over 500 peer-reviewed papers each year. The growing sophistication of the research literature was also reflected in studies of treatments. The ear-

lier literature on well-intended but unproductive psychotherapeutic interventions (Riddle 1987) gave way to more sophisticated research.

Biomedical work, including many of the early reports on pharmacological intervention, first consisted of case studies; studies of larger samples were relatively rare although with some important exceptions, such as the series of increasingly sophisticated studies of pharmacological interventions by Magda Campbell and colleagues (Anderson et al. 1984, 1989). Although pharmacological interventions were commonly used (Anderson et al. 1984), much of the available evidence was of rather limited quality. With some important exceptions (see Chap. 8), clinical trials often used small samples with inadequate subject characterization. Findings often failed to replicate and clinicians were left with relatively minimal guidance, although the advent of the various practice guidelines (Volkmar et al. 1999, in press) have provided some help in this regard. Although many different compounds have now been studied, only two have been approved by the US Food and Drug Administration (FDA) for use in autism (i.e., risperidone and aripiprazole). Unfortunately, in general, the core social-communication problems in autism have not been particularly responsive to pharmacological interventions, although there is some suggestion that combinations of psychopharmacology and behavioral or parent management training may help facilitate learning and adjustment to the school environment (see Chap. 8). In any case, it is important to be sure that pharmacological interventions do not have untoward effects on learning (Aman, Hollway et al. 2008).

As noted by Rogers (1998), much of the behavioral treatment literature in the 1990s had to do with highly focal and specific treatments. This large body of work clearly demonstrated evidence of effectiveness in dealing with problem behaviors, encouraging acquisition of more adaptive skills (Koegel and Koegel 1995; Schreibman 1998) and enhancing communicative abilities (Paul and Sutherland 2005). Many of the comprehensive model programs for children with autism also began to publish data related to the effectiveness of their model although, as Rogers noted (1998), only eight research groups have published studies of treatment efficacy focused on preschool children. Rogers noted weaknesses in the various studies (as well as some important strengths). These issues arose at several different levels. For example, in evaluating the original Lovaas (1987) report of major differences in IQ and school functioning as a result of early intensive behavioral intervention (EIBI), Rogers (1998) noted that strengths of the study included a (relatively) large sample with one treatment and two control groups; a treatment manual and supervision; blinded outcome data; and outcome data from various points in time. Weaknesses that Rogers noted were lack of random assignment to groups; failure to document actual treatment duration, i.e., the results might have been a result of treatment intensity rather than orientation (Dawson and Osterling 1997); issues in measurement selection, and so forth. Subsequent studies (although differing in some ways from the original study) did not demonstrate the same level of benefit as the initial study and at least one subsequent study (Smith et al. 2000) noted some of the difficulties inherent for parents undertaking an intensive treatment program, i.e., treatment fidelity was hard to maintain. Having reviewed eight treatment efficacy studies, Rogers' conclusion was that while positive outcomes were reported "the field does not yet have a treatment that meets the present criteria for well-established or probably efficacious treatment" (Rogers 1998: 168).

Beginning in the late 1990s and continuing today, there has been a veritable explosion in emphasis on evidence-based practice (EBP). To examine how this movement has impacted the treatment of individuals with autism spectrum disorders (ASDs), we first describe the history and components of EBP. Descriptions of various attempts at defining EBP in autism follow and the chapter concludes with our thoughts on the present state of EBP in autism.

WHAT IS EVIDENCE-BASED PRACTICE?

Evidence-Based Medicine

The conceptualization, ideals, and guidelines that have become evidence-based practice emerged first in the medical field as evidence-based medicine (EBM). A commonly cited definition for EBM (Sackett et al. 1996, 2000; Straus et al. 2005) postulates EBM as a multi-step process involving the best current evidence, clinical expertise, and patient choice. Drake et al. (2005) suggest EBM is based on five principles: a foundation of the philosophy and ethics of basic values; the need to consider scientific evidence as an important factor in decision making; the realization and recognition that scientific evidence is complicated, hierarchical, often ambiguous, and usually limited; the recognition that factors other than scientific evidence (including client values) are important in decision making; and the recognition that clinical expertise is an important factor in decision making. The medical definition of EBM has strayed little from this and recently the Institute of Medicine (2008) proposed a similar conceptualization and definition to the one provided by Sackett and colleagues. Although this is a widely accepted conceptualization of EBM, arguments against EBM have been raised (Drake et al. 2005), including lack of consensus opinions concerning the evidence, the lack of or limited quantities of evidence, and the opportunities for practitioner biases to influence decision making.

As conceptualized by Sackett et al. and expanded upon by others (Dawes et al. 2005; Hatcher et al. 2005), EBP is a multistep process. The first step of the process involves formulating a question at the level of the individual or population of concern relating to what one is trying to achieve. Within this step, two acronyms are frequently used to guide the question making: problem, intervention, comparison (if appropriate), outcome (PICO) and patient, exposure to intervention, control group, outcome, and time course (PECOT). The second step of the EBP process involves searching and finding the evidence related to this question. Hatcher et al. (2005) suggest many practitioners accomplish this step by asking other people or by checking textbooks, which are typically out of date. They highlight electronic databases as the most difficult but best method of searching for evidence (see Chap. 14). Helpful guidelines on searching for evidence have been provided by Lucas and Cutspec (2005), McHugo and Drake (2003), Petticrew and Roberts (2006), and Hamilton (2007). The third step of the EBP process involves critically appraising the evidence yielded in the search. Multiple methods have been outlined for accomplishing this process, including evidence grading schemes (Guyatt et al. 2008), systematic reviews (Higgins and Green 2008; Petticrew and Roberts 2006), meta-analysis (Borenstein et al. 2009), best-evidence synthesis (Slavin 1986), reviews of meta-analyses, and other systematic reviews (Becker and Oxman 2008; Hamilton 2007). All of these methods have advantages and disadvantages. The fourth step of the EBP process is taking the results of the synthesis and making a decision for practice. Depending on the context, e.g., planning an IEP for an individual child or provision of a model service delivery program to a school or school

district, this can take various forms. The fifth and final step of the EBP process is an iterative process that involves monitoring the success or failure of the practice that was implemented. This step provides an opportunity to adjust the model depending on feedback and make it increasingly effective and efficient.

Evidence-Based Practice in the Social Sciences

Since moving to the social sciences, the concept of EBP has been adopted and expanded to match the ideologies and traditions of the various disciplines within the social sciences. Most organizations representing individuals practicing in the social sciences now have a definition of EBP. However, reported use of EBP is low (Nelson and Steele 2007; Upton and Upton 2006) and the evidence on practitioner attitudes and perspectives of EBP are varied. Although many practitioners contend that EBP is an important activity that helps ensure sound decision are made, when surveyed practitioners frequently identify many barriers that prevent the practice of EBP (Pagoto et al. 2007; Nelson and Steele 2007; Salmond 2007). When lists of barriers and facilitators of EBP are compared, many factors (e.g., policy and consumer demand) appear on both lists, suggesting divergent attitudes to EBP remain. Pagoto et al. (2007) identified these divergent attitudes as the largest barrier to the implementation of EBP. Lack of training is also frequently identified as a barrier to the practice of EBP (Dulcan 2005; Pagoto et al. 2007; Nelson and Steele 2007; Salmond 2007). In a recent survey of practitioners, Upton and Upton (2006) showed that attitudes vary across fields and that many practitioners do not look for or use evidence from research conducted outside of their field. Because research in autism is conducted across many fields with different theoretical backgrounds and diverse research methods, it is imperative that researchers consider, acquire, and synthesize research across disciplines. Practitioner training programs should consider these and other priorities when designing educational courses and experiences for pre-service personnel (Lerman et al. 2004; Scheuermann et al. 2003); see Chap. 13.

Within psychology, in particular, there has been a strong, and growing, body of research on evidence-based treatments (EBT), sometimes referred to as empirically supported treatments (EST; Hamilton 2007) or evidence-based psychotherapies (Kazdin and Weisz 2003; Weisz and Kazdin 2010), with a focus on both the efficiency and effectiveness of specifically defined psychosocial interventions. In some contrast to the work within the EBM tradition, this body of research has tended to center on the study of specific, and well documented, psychosocial treatments. It might, for example, take the form of examining the efficacy of a specific therapy for depression, anxiety, or conduct disorder. A central concern within this tradition has been the focus on how applicable and generalizable the treatment model is from the (typical) university-based clinic within which it was developed to more "real-world" settings (typically, community mental health clinics or private practitioners).

As has been the case with EBM, the movement to EBP has not been free from debate (Chambless and Ollendick 2001; Sternberg 2006; Westen and Bradley 2005). Many organizations have reported difficulty defining the construct (Chorpita 2003; Hamilton 2007; Kazdin 2001) and have called for EBP definitions to contain greater specificity (Kazdin 2008). Other researchers have expressed a concern as to whether the medical model fits with the processes and goals of social science (Cutspec 2004). Researchers in the social sciences have also pointed out the difficulties of conducting large clinical

trials (Chorpita 2003), which has led to debate on how and if research designs other than the RCT should be included as evidence (Drake et al. 2004; Odom et al. 2005; Smith and Pell 2003). Further concern about the appropriateness and clinical utility of the outcome measures have also been raised (De Los Reyes and Kazdin 2006). These struggles and the divide between clinical knowledge and field practice have led some to question the utility of identifying EBP (Barkham and Mellor-Clark 2003). Ultimately, the EBP movement is a global movement that appears to be gaining strength and shows no signs of abating.

PREVIOUS DEFINITIONS OF EVIDENCE-BASED PRACTICE APPLIED TO RESEARCH IN AUTISM

The following review of definitions and criteria is intended to place EBP in the context of how it has been conceptualized and used with respect to research involving individuals with autism. We include an overview of definitions of EBP from organizations representing practitioners or clinicians who work with individuals who have autism. As stated above, research in autism is conducted by researchers across many fields using diverse scientific research methodologies. Therefore, we felt it necessary to provide an overview of the multiple interpretations of EBP in autism research. This is not intended to provide an exhaustive review of the applications of EBP in autism, but rather a representative sample from medicine, psychology, and education. Accompanying the review of definitions are descriptions of how the respective organizations applied their criteria to interventions for individuals with autism.

Medical Definitions

Although the exact etiology of autism remains unknown, it is frequently considered and treated as a medical condition. Therefore, many individuals within the medical field are involved in the treatment of children with autism. While most fields within medicine follow the definition of EBP outlined by Sackett et al. (2000), many organizations have provided specific criteria for EBP that have been applied to interventions and practices for individuals with autism.

Food and Drug Administration (FDA). In the United States, the FDA is a federal agency that is responsible for protecting and advancing the public's health, including approving and regulating medication. To gain approval from the FDA, a drug must be shown to be safe and effective through a multi-stage clinical trial process. One example of an application of evidence standards to the treatment of autism in the medical field is the recent approval of risperidone for the treatment of irritability (i.e., serious behavioral problems) in children and adolescents with autism between the ages of five and 16 (McDougle et al. 2005; Scahill et al. 2007). Recently, aripiprazole was also approved for the treatment of irritability in individuals with autism aged between six and 17 (Bristol-Myers Squib 2009). Although other medications are commonly used off-label for the treatment of symptoms associated with autism (see Chap. 8), risperidone and aripiprazole are the only medications that have met the evidence standards of the FDA.

American Academy of Neurology. This organization has recently updated its guidelines for evaluating the efficacy of research and treatments (French and Gronseth 2008; Gronseth and French 2008). In these guidelines, randomized control trials are the preferred method for obtaining the top rating for strength of evidence. However, consistent with these guidelines (Gronseth and French 2008), the top strength of recommendation category (standard) could be achieved using evidence from other research designs when randomized clinical trials are not possible. The guidelines also contain a method for quantifying the strength of the evidence for individual articles, which are then integrated into three categories of strength of recommendation (in order from the highest level: standard, guideline, and practice option). Filipek et al. (2000) adopted an earlier version of the guidelines and applied them to the screening and diagnosis of autism. Their practice parameter outlines a two-level process of routine developmental surveillance for all children and diagnostic evaluation for ASD when risk is detected. Two practices, genetic testing and selective metabolic testing, received the highest level of recommendation.

Speech-language pathology. The American Speech–Language–Hearing Association (ASHA) is the professional, scientific, and credentialing organization for individuals working in the speech and hearing sciences. It has defined EBP with an emphasis on the integration of empirical evidence, clinical expertise, and client values (Robey et al. 2004). Mullen (2007) recently outlined ASHA's Level of Evidence System for the appraisal of studies. This presentation emphasized the importance of including and giving equal weight to research conducted using multiple research methodologies and the idea that research can be summarized even when different research methods are used. One contribution to the development of EBP in autism was the recent publication of guidelines for speech–language pathologists (ASHA 2006). Although written for speech–language pathologists, the guidelines provide a nice summary of many aspects of working with individuals with autism that bridges disciplines including assessment, screening, diagnosis, intervention, and program planning.

Medical insurance companies. Recently two major US medical insurance companies have conducted systematic reviews (Blue Cross and Blue Shield 2009; Cigna 2008) with respect to interventions for children with ASD. The reports do not provide an exhaustive review of insurance company reports on ASD but they highlight the increasing oversight by these companies to ensure that practices for children with ASD are EBP. As the EBP movement continues to gain momentum, this trend is likely to increase. A specific question addressed in the report from Blue Cross and Blue Shield (2009) centered on the efficacy of early intensive behavioral intervention. After conducting a review of 16 intervention studies, the company determined that the quality of the research and inconsistent results did not permit conclusions about the efficacy of the intervention to be drawn. The coverage guidelines provided by Cigna were more comprehensive in scope and covered a broad range of diagnostic, assessment, and treatment issues. The summary of the guidelines conclude that no medical cure has been established for autism; that educational and psychosocial services can be helpful; and that a number of treatments have no empirical support for their efficacy (these treatments are listed in the guidelines). Because Cigna has many different insurance plans, specific declarations about which treatments would or would not be covered could not be made (individuals were referred to their specific plan documents).

The emphasis placed on EBP in the medical fields involved with autism is large. Unfortunately, much discrepancy exists in how "evidence" has been defined. Part of this discrepancy is likely due to the large area of science covered in the medical field (e.g., allied health services, surgery, genetics, basic sciences). In their discussions of EBP, Sackett and colleagues emphasized that the process of EBP should not be restricted to evidence obtained from randomized trials and meta-analyses. Additional researchers have also called for a broader inclusion of multiple research methods (Drake et al. 2004). However, some individuals in the medical field cling to a reliance, for their highest levels of recommendation, on a definition of EBP limited to demonstration of superiority to a control condition in two randomized clinical trials conducted by independent research teams. As such, differing opinions exist on what treatments are considered EBP. Because few interventions have been evaluated using RCTs, the reliance on this type of evidence is likely to lead to inaccurate conclusions.

Mental Health Definitions

Child and adolescent psychiatry. The American Academy of Child and Adolescent Psychiatry has a long standing commitment to inclusion of EBP in its series of practice parameters – essentially evidence-based guidelines for practicing clinicians. These guidelines, including those published, focus on a range of disorders including autism (Volkmar et al. 1999, in press) as well as on specific interventions including drug treatments (Walkup et al. 2009). Although EBP is emphasized in many psychiatric training programs and texts (Hamilton 2007) and many individuals with autism encounter psychiatrists in diagnosis or treatment, the impact and presence of EBP has been less visible and influential than in other disciplines, such as psychology.

Psychology. To address evidence-based practices in psychology, the American Psychological Association (APA) formed the Task Force on Psychological Interventions to determine a set of guidelines that could be used to evaluate psychotherapies for children (Chambless et al. 1996; Chambless and Hollon 1998). The guidelines established three levels of EBP (in order from the highest level: well-established, probably efficacious, and experimental).

The subsequent guidelines marked one of the first definitions of EBP in a social science and formed a foundation from which other divisions within the APA would use to define EBP. The definition of EBP in psychology has an emphasis on the triad of elements from Sackett et al. (2000). The original guidelines (Chambless et al. 1996) have undergone constant scrutiny and debate (Norcross et al. 2005; Stuart and Lilienfeld 2007; Wampold et al. 2007; Wendt and Slife 2007) and were recently updated (APA Presidential Task Force on Evidence-Based Practice 2006).

Lonigan et al. (1998) incorporated and modified the APA guidelines for the Society of Clinical Child and Adolescent Psychology (currently APA Division 53). Their guidelines were very similar to the guidelines of the APA Task Force except for two key issues: a manual was not required for a treatment to receive the top rating of efficacy and they quantified the number of participants from SSED necessary for a treatment to be an evidence-based practice (e.g., three separate studies with at least nine participants). It should be noted that the third level (possibly efficacious) can be reached with evidence from one empirical investigation.

An early application of APA EBP standards to interventions for children with autism was conducted by Rogers (1998). The review noted that there were no RCTs that had been conducted on interventions for young children with autism and ultimately concluded that none of the eight comprehensive programs reviewed demonstrated the evidence needed to meet the criteria of EBP. Recently, Rogers and Vismara (2008) have provided an updated review of early intervention programs for the 10-year follow up (Silverman and Hinshaw 2008). Rogers and Vismara noted that several RCTs had demonstrated both short and longer term effects and that these included both improved functioning overall as well as lower levels of maladaptive behavior. On the other hand, they noted that, given the limited data available, the issues of which interventions had most effect, which variables moderate these effects, and the degree to which improvement could be expected remained areas of controversy. Rogers and Vismara (2008) reviewed five RCTs and evidence from several quasi-experimental studies on early interventions for young children with autism. Using the typology from the studies of Nathan and Gorman (2002, 2007), which range from Type 1 (RCTs) to Type 6 (case reports), Rogers and Vismara noted that most studies did not meet the highest criteria (Type 1) for rigor; most were classified as Type 2, which was expanded to include SSEDs, or Type 3. Based on their review, treatments based on the ABA model of Lovaas (1987) received the highest level of recommendation (well-established), pivotal response treatments (Koegel and Koegel 2006) received the second level of recommendation (probably efficacious), and three interventions received the third level of recommendation (possibly efficacious). It should be noted that those three treatments (a direct service model with parent training component (Jocelyn et al. 1998); a home-based, parent-delivered, developmental intervention (Drew et al. 2002); and a parent-delivered, pragmatic language treatment (Aldred et al. 2004)) were given this status based on the results of one study each; further replication is needed before more confident conclusions can be reached.

APA Division 16 and the Society for the Study of School Psychology expanded the guidelines of the APA Task Force, and created the *Procedural and Coding Manual for Review of Evidence-Based Interventions* (Kratochwill and Stoiber 2002). These guidelines were noteworthy because they contained separate guidelines for four different research methodologies: group-design research (Lewis-Snyder et al. 2002); single subject research (Shernoff et al. 2002); qualitative research;

and confirmatory program evaluation. Additionally, the school psychology guidelines broadened the scope of EBP with the inclusion of qualitative research methods and confirmatory program evaluations; previous definitions of EBP by the APA had limited the research methodologies to group experimental and SSED. The procedural manual provided very clear guidelines and templates on evaluating individual treatments; however, it did not specify how to synthesize the evaluations to determine a study's quality.

Hawaii Empirical Basis to Services Task Force. A direct application of an adaptation of APA guidelines to practices for children with autism was completed in 2002 and updated on a biennial cycle (Chorpita et al. 2002; Chorpita and Daleiden 2007). In their review of empirically supported treatments, the Hawaii Task Force used five levels of evidence (in order from the highest level: best evidence, good support, moderate support, minimal support, and no support). The initial results (2002) did not show any comprehensive program meeting the criteria for EBP. Two focal interventions, functional communication training or ABA and the Caregiver-Based Intervention Program, received a Level 3 rating. However, it was supported by evidence from only one study. The 2007 update indicated that two practices, intensive behavioral treatment and intensive communication training, have the highest rating (i.e., best support). The committee also determined that one treatment (auditory integration training) is at Level 5 and one treatment (the Caregiver Psychoeducational Program) is at Level 4. Collectively, the initial review of the task force and the biennial updates of interventions for many childhood disorders provide a model for large-scale implementation of EBP.

Professionals in the mental health fields continue to be an integral part in the treatment of individuals with autism. Hence, the continued development of EBP in psychology continues to be of great interest to practitioners working with children with autism. Many of the most thorough reviews of autism interventions have been conducted by psychologists or published in psychological journals. Additionally, as outlined above, some interventions are now identified as EBP in psychology; they have been identified using well-defined and widely accepted standards. Even though there are many treatments for individuals with autism recognized as EBP, texts on EBP for mental health professionals often omit information on autism (Drake et al. 2005; Norcross et al. 2008). Finally, the inclusion of interventions shown to have efficacy in only one study in some EBP standards is worrisome. Science is built on the logic of replication and the designation of practices without replicated effects might result in less than optimal practice. This reinforces the need to examine the criteria being used when searching for EBP.

Educational Definitions

General education. No Child Left Behind (Public Law 107–110, § 115 Stat 1425) requires teachers to use instructional strategies based on "scientifically based research," which is a phrase that appears 111 times in the legislation. Since the passage of this law, educational agencies have become increasingly responsible for identifying and implementing EBP in classrooms and many definitions of "scientifically based" have been applied (Eisenhart and Towne 2003). The National Research Council (NRC) convened the Committee on Scientific Principles for Education Research to examine the state of the science in educational research and it released guidelines for the evaluation of scientific evidence in educational research (Shavelson and Towne 2002). The report strongly emphasized that educational research should examine many different types of research question using a variety of research methods that were appropriate to the research question being asked. However, this broader definition of evidence is not used by all organizations in education. This is most evident in the guidelines of the What Works Clearinghouse, which limits the highest level of recommendation to studies conducted using RCTs. Studies conducted using SSED or qualitative research methods, two common methods in educational research, do not currently meet inclusion criteria, which has likely contributed to the omission of autism interventions from the What Works Clearinghouse.

Special education. The reauthorization of IDEA (Public Law 108–446, § 118 Stat 2647) aligned the standards of education for individuals with disabilities to have scientifically based research support. The field of special education has used a broad view of evidence, which was shown in the guidelines for EBP created by the task force from the Division for Research of the Council for Exceptional Children (Odom et al. 2005). These guidelines provided definitions and criteria for four frequently used research methodologies in special education research: experimental group research (Gersten et al. 2005); SSED (Horner et al. 2005); correlational research (Thompson et al. 2005); and qualitative research (Brantlinger et al. 2005). With respect to autism research, the guidelines for SSED have recently been applied to the Picture Exchange Communication System (Preston and Carter 2009) and video modeling (Bellini and Akullian 2007).

Because many individuals with autism are served in both regular education classrooms and special education settings, multiple definitions of EBP have been and will continue to be applied to the education of children with autism. The continued debate over what constitutes evidence (Slavin 2008) will continue to hinder practitioners using EBP in schools and other educational settings.

Other Applications of Evidence-Based Practice Standards

Committee on educational interventions for children with autism. Probably the most single influential review of treatments has been the one provided by the National Research Council (NRC 2001). This report[1] was conducted in response to an inquiry from the US Department of Education about the efficacy of early intervention in young (preschool and early school age) children with autism. The NRC formed a Committee on Educational Interventions for Children with Autism and charged it with integrating the existing literature and developing a framework for evaluating the available scientific evidence concerning effects of educational interventions. As part of this process, the committee engaged in a series of reviews (integrated in the final report) on issues of diagnosis, assessment and prevalence, the role of families, goals for educational services, characteristics of effective intervention programs, public policy issues, personnel preparation issues, and research. The report specifically addresses areas of development and behavior that are appropriate concerns for intervention programs in autism, i.e., communication, social, cognitive, sensory, and motor development as well as adaptive skills and problem behaviors.

This report was a watershed in many respects. It provided a clear answer, based on its review of the available literature, that early intervention does make an important difference in the lives of young children with autism. Its review and overview of the many areas of similarity (and some areas of difference) between the ten model comprehensive programs has been particularly important, as has been the focus on policy and research needs and implications. Its final chapter presented a summary and

---

[1] Fred R. Volkmar was an author of this report.

recommendations for intervention and program strategies and educational content. Several of the NRC's conclusions (National Research Council 2001) deserve special emphasis. In the first place, it noted that, on balance, about 25 h a week of year-round programming seemed effective (this represents a somewhat unusual combination of "hours per week" as described by the very different model programs reviewed). The observation that some children do not improve, even in the best of programs, highlighted the need to study the interaction of treatment efficacy and "dose" effects with child characteristics. The review of methodological issues presaged many of the issues noted in this volume, e.g., the diversity and separate nature of the various intervention literatures, issues of early screening and diagnosis, the importance of careful subject characterization, and the role of various strategies including RCTs and SSEDs in designing effective treatments. The report also emphasized the power of developmental and "nonspecific" effects, the interaction of treatment with child and family characteristics, and the importance of replication and measurement of treatment effects. To this end, the relevance of such important research issues as treatment fidelity and modeling of growth and intervention effects was also highlighted. The problem of moving from research to real-world settings and of integrating evidence-based approaches into school settings was also emphasized. In the final report, the committee proposed that the only way to achieve its top rating was through the use of randomized control trials (National Research Council 2001; Lord et al. 2002). Although the NRC report on autism is starting to become dated, it remains a standard reference for interventions for young children with ASD.

Several flaws in the design of the NRC's review may have weakened its conclusions. Probably most important, the issue of which programs were included or not included was determined based on a set of criteria. These included federal funding, peer-reviewed publications, and overall program orientation. Twelve such programs were identified in the United States and program directors or developers were asked to respond; ten did so and their programs were reviewed in detail. As might be expected given the relatively broad inclusion criteria, the research basis for these programs was widely varied and includes some programs with literally a handful of related peer-reviewed publications up to programs with many such publications. Given the emphasis on peer-reviewed papers and federal funding, unsurprisingly, all programs reviewed were based in a university in some respect. Some of the programs, particularly those with longer histories, had undergone major changes in location or method over time, e.g., moving from center-based to home-based instruction or moving from one university affiliation to another. There was no attempt to develop more detailed approaches to quantifying or scoring the quality of the programs (see Chap. 2). Obstacles to treatment effectiveness were also not a major focus of the report (although some were noted at least in passing). Reflecting the state of science at the time, issues of EBT, EBM, and EBP were not explicitly highlighted (e.g., the index carries no entry for any of these terms). Given the focus on educational programs and interventions for younger children, drug treatments were only briefly discussed and no attention was paid to programs for older school-aged children, adolescents, and adults with autism. Despite these, for the time, relatively minor limitations, this report marked a major improvement in the attempt to delineate evidence-based treatments or practices in autism and related disorders.

Scottish Intercollegiate Guidelines Network. In 2007, the Scottish Intercollegiate Guidelines Network published Clinical Guidelines (SIGN 2007a) and a Quick

Reference Guide (SIGN 2007b) for the assessment, diagnosis, and treatment of young children with ASD. The guidelines were created through a review of empirical studies published between 1996 and 2006 and provide comprehensive coverage of issues surrounding assessment, diagnosis, and interventions for autism and quantifications of the quality of evidence. The quality of evidence for each practice is aggregated into four grades of recommendation (A, B, C, or D, where A is the highest level). As with many guidelines, the top ratings are restricted to studies conducted using RCT designs. In addition to the grade of recommendation, a statement about the recommendation is provided and "good practice points" (indicated by a check-mark in a box in the manuscript) are inserted to assist clinicians and practitioners in using best practice. The Lovaas program was the only practice receiving the highest grade. Five practices (education and skills intervention for parents of preschool children, risperidone, methylphenidate, melatonin, and behavioral intervention) received the second level. The comprehensive and user-friendly nature of the guidelines (especially the Quick Reference Guide) makes them an excellent resource for individuals using EBP with children with autism.

National Autism Center. Recently, researchers from the National Autism Center published a report (National Autism Center 2009a) for which hundreds of research articles on autism interventions were reviewed by experts who rated multiple dimensions of methodology. These ratings were compiled to obtain a scientific merit rating for each article and the strength of evidence for a specific treatment was classified as one of four categories (from the highest level: established, emerging, unestablished, and ineffective or harmful). As with the evaluation tool developed by Reichow et al. (2008), see Chap. 2, evidence obtained from studies using group research designs and SSED could

be combined to evaluate a specific treatment. Eleven interventions were identified as established treatments, 22 interventions were identified as emerging treatments, and five interventions were identified as unestablished treatments. A guide centered on issues associated with EBP in school settings associated with the findings from the *National Standards Report* was recently released (National Autism Center 2009b).

Conclusion

Multiple organizations and groups have now produced practice guidelines concerning the treatment or identification of ASD. These organizations have proposed methods for appraising empirical evidence in search of EBP. However, the resulting definitions have varied across, and sometimes within, divisions of professions; a universal definition remains elusive. The evaluative method described in Chap. 2 is but one example of an evidence grading scheme. With the increasing emphasis being placed on EBP, multiple organizations have developed conceptually similar schemes. The use of an evidence grading scheme is intended to decrease bias and increase agreement (Boruch and Rui 2008; Guyatt et al. 2008), however, examination of various grading schemes suggests differences between raters using the same scheme and differences in one rater using different schemes are plausible (Leff and Conley 2006). Direct evidence of differences between raters using one scheme is likely a factor in this volume, and if multiple systems had been used by one author, it is likely that problems with the second type of error (i.e., inconsistencies between schemes) would have occurred. Having multiple definitions of EBP can create confusion since an intervention might be considered an EBP under one definition and not under another (Tankersly et al. 2008;

Slavin 2008). Furthermore, the difficulties faced in doing research on children with autism (Lord et al. 2005; Smith et al. 2007) frequently limits or hinders the ability of research to achieve the highest levels of evidence. Standardization and training, such as that done by the National Autism Center (National Autism Center 2009a), can help reduce though not eliminate these risks and such inconsistencies may well inhibit the widespread adoption of any one system (Atkins et al. 2004). Furthermore, others have questioned whether patients and policy makers will ever find such evidence-grading schemes useful (Atkins et al. 2004; Upshur 2003). The full potential of evidence-grading schemes and systems will never be realized unless great attention is paid to barriers to their use.

The evaluative method that is presented in Chap. 2 was developed to address these concerns (Reichow et al. 2008). Since the focus of this book is EBP, the authors of the other chapters were asked to review the evidence and make determinations about which practices might or might not be considered EBP. The evaluative method described in Chap. 2 was provided to the authors, but they were not required to use it; some authors used the method and some did not. The resulting treatment reviews presented in Part II provide a snapshot of the empirical evidence supporting certain treatments for individuals with autism. The book concludes with four chapters focused on the future of EBP in autism.

REFERENCES

Aldred, C., Green, J., & Adams, C. (2004). A new social communication intervention for children with autism: Pilot randomized controlled treatment study suggesting effectiveness. *Journal of Child Psychology and Psychiatry, 45*, 1420–1430.

Aman, M. G., Hollway, J. A., et al. (2008). Cognitive effects of risperidone in children with autism and irritable behavior. *Journal of Child and Adolescent Psychopharmacology, 18*(3), 227–236.

American Speech–Language–Hearing Association. (2006). Guidelines for speech-language pathologists in assessment, diagnosis, and treatment of autism spectrum disorders across the life span. http://www.asha.org/docs/html/GL2006-00049.html. Accessed 20 July 2009.

Anderson, L. T., Campbell, M., Grega, D. M., Perry, R., Small, A. M., et al. (1984). Haloperidol in the treatment of infantile autism: Effects on learning and behavioral symptoms. *The American Journal of Psychiatry, 141*(10), 1195–1202.

Anderson, L. T., Campbell, M., Adams, P., Small, A. M., Perry, R., et al. (1989). The effects of haloperidol on discrimination learning and behavioral symptoms in autistic children. *Journal of Autism and Developmental Disorders, 19*(2), 227–239.

American Psychiatric Association. (1980). *Diagnostic and statistical manual of mental disorders* (3rd ed.). Washington, DC: Author.

American Psychiatric Association. (1994). *Diagnostic and statistical manual of mental disorders* (4th ed.). Washington, DC: Author.

APA Presidential Task Force on Evidence-Based Practice. (2006). Evidence-based practice in psychology. *The American Psychologist, 61*, 271–285.

Atkins, D., Eccles, M., Flottorp, S., Guyatt, G. H., Henry, D., et al. (2004). Systems for grading the quality of evidence and the strength of recommendations I: Critical appraisal of existing approaches. *BMC Health Services Research, 4*, e38.

Barkham, M., & Mellor-Clark, J. (2003). Bridging evidence-based practice and practice-based evidence: Developing a rigorous and relevant knowledge for the psychological therapies. *Clinical Psychology & Psychotherapy, 10*, 319–327.

Bartak, L., & Rutter, M. (1973). Special educational treatment of autistic children: A comparative study: 1 design of study and characteristics of units. *Journal of Child Psychology and Psychiatry, 14*(3), 161–179.

Becker, L. A., & Oxman, A. D. (2008). Overviews of reviews. In J. P. T. Higgins & S. Green (Eds.), *Cochrane handbook for systematic reviews of interventions* (pp. 602–631). West Sussex: Wiley.

Bellini, S., & Akullian, J. (2007). A meta-analysis of video modeling and video self-modeling interventions for children and adolescents with autism spectrum disorders. *Exceptional Children, 73*, 264–287.

Berkman, M. (1997). The legal rights of children with disabilities to education and developmental services. In D. J. Cohen & F. R. Volkmar

(Eds.), *Handbook of autism and pervasive developmental disorders* (2nd ed., pp. 808–827). New York: Wiley.

Bettelheim, B. (1950). *Love is not enough: The treatment of emotionally disturbed children*. Glencoe: Free.

Blue Cross & Blue Shield. (2009). Special report: Early intensive behavioral intervention based on applied behavior analysis among children with autism spectrum disorders. http://www.bcbs.com/blueresources/tec/vols/23/23_09.pdf. Accessed from 28 August 2009.

Borenstein, M., Hedges, L. V., Higgins, J. P. T., & Rothstein, H. R. (2009). *Introduction to meta-analysis*. West Sussex: Wiley.

Boruch, R., & Rui, N. (2008). From randomized controlled trials to evidence grading schemes: Current state of evidence-based practice in social sciences. *Journal of Evidence-Based Medicine, 1*, 41–49.

Brantlinger, E., Jimenez, R., Klingner, J., Pugach, M., & Richardson, V. (2005). Qualitative studies in special education. *Exceptional Children, 71*, 195–207.

Bristol-Myers Squib. (2009). US Food and Drug Administration approves Abilify (aripiprazole) for the treatment of irritability associated with autistic disorder in pediatric patients (ages 6 to 17 years). Press release. http://www.businesswire.com/news/bms/20091120005816/en/U.S.-Food-Drug-Administration-Approves-ABILIFY%C2%AE-aripiprazole. Accessed 1 January 2010.

Carr, E. G., & Carlson, J. I. (1993). Reduction of severe behavior problems in the community using a multicomponent treatment approach. *Journal of Applied Behavior Analysis, 26*(2), 157–172.

Chambless, D. L., & Hollon, S. D. (1998). Defining empirically supported therapies. *Journal of Consulting and Clinical Psychology, 66*, 7–18.

Chambless, D. L., & Ollendick, T. H. (2001). Empirically supported psychological interventions: Controversies and evidence. *Annual Review of Psychology, 52*, 685–716.

Chambless, D. L., Sanderson, W. C., Shoham, V., Bennett Johnson, S., Pope, K. S., et al. (1996). An update on empirically validated therapies. *The Clinical Psychologist, 49*(2), 5–18.

Charlop, M. H., Schreibman, L., & Tryon, A. S. (1983). Learning through observation: The effects of peer modeling on acquisition and generalization in autistic children. *Journal of Abnormal Child Psychology, 11*(3), 355–366.

Chorpita, B. F. (2003). The frontier of evidence-based practice. In A. E. Kazdin & J. R. Weisz (Eds.), *Evidence-based psychotherapies for children and adolescents* (pp. 42–59). New York: Guilford.

Chorpita, B. F., & Daleiden, E. L. (2007). *Biennial report: Effective psychosocial interventions for youth with behavioral and emotional needs*. Honolulu: Child and Adolescent Mental Health Division, Hawaii Department of Health.

Chorpita, B. F., Yim, L. M., Conkervoet, J. C., Arensdorf, A., Amundsen, M. J., et al. (2002). Toward large-scale implementation of empirically supported treatments for children: A review and observations by the Hawaii empirical basis to services task force. *Clinical Psychology: Science and Practice, 9*, 165–190.

Cigna. (2008). Cigna medical coverage policy, autism spectrum disorders/pervasive developmental disorders: Assessment and treatment. http://www.cigna.com/customer_care/healthcare_professional/coverage_positions/medical/mm_0447_coveragepositioncriteria_autism_pervasive_developmental_disorders.pdf. Accessed 28 August 2009.

Cohen, D., & Young, G. (1977). Neurochemistry and child psychiatry. *Journal of the American Academy of Child Psychiatry, 16*, 353–411.

Cutspec, P. A. (2004). Bridging the research-to-practice gap: Evidence-based education. *Centerscope, 2*(2), 1–8.

Dawes, M., Summerskill, W., Glasziou, P., Cartabellotta, A., Martin, J., et al. (2005). Sicily statement on evidence-based practice. *BMC Medical Education, 5*, 1.

Dawson, G., & Osterling, J. (1997). Early intervention in autism: Effectiveness of common elements of current approaches. In M. J. Guralnick (Ed.), *The effectiveness of early intervention: Second generation research* (pp. 302–326). Baltimore: Brooks.

De Los Reyes, A., & Kazdin, A. E. (2006). Conceptualizing changes in behavior in intervention research: The range of possible changes model. *Psychological Review, 113*, 554–583.

Despert, J. L. (1971). Reflections on early infantile autism. *Journal of Childhood Autism and Schizophrenia, 1*, 363–367.

Drake, R. E., Latimer, E. A., Leff, H. S., McHugo, G. J., & Burns, B. J. (2004). What is evidence? *Child and Adolescent Psychiatric Clinics of North America, 13*, 717–728.

Drake, R. E., Merrens, M. R., & Lynde, D. W. (Eds.). (2005). *Evidence-based mental health practice: A textbook*. New York: W. W. Norton.

Drew, A., Baird, G., Baron-Cohen, S., Cox, A., Slonims, V., et al. (2002). A pilot randomized control trial of a parent training intervention for pre-school children with autism: Preliminary findings and methodological challenges. *European Child & Adolescent Psychiatry, 11*, 266–272.

Dulcan, M. K. (2005). Practitioner perspectives on evidence-based practice. *Child and Adolescent Psychiatric Clinics of North America, 14,* 225–240.

Dunlap, G., & Fox, L. (1999). A demonstration of behavioral support for young children with autism. *Journal of Positive Behavior Interventions, 1*(2), 77–87.

Eisenhart, M., & Towne, L. (2003). Contestation and change in national policy on "scientifically based" education research. *Educational Researcher, 32*(7), 31–38.

Farrell, M. (2009). *Foundations of special education: An introduction.* Chichester: Wiley-Blackwell.

Fenton, G., D'Ardia, C., Valente, D., Del Vecchio, I., Fabrizi, A., et al. (2003). Vineland adaptive behavior profiles in children with autism and moderate to severe developmental delay. *Autism, 7*(3), 269–287.

Ferster, C. B. (1961). Positive reinforcement and behavioral deficits of autistic children. *Child Development, 32,* 251–264.

Filipek, P. A., Accardo, P. J., Ashwal, S., Baranek, G. T., Cook, E. H., Jr., et al. (2000). Practice parameter: Screening and diagnosis of autism. *Neurology, 55,* 468–479.

Folstein, S., & Rutter, M. J. (1977). Infantile autism: A genetic study of 21 twin pairs. *Journal of Child Psychology and Psychiatry, 18,* 297–321.

French, J., & Gronseth, G. (2008). Lost in a jungle of evidence: We need a compass. *Neurology, 71,* 1634–1638.

Gersten, R., Fuchs, L. S., Coyne, M., Greenwood, C., & Innocenti, M. S. (2005). Quality indicators for group experimental and quasi-experimental research in special education. *Exceptional Children, 71,* 149–164.

Greden, J., & Groden, G. (1997). Initiating and administering programs: Alternative settings. In D. J. Cohen & F. R. Volkmar (Eds.), *Handbook of autism and pervasive developmental disorders* (2nd ed., pp. 676–690). New York: Wiley.

Gronseth, G., & French, J. (2008). Practice parameters and technology assessments: What they are, what they are not, and why you should care. *Neurology, 71,* 1639–1643.

Guyatt, G. H., Oxman, A. D., Vist, G., Kunz, R., Falck-Ytter, Y., et al. (2008). GRADE: An emerging consensus on rating quality of evidence and strength of recommendations. *British Medical Journal, 336,* 925–926.

Hamilton, J. (2007). Evidence-based practice as a conceptual framework. In A. Martin & F. R. Volkmar (Eds.), *Lewis' child and adolescent psychiatry: A comprehensive approach* (4th ed., pp. 124–140). Philadelphia: Wolters Kluwer.

Harris, S. L., & Handleman, J. S. (1997). Helping children with autism enter the mainstream. In D. J. Cohen & F. R. Volkmar (Eds.), *Handbook of autism and pervasive developmental disorders* (2nd ed., pp. 665–675). New York: Wiley.

Harris, S. L., Handleman, J. S., & Jennett, H. K. (2005). Models of educational intervention for students with autism: Home, center, and school-based programming. In F. R. Volkmar, R. Paul, A. Klin, & D. J. Cohen (Eds.), *Handbook of autism and pervasive developmental disorders* (3rd ed., pp. 1043–1054). Hoboken: Wiley.

Hatcher, S., Butler, R., & Oakley-Browne, M. (2005). *Evidence-based mental health care.* Edinburgh: Elsevier Churchill Livingstone.

Higgins, J. P. T., & Green, S. (2008). *Cochrane handbook for systematic reviews of interventions.* West Sussex: Wiley-Blackwell.

Horner, R. H., Carr, E. G., Halle, J., McGee, G., Odom, S., & Wolery, M. (2005). The use of single subject research to identify evidence-based practice in special education. *Exceptional Children, 71,* 165–179.

Howlin, P. (2005). Outcomes in autism spectrum disorders. In F. R. Volkmar, R. Paul, A. Klin, & D. J. Cohen (Eds.), *Handbook of autism and pervasive developmental disorders* (3rd ed., pp. 201–222). Hoboken: Wiley.

Institute of Medicine. (2008). *Evidence-based medicine and the changing nature of health care.* Washington, DC: National Academies.

Jocelyn, L. J., Casiro, O. G., Beattie, D., Bow, J., & Kneisz, J. (1998). Treatment of children with autism: A randomized controlled trial to evaluate a caregiver-based intervention program in community day-care centers. *Developmental and Behavioral Pediatrics, 19,* 326–334.

Kanner, L. (1943). Autistic disturbances of affective contact. *The Nervous Child, 2,* 217–250.

Kazdin, A. E. (2001). Bridging the enormous gaps of theory with therapy research and practice. *Journal of Clinical Child Psychology, 30,* 59–66.

Kazdin, A. E. (2008). Evidence-based treatments and delivery of psychological services: Shifting our emphases to increase impact. *Psychological Services, 5,* 201–215.

Kazdin, A. E., & Weisz, J. R. (Eds.). (2003). *Evidence-based psychotherapies for children and adolescents.* New York: Guilford.

Klin, A., Saulnier, C. A., Sparrow, S. S., Cicchetti, D. V., Volkmar, F. R., et al. (2007). Social and communication abilities and disabilities in higher functioning individuals with autism spectrum disorders: The Vineland and the ADOS. *Journal of Autism and Developmental Disorders, 37*(4), 748–759.

Koegel, R. L., & Koegel, L. K. (Eds.). (1995). *Teaching children with autism: Strategies for initiating positive interactions and improving learning opportunities.* Baltimore: Brookes.

Koegel, R. L., & Koegel, L. K. (Eds.). (2006). *Pivotal response treatments for autism: Communication, social, and academic development.* Baltimore: Brookes.

Koegel, L. K., Harrower, J. K., & Koegel, R. L. (1999). Support for children with developmental disabilities in full inclusion classrooms through self-management. *Journal of Positive Behavior Interventions, 1*(1), 26–34.

Kolvin, I. (1971). Studies in the childhood psychoses: Diagnostic criteria and classification. *The British Journal of Psychiatry, 118*, 381–384.

Kratochwill, T. R., & Stoiber, K. C. (2002). Evidence-based interventions in school psychology: Conceptual foundations of the procedural and coding manual of Division 16 and the Society for the Study of School Psychology task force. *School Psychology Quarterly, 17*, 341–389.

Leff, H. S., & Conley, J. A. (2006). Desired attributes of evidence assessments for evidence-based practices. *Administration and Policy in Mental Health and Mental Health Services Research, 33*, 648–658.

Lerman, D. C., Vorndran, C. M., Addison, L., & Kuhn, S. C. (2004). Preparing teachers in evidence-based practices for young children with autism. *School Psychology Review, 33*, 510–526.

Lettick, A. L. (1981). The first use of total communication. *Journal of Autism and Developmental Disorders, 11*(3), 361.

Lewis-Snyder, G., Stoiber, K. C., & Kratochwill, T. R. (2002). Evidence-based interventions in school psychology: An illustration of task force coding criteria using group-based research design. *School Psychology Quarterly, 17*, 423–465.

Lonigan, C. J., Elbert, J. C., & Johnson, S. B. (1998). Empirically supported psychosocial interventions for children: An overview. *Journal of Clinical Child Psychology, 27*, 138–145.

Lord, C., Bristol-Power, M., Cafiero, J. M., Filipek, P. A., Gallagher, J. J., et al. (2002). Special issue (October): Editorial preface. *Journal of Autism and Developmental Disorders, 32*(5), 349–350.

Lord, C., Wagner, A., Rogers, S., Szatmari, P., Aman, M., et al. (2005). Challenges in evaluating psychosocial interventions for autistic spectrum disorders. *Journal of Autism and Developmental Disorders, 35*, 695–711.

Lovaas, O. I. (1987). Behavioral treatment and normal educational and intellectual functioning in young autistic children. *Journal of Consulting and Clinical Psychology, 55*, 3–9.

Lovaas, O. I., & Smith, T. (1988). Intensive behavioral treatment for young autistic children.

In B. B. Lahey & A. E. Kazdin (Eds.), *Advances in clinical child psychology* (11, pp. 285–324). New York: Plenum.

Lovaas, O. I., Berberich, J. P., Perloff, B. F., & Schaeffer, B. (1966a). Acquisition of imitative speech by schizophrenic children. *Science, 151*, 705–707.

Lovaas, O. I., Freitag, G., Kinder, M. I., Rubenstein, B. D., Schaeffer, B., et al. (1966b). Establishment of social reinforcers in two schizophrenic children on the basis of food. *Journal of Experimental Child Psychology, 4*(2), 109–125.

Lovaas, O., Schreibman, L., Koegel, R. L., & Rehm, R. (1971). Selective responding by autistic children to multiple sensory input. *Journal of Abnormal Psychology, 77*(3), 211–222.

Lucas, S. M., & Cutspec, P. A. (2005). The role and process of literature searching in the preparation of a literature synthesis. *Centerscope, 4*(3), 1–26.

Mandlawitz, M. R. (2005). Educating children with autism: Current legal issues. In F. R. Volkmar, R. Paul, A. Klin, & D. J. Cohen (Eds.), *Handbook of autism and pervasive developmental disorders* (3rd ed., pp. 1161–1173). Hoboken: Wiley.

McDougle, C. J., Scahill, L., Aman, M. G., McCracken, J. T., Tierney, E., et al. (2005). Risperidone for the core symptom domains of autism: Results from the RUPP Autism Network study. *The American Journal of Psychiatry, 162*, 1142–1148.

McGee, G. G., Morrier, M. J., & Daly, T. (1999). An incidental teaching approach to early intervention for toddlers with autism. *Journal of the Association for Persons with Severe Disabilities, 24*, 133–146.

McHugo, G. J., & Drake, R. E. (2003). Finding and evaluating the evidence: A critical step in evidence-based medicine. *The Psychiatric Clinics of North America, 26*, 821–831.

Mesibov, G. B., Shea, V., & Schopler, E. (2005). *The TEACCH approach to autism spectrum disorders.* New York: Springer.

Mullen, R. (2007). The state of the evidence: ASHA develops levels of evidence for communication sciences and disorders. *The ASHA Leader, 12*(3), 8–9 and 24–25.

Nathan, P., & Gorman, J. M. (2002). *A guide to treatments that work* (2nd ed.). New York: Oxford.

Nathan, P., & Gorman, J. M. (2007). *A guide to treatments that work* (3rd ed.). New York: Oxford.

National Autism Center. (2009a). *National standards report.* Randolph: National Autism Center.

National Autism Center. (2009b). *Evidence-based practice and autism in the schools: A guide to providing appropriate interventions to students with autism spectrum disorders.* Randolph: Author.

National Research Council. (2001). *Educating young children with autism.* Washington, DC: National Academy.

Nelson, T. D., & Steele, R. G. (2007). Predictors of practitioner self-reported use of evidence-based practices: Practitioner training, clinical setting, and attitudes toward research. *Administration and Policy in Mental Health and Mental Health Services Research, 34*, 319–330.

Norcros, J. C., Koocher, G. P., & Hogan, T. P. (Eds.). (2008). *Clinician's guide to evidence-based practices: Mental health and the addictions.* Oxford: Oxford University Press.

Norcross, J., Beutler, L., & Levant, R. (Eds.). (2005). *Evidence-based practices in mental health: Debate and dialogue on the fundamental questions.* Washington, DC: American Psychological Association.

Odom, S. L., Brantlinger, E., Gersten, R., Horner, R. H., Thompson, B., & Harris, K. R. (2005). Research in special education: Scientific methods and evidence-based practices. *Exceptional Children, 71*, 137–148.

Pagoto, S. L., Spring, B., Coups, E. J., Mulvaney, S., Coutu, M. F., & Ozakinci, G. (2007). Barriers and facilitators of evidence-based practice perceived by behavioral science professionals. *Journal of Clinical Psychology, 63*, 695–705.

Paul, R., & Sutherland, D. (2005). Enhancing early language in children with autism spectrum disorders. In F. R. Volkmar, R. Paul, A. Klin, & D. J. Cohen (Eds.), *Handbook of autism and pervasive developmental disorders* (3rd ed., pp. 946–976). Hoboken: Wiley.

Petticrew, M., & Roberts, H. (2006). *Systematic reviews in the social sciences.* Malden: Blackwell.

Preston, D., & Carter, M. (2009). A review of the efficacy of the Picture Exchange Communication System intervention. *Journal of Autism and Developmental Disorders, 39*, 1471–1486.

Public Law 101–336, §12101 Stat. 327 (1990). Americans with Disabilities Act of 1990.

Public Law 107–110, § 115 Stat. 1425 (2002). No Child Left Behind Act of 2001.

Public Law 108–446, § 118 Stat. 2647 (2004). Individuals with Disabilities Education Improvement Act of 2004.

Public Law 94–142 (1975). Education for All Handicapped Children Act of 1975.

Reichow, B., Volkmar, F. R., & Cicchetti, D. V. (2008). Development of an evaluative method for determining the strength of research evidence in autism. *Journal of Autism and Developmental Disorders, 38*, 1311–1319.

Riddle, M. A. (1987). Individual and parental psychotherpay in autism. In D. J. Cohen & A. Donnellan (Eds.), *Handbook of autism and pervasive developmental disorders* (pp. 528–544). New York: Wiley.

Rimland, B. (1964). *Infantile autism: The syndrome and its implication for a neural theory of behavior.* New York: Appleton-Century-Crafts.

Robey, R., Apel, K., Dollaghan, C., Ellmo, W., Hall, N., et al. (2004). Report of the joint coordinating committee on evidence-based practice. American Speech–Language–Hearing Association. http://www.asha.org/uploaded-Files/members/ebp/JCCEBPReport04.pdf. Accessed 4 January 2010.

Rogers, S. J. (1998). Empirically supported comprehensive treatments for young children with autism. *Journal of Clinical Child Psychology, 27*, 168–179.

Rogers, S. J., & Vismara, L. A. (2008). Evidence-based comprehensive treatments for early autism. *Journal of Clinical Child and Adolescent Psychology, 37*, 8–38.

Rogers, S. J., Hall, T., Osaki, D., Reaven, J., & Herbison, J. (2000). The Denver Model: A comprehensive, integrated educational approach to young children with autism and their families. In J. S. Handleman & S. L. Harris (Eds.), *Preschool education programs for children with autism* (2nd ed., pp. 95–133). Austin: Pro-Ed.

Rutter, M. (1972). Childhood schizophrenia reconsidered. *Journal of Autism and Childhood Schizophrenia, 2*(4), 315–337.

Sackett, D. L., Rosenberg, W. M. C., Gray, J. A. M., Haynes, R. B., & Richardson, W. S. (1996). Evidence-based medicine: What it is and what it isn't. *British Medical Journal, 312*, 71–72.

Sackett, D. L., Straus, S. E., Richardson, W. S., Rosenberg, W., & Haynes, R. B. (2000). *Evidence-based medicine: How to practice and teach EBM* (2nd ed.). London: Churchill Livingstone.

Salmond, S. W. (2007). Advancing evidence-based practice: A primer. *Orthopaedic Nursing, 26*(2), 114–123.

Scahill, L., Koenig, K., Carrol, D. H., & Pachler, M. (2007). Risperidone approved for the treatment of serious behavioral problems in children with autism. *Journal of Child and Adolescent Psychiatric Nursing, 20*, 188–190.

Scheuermann, B., Webber, J., Boutot, E. A., & Goodwin, M. (2003). Problems with personnel preparation in autism spectrum disorders. *Focus on Autism and Developmental Disabilities, 18*, 197–206.

Schopler, E. (1997). Implementation of TEACCH philosophy. In D. J. Cohen & F. R. Volkmar (Eds.), *Handbook of autism and pervasive developmental disorders* (2nd ed., pp. 767–795). New York: Wiley.

Schopler, E., Brehm, S. S., Kinsbourne, M., & Reichler, R. J. (1971). Effect of treatment structure on development in autistic chldren. *Archives of General Psychiatry, 24*, 415–421.

Schreibman, L. (1998). *Autism.* Newbury Park: Sage.

Schreibman, L., & Ingersoll, B. (2005). Behavioral interventions to promote learning in individuals with autism. In F. R. Volkmar, R. Paul, A. Klin, & D. J. Cohen (Eds.), *Handbook of autism and pervasive developmental disorders* (3rd ed., pp. 882–896). Hoboken: Wiley.

Schreibman, L., & Koegel, R. L. (1996). Fostering self-management: Parent-delivered pivotal response training for children with autistic disorder. In E. D. Hibbs & P. S. Jensen (Eds.), *Psychosocial treatments for child and adolescent disorders: Empirically based strategies for clinical practice* (2nd ed., pp. 525–552). Washington, DC: American Psychological Association.

Schreibman, L., & Koegel, R. L. (2005). Training for parents of children with autism: Pivotal responses, generalization, and individualization of interventions. In E. D. Hibbs & P. S. Jensen (Eds.), *Psychosocial treatments for child and adolescent disorders: Empirically based strategies for clinical practice* (2nd ed., pp. 605–631). Washington, DC: American Psychological Association.

Scottish Intercollegiate Guidelines Network. (2007a). Assessment, diagnosis and clinical interventions for children and young people with autism spectrum disorders: A national clinical guideline. http://www.sign.ac.uk/pdf/sign98.pdf. Accessed 5 January 2010.

Scottish Intercollegiate Guidelines Network. (2007b). Assessment, diagnosis and clinical interventions for children and young people with autism spectrum disorders: Quick reference guide. http://www.sign.ac.uk/pdf/qrg98.pdf. Accessed 5 January 2010.

Shavelson, R. J., & Towne, L. (Eds.). (2002). *Scientific research in education*. Washington, DC: National Academy.

Shernoff, E. S., Kratochwill, T. R., & Stoiber, K. C. (2002). Evidence-based interventions in school psychology: An illustration of task force coding criteria using single-participant research design. *School Psychology Quarterly, 17*, 390–422.

Silverman, W. K., & Hinshaw, S. P. (2008). The second special issue on evidence-based psychosocial treatments for children and adolescents: A 10-year update. *Journal of Clinical Child and Adolescent Psychology, 37*, 1–7.

Simonson, L. R., Simonson, S. M., & Volkmar, F. R. (1990). Benhaven's residential program. *Journal of Autism and Developmental Disorders, 20*(3), 323–337.

Slavin, R. E. (1986). Best evidence synthesis: An alternative to meta-analytic and traditional reviews. *Educational Researcher, 15*, 5–11.

Slavin, R. E. (2008). Perspectives on evidence-based research in education: What works? Issues in synthesizing educational program evaluations. *Educational Researcher, 37*, 5–14.

Smith, G. C. S., & Pell, J. P. (2003). Parachute use to prevent death and major trauma related to gravitational challenge: Systematic review of randomised controlled trials. *British Medical Journal, 327*, 1459–1461.

Smith, T., Groen, A. D., & Wynn, J. W. (2000). Randomized trial of intensive early intervention for children with pervasive developmental disorder. *American Journal of Mental Retardation, 105*(4), 269–285.

Smith, T., Scahill, L., Dawson, G., Guthrie, D., Lord, C., et al. (2007). Designing research studies on psychosocial interventions in autism. *Journal of Autism and Developmental Disorders, 37*, 354–366.

Sternberg, R. J. (2006). Evidence-based practice: Gold standard, gold plated, or fool's gold. In C. D. Goodheart, A. E. Kazdin, & R. J. Sternberg (Eds.), *Evidence-based psychotherapy: Where practice and research meet* (pp. 261–271). Washington, DC: American Psychological Association.

Strain, P. S. (2001). Empirically based social skill intervention: A case for quality-of-life improvement. *Behavioral Disorders, 27*(1), 30–36.

Strain, P. S., & Hoyson, M. (2000). The need for longitudinal, intensive social skill intervention: LEAP follow-up outcomes for children with autism. *Topics in Early Childhood Special Education, 20*(2), 116–122.

Straus, S. E., Richardson, W. S., Glasziou, P., & Haynes, R. B. (2005). *Evidence-based medicine: How to practice and teach EBM* (3rd ed.). Edinburgh: Elsevier.

Stuart, R. B., & Lilienfeld, S. O. (2007). The evidence missing from evidence-based practice. *The American Psychologist, 62*, 615–616.

Sullivan, R. C. (2005). Community-integrated residential services for adults with autism: A working model (based on a mother's odyssey). In F. R. Volkmar, R. Paul, A. Klin, & D. J. Cohen (Eds.), *Handbook of autism and pervasive developmental disorders* (3rd ed., pp. 1255–1264). Hoboken: Wiley.

Tankersly, M., Cook, B. G., & Cook, L. (2008). A preliminary examination to identify the presence of quality indicators in single subject research. *Education and Treatment of Children, 31*, 523–548.

Thompson, B., Diamond, K. E., McWilliam, R., Snyder, P., & Snyder, S. (2005). Evaluating the quality of evidence from correlational research for evidence-based practice. *Exceptional Children, 71*, 181–194.

Upshur, R. E. G. (2003). Are all evidence-based practices alike? Problems in the ranking of evidence. *Canadian Medical Association Journal, 169*(7), 672–673.

Upton, D., & Upton, P. (2006). Knowledge and use of evidence-based practice by allied health and health science professionals in the United Kingdom. *Journal of Allied Health, 35*(3), 127–133.

Volkmar, F. (in press). Looking back and moving forward: A decade of research on autism. *Journal of Child Psychology and Psychiatry*.

Volkmar, F. R., & Wiesner, L. A. (2009). *A practical guide to autism*. Hoboken: Wiley.

Volkmar, F., Cook, E. H., Jr., Pomeroy, J., Realmuto, G., & Tanguay, P. (1999). Summary of the practice parameters for the assessment and treatment of children, adolescents, and adults with autism and other pervasive developmental disorders. American Academy of Child and Adolescent Psychiatry Working Group on quality issues. *Journal of the American Academy of Child and Adolescent Psychiatry, 38*(12), 1611–1616 [erratum in Journal of the American Academy of Child & Adolescent Psychiatry, 39(7):938].

Volkmar, F. R., State, M., & Klin, A. (2009). Autism and autism spectrum disorders: Diagnostic issues for the coming decade. *Journal of Child Psychology and Psychiatry, 50*(1–2), 108–115.

Volkmar, F. R., Woodbury-Smith, M., *et al.* (in press). Practice parameters for the assessment and treatment of children and adolescents with autism and pervasive developmental disorders. *Journal of the American Academy of Child & Adolescent Psychiatry*.

Walkup, J., Bernet, W., Bukstein, O., Walter, H., Arnold, V., et al. (2009). Practice parameter on the use of psychotropic medication in children and adolescents American Academy of Child & Adolescent Psychiatry Working Group on Quality Issues. *Journal of the American Academy of Child & Adolescent Psychiatry, 48*(9), 961–973.

Wampold, B. E., Goodheart, C. D., & Levant, R. F. (2007). Clarification and elaboration on evidence-based practice in psychology. *The American Psychologist, 62*, 616–618.

Weisz, J. R., & Kazdin, A. E. (Eds.). (2010). *Evidence-based psychotherapies for children and adolescents* (2nd ed.). New York: Guilford.

Wendt, D. C., Jr., & Slife, B. D. (2007). Is evidence-based practice diverse enough? Philosophy of science considerations. *The American Psychologist, 62*, 613–614.

Westen, D., & Bradley, R. (2005). Empirically supported complexity: Rethinking evidence-based practice in psychotherapy. *Current Directions in Psychological Science, 14*, 266–271.

Wolery, M., Werts, M. G., et al. (1995). Experienced teachers' perceptions of resources and supports for inclusion. *Education and Training in Mental Retardation and Developmental Disabilities, 30*(1), 15–26.

World Health Organization. (1992). *International classification of diseases and related health problems*, 10th ed. Geneva, Switzerland.

CHAPTER 2

Development, Procedures, and Application of the Evaluative Method for Determining Evidence-Based Practices in Autism

Brian Reichow

ABBREVIATIONS

ASDs   Autism spectrum disorders
EBP   Evidence-based practice
SSED   Single subject experimental
        design

BACKGROUND

Recently, we sought to review the empirical evidence on interventions for children with autism spectrum disorders (ASDs) in search of interventions meeting the criteria of evidence-based practice (EBP). As outlined in Chap. 1, EBP is defined differently by different disciplines. Although many of these definitions were quite good, it quickly became apparent that locating and defining EBP for children with ASDs using the available definitions and procedures would be difficult. Therefore, we decided to create a new

method for evaluating empirical evidence to determine if a practice could be considered an EBP. This decision was made only after determining that existing methods were not well suited for our specific needs; when possible, elements and standards from existing methods were adopted into the evaluative method presented in this chapter.

The evaluative method (Reichow et al. 2008) was created to assist with the identification of practices that could be considered EBPs for children with ASDs. It provides a method of evaluating intervention research and includes three instruments: rubrics for the evaluation of research report rigor; guidelines for the evaluation of research report strength; and criteria for determining if an intervention has the evidence needed to be considered an EBP. Initial assessments suggest that the evaluative method is a tool that can be used reliably to review intervention research to produce valid assessments of the empirical evidence on practices for children with ASDs (see Chap. 3).

B. Reichow et al. (eds.), *Evidence-Based Practices and Treatments for Children with Autism*, DOI 10.1007/978-1-4419-6975-0_2, © Springer Science+Business Media, LLC 2011

This chapter expands upon previous presentations of the evaluative method in two ways. First, it provides operationalized definitions and rating criteria for the primary and secondary quality indicators for the rubrics. Secondly, it provides a formula (i.e., an algorithm) that can be used to apply the EBP criteria to a set of studies to determine the EBP status of an intervention.

RESEARCH REPORT RIGOR

To evaluate the rigor of research reports, two rubrics were developed, one for research conducted using group research methods and one for research conducted using single subject experimental designs (SSED). These rubrics provide a grading scheme that evaluates the quality (i.e., the rigor) of methodological elements of individual research reports. Two levels of methodological element are included in the rubrics (Table 2.1): primary quality indicators and secondary quality indicators. Primary quality indicators are elements of the research methodology deemed critical for demonstrating the validity of a study. They are operationally defined and graded on a trichotomous ordinal scale (high quality, acceptable quality, and unacceptable quality). The secondary quality indicators are elements of research design that, although important, are not deemed necessary for the establishment of the validity of a study. They are operationally defined on a dichotomous scale (the report either contains or does not contain evidence of each indicator).

Because high-integrity experiments of group research designs and SSED share many characteristics, attempts were undertaken to retain similar definitions across rubrics. However, indicators specific to one type of research method are needed due to the differences in research methodologies (see Table 2.1).

When using the rubrics to evaluate research reports, we have found it helpful to create separate scoring sheets for each type of research methodology. Examples

TABLE 2.1 Primary and secondary quality indicators by type of experimental design

Group research designs	Single subject experimental design
Primary quality indicators	
• Participant characteristics	• Participant characteristics
• Independent variable	• Independent variable
• Comparison condition	• Dependent variable
• Dependent variable	• Baseline condition
• Link between research question and data analysis	• Visual analysis
• Statistical analysis	• Experimental control
Secondary quality indicators	
• Random assignment	• Interobserver agreement
• Interobserver agreement	• Kappa
• Blind raters	• Blind raters
• Fidelity	• Fidelity
• Attrition	• Generalization or maintenance
• Generalization or maintenance	• Social validity
• Effect size	
• Social validity	

of these scoring sheets are shown in Appendices 1 and 2 for group research designs and SSED, respectively. The following sections discuss the criteria for allocating a rating under each indicator.

Primary Quality Indicators for Group Research Design

Participant characteristics (PART) A high (H) quality rating is awarded to a study that meets the following criteria:

1. Age and gender are provided for all participants (mean age is acceptable).

2. All participants' diagnoses are operationalized by including the specific diagnosis and diagnostic instrument (acceptable instruments include ADOS, ADI-R, CARS, DSM-IV, and ICD-10) used to make the diagnosis or an operational definition of behaviors and symptoms of the participants.
3. Information on the characteristics of the interventionist are provided (the ability to determine who did the intervention is minimal a criterion) and information on any secondary participants (e.g., peers) is provided.
4. If a study provides standardized test scores, the measures used to obtain those scores are indicated.

An acceptable (A) quality rating is awarded to a study that meets criteria 1, 3 and 4. A study that does not meet all of criteria 1, 3, and 4 is of unacceptable quality and is awarded a U rating.

Independent variable (IV) (e.g., *intervention*) An H rating is awarded to a study that defines independent variables with replicable precision (i.e., one could reproduce the intervention given the description provided). If a manual is used, the study passes this criterion. An A rating is awarded to a study that defines many elements of the independent variable but omits specific details. A U rating is awarded to a study that does not sufficiently define the independent variables.

Comparison condition (CC) An H rating is awarded to a study that defines the conditions for the comparison group with replicable precision, including a description of any other interventions participants receive. An A rating is awarded to a study that vaguely describes the conditions for the comparison group; information on other interventions may not be reported. A U rating is awarded to a study that does not report the conditions for the comparison group or has no control or comparison group.

Dependent variable (DV) or outcome measure An H rating is awarded to a study that meets the following criteria:

- The variables are defined with operational precision.
- The details necessary to replicate the measures are provided.
- The measures are linked to the dependent variables.
- The measurement data is collected at appropriate times during the study for the analysis being conducted.

An A rating is awarded to a study that meets three of the four criteria. A U rating is awarded to a study that meets fewer criteria.

Link between research question and data analysis (LRQ) An H rating is awarded to a study in which data analysis is strongly linked to the research questions and uses correct units of measure (i.e., child level, teacher level, etc.) on all variables. An A rating is awarded to a study in which data analysis is poorly linked to the research questions but uses correct units for a majority of the outcome measures. A U rating is awarded to a study in which data analysis is linked weakly or not at all to the research questions and uses the correct unit for only a minority of the outcome measures.

Statistical analysis (STAT) An H rating is awarded to a study in which proper statistical analyses were conducted with an adequate power and sample size ($n > 10$) for each statistical measure. An A rating is awarded to a study in which proper statistical analyses were conducted for at least 75% of the outcome measures or in which proper statistical analyses were conducted on 100% of outcome measures but with inadequate power or a small sample size. A U rating is awarded to a study in which statistical analysis was not done correctly, the sample size was too small or the power was inadequate.

Secondary Quality Indicators for Group Research Design

These indicators are rated on a dichotomous scale (there either is, or is not, evidence of the indicator).

Random Assignment (RA) This indicator is positive if participants are assigned to groups using a random assignment procedure.

Interobserver Agreement (IOA) This indicator is positive if IOA is collected across all conditions, raters, and participants with reliability >.80 (Kappa >.60) or psychometric properties of standardized tests are reported and are >.70 agreement with a Kappa >.40.

Blind Raters (BR) This indicator is positive if raters are blind to the treatment condition of the participants.

Fidelity (FID) This indicator is positive if treatment or procedural fidelity is continuously assessed across participants, conditions, and implementers, and if applicable, has measurement statistics >.80.

Attrition (ATR) This indicator is positive if articulation is comparable (does not differ between groups by more than 25%) across conditions and less than 30% at the final outcome measure.

Generalization or Maintenance (G/M) This indicator is positive if outcome measures are collected after the final data collection to assess generalization or maintenance.

Effect Size (ES) This indicator is positive if effect sizes are reported for at least 75% of the outcome measures and are >.40.

Social Validity (SV) This indicator is positive if the study contains at least four of the following features:

- Socially important DVs (i.e., society would value the changes in outcome of the study)
- Time- and cost-effective intervention (i.e., the ends justify the means)
- Comparisons between individuals with and without disabilities
- A behavioral change that is large enough for practical value (i.e., it is clinically significant)

- Consumers who are satisfied with the results
- IV manipulation by people who typically come into contact with the participant
- A natural context

Primary Quality Indicators for SSEDs

Participant Characteristics (PART) A high (H) quality rating is awarded to a study that meets the following criteria:

1. Age and gender are provided for all participants.
2. All participants' diagnoses are operationalized by including the specific diagnosis and diagnostic instrument (acceptable instruments include ADOS, ADI-R, CARS, DSM-IV, and ICD-10) used to make the diagnosis or an operational definition of behaviors and symptoms of the participants.
3. Information on the characteristics of the interventionist are provided (the ability to determine who did the intervention is a minimal criterion) and information on any secondary participants (e.g., peers) is provided.
4. If a study provides standardized test scores, the measures used to obtain those scores are indicated.

An acceptable (A) quality rating is awarded to a study that meets criteria 1, 3, and 4. A study that does not meet all of criteria 1, 3, and 4 is of unacceptable quality and is awarded a U rating.

Independent Variable (IV) (e.g., *intervention*) An H rating is awarded to a study that defines independent variables with replicable precision (i.e., you could reproduce the intervention given the description provided). If a manual is used, the study passes this criterion. An A rating is awarded to a study that defines many elements of the independent variable but omits specific details. A U rating is awarded to a study that does not sufficiently define the independent variables.

Baseline Condition (BSLN) An H rating is awarded to a study in which 100% of baselines:

- Encompass at least three measurement points
- Appear through visual analysis to be stable
- Have no trend or a counter-therapeutic trend
- Have conditions that are operationally defined with replicable precision

An A rating is awarded to a study in which at least one of the above criteria was not met in at least one, but not more than 50%, of the baselines. A U rating is awarded to a study in which two or more of the above criteria were not met in at least one baseline or more than 50% of the baselines do not meet three of the criteria.

Dependent variable (DV) or outcome measure An H rating is awarded to a study that meets the following criteria:

- The variables are defined with operational precision.
- The details necessary to replicate the measures are provided.
- The measures are linked to the dependent variables.
- The measurement data is collected at appropriate times during the study for the analysis being conducted.

An A rating is awarded to a study that meets three of the four criteria. A U rating is awarded to a study that meets fewer criteria.

Visual Analysis (VIS ANAL) An H rating is awarded to a study in which 100% of graphs (i.e., tiers within a figure):

- Have data that are stable (level or trend)
- Contain less than 25% overlap of data points between adjacent conditions, unless behavior is at ceiling or floor levels in the previous condition

- Show a large shift in level or trend between adjacent conditions that coincide with the implementation or removal of the IV. If there was a delay in change at the manipulation of the IV, the study is accepted as high quality if the delay was similar across different conditions or participants (+/–50% of delay)

An A rating is awarded to a study in which two of the criteria were met on at least 66% of the graphs. A U rating is awarded to a study in which two or fewer criteria were met on less than 66% of the graphs.

Experimental Control (EXP CON) An H rating is awarded to a study that contains at least three demonstrations of the experimental effect, occurring at three different points in time and changes in the DVs vary with the manipulation of the IV in all instances of replication. If there was a delay in change at the manipulation of the IV, the study is accepted as high quality if the delay was similar across different conditions or participants (+/–50% of delay). An A rating is awarded to a study in which at least 50% of the demonstrations of the experimental effect meet the above criteria, there are two demonstrations of the experimental effect at two different points in time and changes in the DVs vary with the manipulation of the IV. A U rating is awarded to a study in which less than 50% of the demonstrations of the experimental effect meet the above criteria, there are fewer than two demonstrations of the experimental effect occurring at two different points in which changes in the DVs vary with the manipulation of the IV.

Secondary Quality Indicators for SSEDs

These indicators are rated on a dichotomous scale (there either is, or is not, evidence of the indicator).

Interobserver Agreement (IOA) This indicator is positive if IOA is collected across all conditions, raters, and participants with reliability >.80.

Kappa (KAP) This indicator is positive if Kappa is calculated on at least 20% of sessions across all conditions, raters, and participants with a score >.60.

Blind Raters (BR) This indicator is positive if raters are blind to the treatment condition of the participants.

Fidelity (FID) This indicator is positive if treatment or procedural fidelity is continuously assessed across participants, conditions, and implementers, and if applicable, has measurement statistics >.80.

Generalization or Maintenance (G/M) This indicator is positive if outcome measures are collected after the final data collection to assess generalization or maintenance.

Social Validity (SV) This indicator is positive if the study contains at least four of the following features:

- Socially important DVs (i.e., society would value the changes in outcome of the study)
- Time- and cost-effective intervention (i.e., the ends justify the means)
- Comparisons between individuals with and without disabilities

- A behavioral change that is large enough for practical value (i.e., it is clinically significant)
- Consumers who are satisfied with the results
- IV manipulation by people who typically come into contact with the participant
- A natural context

RESEARCH REPORT STRENGTH RATINGS

The second instrument of the evaluative method provides scoring criteria to synthesize the ratings from the rubrics into a rating of the strength of the research report. There are three levels of research report strength: strong, adequate, and weak. The requirements for each strength rating are shown in Table 2.2. Research reports with a strong rating demonstrate concrete evidence of high quality. These reports received high quality grades on all primary indicators and contained evidence of multiple secondary quality indicators.

TABLE 2.2   Guidelines for the determination of research report strength ratings (Adapted from Reichow et al. 2008. With permission)

Strength rating	Group research	Single subject research
Strong	Received high quality grades on all primary quality indicators and showed evidence of four or more secondary quality indicators	Received high quality grades on all primary quality indicators and showed evidence of three or more secondary quality indicators
Adequate	Received high quality grades on four or more primary quality indicators with no unacceptable quality grades on any primary quality indicators, and showed evidence of at least two secondary quality indicators	Received high quality grades on four or more primary quality indicators with no unacceptable quality grades on any primary quality indicators, and showed evidence of at least two secondary quality indicators
Weak	Received fewer than four high quality grades on primary quality indicators or showed evidence of less than two secondary quality indicators	Received fewer than four high quality grades on primary quality indicators or showed evidence of less than two secondary quality indicators

An adequate rating designates research showing strong evidence in most, but not all areas. Elements of reports achieving an adequate rating might have received acceptable grades on up to two primary quality indicators and must have shown evidence of at least two secondary quality indicators. A study receiving an adequate strength rating cannot receive an unacceptable grade on any primary quality indicator. A weak rating indicates that the research report has many missing elements or fatal flaws. Reports receiving one or more unacceptable grades on primary quality indicators or evidence of one or fewer secondary quality indicators receive a weak rating. Because conclusions about the results of a study receiving a weak rating are tentative at best, studies receiving this rating are not used when determining the EBP status of an intervention.

CRITERIA FOR LEVELS OF EBP

The final instrument provides the criteria for the aggregation of research reports with respect to their strength rating across studies to determine whether a practice has amassed enough empirical support to be classified as an EBP. The criteria for two levels of EBP, established and promising (see Table 2.3), have been guided by

TABLE 2.3   Criteria for treatments to be considered EBP (Adapted from Reichow et al. 2008. With permission)

Level of EBP	Example criteria
Established (≥ 60 points from the EBP status formula)	• Five SSED studies of strong research report strength with a total sample size of at least 15 participants across studies conducted by at least three research teams in three different geographic locations • Ten SSED studies of adequate research report strength with a total sample size of at least 30 different participants across studies conducted by at least three research teams in three different geographic locations • Two group design studies of strong research report strength conducted by in different geographic locations • Four group design studies of at least adequate research report strength conducted in at least two different research teams • One group design study of strong research report strength and three SSED studies of strong research report strength with at least 8 different participants • Two group design studies of at least adequate research report strength and six SSED studies of at least adequate research report strength with at least 16 different participants
Promising (> 30 points from the EBP status formula)	• Five SSED studies of at least adequate research report strength with a total sample size of at least 16 different participants across studies conducted by at least two research teams in two different geographic locations • Two group design studies of at least adequate research report strength • One group research report of at least adequate research report strength rating and at least three SSED studies of at least adequate strength rating with at least 8 participants

previous EBP criteria (Filipek et al. 2000; Gersten et al. 2005; Horner et al. 2005; Kratochwill and Stoiber 2002; Lonigan et al. 1998) and contain an operalization for documenting the evidence needed to meet the criteria of the two levels. A treatment must meet at least one example criterion; it can meet multiple criteria.

An established EBP is a treatment shown to be effective across multiple methodologically sound studies conducted by at least two independent research groups in separate geographical locations. Practices meeting this requirement have demonstrated enough evidence for confidence in the treatment's efficacy. A promising EBP is also a treatment shown to be effective across multiple studies but for which the evidence is limited by weaker methodological rigor, fewer replications, and/or an inadequate number of independent researchers demonstrating the effects.

The two levels of EBP status can be obtained only using studies conducted using group research designs, only using studies conducted using SSED, or by using a combination of studies conducted using group research designs and SSED. When determining the EBP status of an intervention in which the evidence was obtained using group research designs, it is necessary to look at how many studies have been conducted. When determining the EBP status of an intervention in which the evidence was obtained using SSED, it is necessary to examine both the number of studies that were conducted and the number of participants with whom the procedures have been replicated. When examining the number of participants, an adaptation of the success estimate created by Reichow and Volkmar (in press) is recommended. The adapted success estimate should be estimated using visual analysis (Gast and Spriggs 2010); it provides an estimate of the number of participants for whom the intervention was successful within each study. Using the adapted success estimate

should provide a more accurate appraisal of the number of participants for whom the intervention has worked than using the total number of participants from a study, as has been suggested in previous definitions of EBP (Horner et al. 2005; Lonigan et al. 1998).

The EBP status formula (2.1) provides a tool that can be used to assess all possible combinations of evidence that can be pooled to demonstrate the efficacy of a practice with respect to its status as an EBP.

$$(\text{Group}_S * 30) + (\text{Group}_A * 15) + (\text{SSED}_S * 4) + (\text{SSED}_A * 2) = Z \quad (2.1)$$

Group_S is the number of studies conducted using group research designs earning a strong rating, Group_A is the number of studies conducted using group research designs earning an adequate rating, SSED_S is the number of participants for whom the intervention was successful from SSED studies earning a strong rating, SSED_A is the number of participants for whom the intervention was successful from SSED studies earning an adequate rating, and Z is the total number of points for an intervention. It was determined that eight participants from strong SSED studies were equivalent to one strong group study by averaging two previous definitions of EBP providing a quantification of the number of SSED participants needed to achieve the highest level of evidence (Horner et al. 2005; Lonigan et al. 1998). When using the formula, 31 points are required for an intervention to meet the criteria of a promising EBP and 60 points are required for an intervention to meet the criteria of an established EBP. The criterion point levels are set such that there must be at least two studies for a practice to meet either EBP criterion and the formula is weighted such that studies with strong ratings contribute twice as much as studies receiving adequate rigor ratings. A reproducible worksheet containing blanks in which to place the necessary information to calculate the EBP status formula is provided in Appendix 3. Table 2.3 presents a sample, but not an exhaustive list, of ways in which the criteria for EBP can be met with studies conducted using only group research designs, using only SSED, and through combinations of the two research methodologies. Because this is an early attempt at synthesizing studies conducted using group research designs and SSED, empirical validation of the criteria is needed.

APPLICATION OF THE EBP STATUS FORMULA AND EBP CRITERIA

This section provides three examples of synthesizing multiple research report strength ratings for an intervention to determine whether the intervention has demonstrated the quantity and quality of

evidence to be considered an EBP. The first two examples are taken from a recent review of interventions for increasing prosocial behavior by Reichow and Volkmar (in press). Based on the results of their review, two interventions for school-aged children met the criteria of EBP.

Synthesizing Group Results

Table 2.4 provides an example of using the EBP status formula and applying the criteria of EBP using the results for social skills group interventions. As shown in the table, two studies using group research methodology received strong rigor ratings, thus $Group_S = 2$. Using Formula (2.1), social skills groups amassed 60 points, which meets the level for an established EBP and so social skills groups for school-aged children can be classified as an established EBP. Note, because only group studies were used, the number of participants in each study was not applicable and did not affect the calculation.

TABLE 2.4   EBP status of social skills groups for school-aged children (As reviewed by Reichow and Volkmar in press)

Study	Research method	Rigor rating	Successful N
Lopata et al. (2008)	Group	Strong	N/A
Owens et al. (2008)	Group	Strong	N/A
Number of group *studies* with strong rigor ratings	2		$= Group_S$
Number of group *studies* with adequate rigor ratings	0		$= Group_A$
Number of *participants* from SSED studies with strong rigor ratings	0		$= SSED_S$
Number of *participants* from SSED studies with adequate rigor ratings	0		$= SSED_A$

Formula for determining EBP status

$$(Group_S * 30) + (Group_A * 15) + (SSED_S * 4) + (SSED_A * 2) = Z$$
$$(2 * 30) + (0 * 15) + (0 * 4) + (0 * 2) = Z$$
$$60 = Z$$

Points (Z)	0	10	20	30	31	40	50	59	60+
EBP status	Not an EBP				Probable EBP				Established EBP

Synthesizing SSED Results

The application of the results of the Reichow and Volkmar (in press) synthesis is presented for video modeling for school-aged children in Table 2.5. As shown, five studies using SSED methods received adequate rigor ratings. Because there were a total of 16 participants across the five studies, $SSED_A = 16$. Using Formula (2.1), video modeling amassed 32 points, which is below the criteria for either level of EBP. Thus, video modeling for school-aged children can be classified as a promising EBP. Note, in contrast to the first example, which used only group design studies, the second example used only SSED studies; thus, all calculations involved the number participants for whom the intervention was successful from each of the studies.

Synthesizing Group and SSED Results

An example of synthesizing results across studies conducted using both group research designs and SSED is illustrated from the analysis of behavioral interventions to improve joint attention behaviors by Ferraioli and Harris (see Chap. 6). As shown in Table 2.6, one group research study received a strong rigor rating ($Group_S = 1$). The remaining studies were conducted using SSED; four studies with 15 participants for whom the interventions were successful received strong rigor ratings ($SSED_S = 15$) and one study with two participants for whom the intervention was successful received an adequate rigor rating ($SSED_A = 2$). In summing the values, behavioral interventions for increasing joint attention behav-

TABLE 2.5   EBP status of video modeling for school-aged children (As reviewed by Reichow and Volkmar in press)

Study	Research method	Rigor rating	Successful N
Buggey (2005)	SSED	Adequate	2
Charlop-Christy and Daneshvar (2003)	SSED	Adequate	3
Nikopoulous and Keenan (2004)	SSED	Adequate	3
Nikopoulous and Keenan (2007)	SSED	Adequate	3
Sherer et al. (2001)	SSED	Adequate	5
Number of group *studies* with strong rigor ratings		0	= $Group_S$
Number of group *studies* with adequate rigor ratings		0	= $Group_A$
Number of *participants* from SSED studies with strong rigor ratings		0	= $SSED_S$
Number of *participants* from SSED studies with adequate rigor ratings		16	= $SSED_A$

Formula for determining EBP status

$$(Group_S * 30) + (Group_A * 15) + (SSED_S * 4) + (SSED_A * 2) = Z$$
$$(0 * 30) + (0 * 15) + (0 * 4) + (16 * 2) = Z$$
$$32 = Z$$

Points (Z)	0	10	20	30	31	40	50	59	60+
EBP status	Not an EBP				Probable EBP				Established EBP

TABLE 2.6 EBP status of behavioral interventions to increase joint attention behaviors (As reviewed by Ferraioli and Harris in Chap. 6)

Study	Research method	Rigor rating	Successful N
Kasari et al. (2006)	Group	Strong	N/A
Martins and Harris (2006)	SSED	Strong	3
Rocha et al. (2007)	SSED	Strong	3
Whalen and Schreibman (2003)	SSED	Strong	5
Whalen et al. (2006)	SSED	Strong	4
Zercher et al. (2001)	SSED	Adequate	2

Number of group *studies* with strong rigor ratings	1	= $Group_S$
Number of group *studies* with adequate rigor ratings	0	= $Group_A$
Number of *participants* from SSED studies with strong rigor ratings	15	= $SSED_S$
Number of *participants* from SSED studies with adequate rigor ratings	2	= $SSED_A$

Formula for Determining EBP Status

$$(Group_S * 30) + (Group_A * 15) + (SSED_S * 4) + (SSED_A * 2) = Z$$
$$(1 * 30) + (0 * 15) + (15 * 4) + (2 * 2) = Z$$
$$94 = Z$$

Points (Z)	0	10	20	30		31	40	50	59		60+
EBP Status	Not an EBP					Probable EBP					Established EBP

iors amassed 94 points, which exceeds the criterion for an established EBP. Because the number of participants for whom the interventions were successful in each study was a factor in the calculations for the SSED variables, the number of participants did factor into the determination of EBP status.

DISCUSSION

In principle, the arrangement of identifying educational practices based on scientific evidence is admirable; using scientific evidence to inform practice should increase the likelihood of providing effective treatments. However, researchers have established few EBP for young children with ASDs through the application of established operationalized criteria (Reichow and Volkmar in Chap. 1;

Rogers and Vismara 2008). The evaluative method outlined in this chapter was created to address the need to identify EBP for young children with ASDs. The method has been used to examine the state of the science in research involving young children with ASDs (Reichow et al. 2007); to evaluate the empirical evidence on the Picture Exchange Communication System (Doehring et al. 2007); to determine the methodological rigor of studies included in research syntheses (Reichow and Volkmar in press; Reichow and Wolery 2009); and to determine the EBP status of interventions to increase the prosocial behavior of individuals with ASDs (Reichow and Volkmar in press). Collectively, the applications of the evaluative method have led to a number of practices being identified as EBP.

One particularly noteworthy characteristic of the criteria of EBP is the combination of multiple research methodologies.

The evaluative method of Reichow et al. (2008) was one of the first conceptualizations of EBP to provide an operationalized method for combining multiple research methods to investigate a single practice. The National Standards Project (National Autism Center 2009) described in Chap. 1 is a second example of synthesizing studies across research designs. Although the innovation of operationalizing a method of combining group research designs and SSED is noteworthy, the inclusion of only these research methodologies is limiting. However, our experience of reviewing the intervention literature for individuals with ASDs leads us to believe that the overwhelming majority of studies have been and continue to be conducted using the two methodologies for which the evaluative method was designed (i.e., group research designs and SSED). Thus, apart from a philosophical objection, it is unclear how much this limitation affects the results of a review conducted using the evaluative method.

The evaluative method has boundaries to its use and is not without limitations. With respect to the boundaries, the method was designed to evaluate research reports of specific interventions (e.g., focal interventions), not comprehensive programs. Second, the method was designed to evaluate individual experimental research reports; thus, the method is not appropriate for evaluating the methodological rigor of systematic reviews or meta-analyses. Since many hierarchies of evidence consider findings from multiple systematic reviews to be the highest level of evidence (Straus et al. 2005), this is a limitation that needs to be addressed in the future. Finally, some of the quality indicators on the rubrics are weighted toward studies demonstrating positive effects (e.g., effect size, visual analysis, and experimental control). Because the rubric for SSED contains these elements as primary quality indicators, a study

failing to demonstrate a positive effect would most likely receive an unacceptable grade on these elements and thus be rated as a weak study. Some definitions of EBP have created categories and grading schemes for treatments that do not work (Hawley and Wiesz 2002; Lilienfied 2005) or for which there is conflicting evidence (De Los Reyes and Kazdin 2008). Making recommendations on ineffective practices was not a goal of the initial project and it is unlikely that the evaluative method in its current state is appropriate for evaluating research with null or negative results. Thus, the evaluative method is best suited for evaluating empirical research on interventions for individuals with ASDs conducted using group research designs or SSED in which the desired change in behavior was achieved.

Five additional limitations should be acknowledged. First, it is likely that there is a minimum set of competencies or knowledge base for using the evaluative method. Because the evaluative method is still relatively new and has not been widely tested, the extent of this limitation is not known. However, we can report that it has been successfully used and adopted by professionals not involved in this project (Children's Services Evidence-Based Practice Advisory Committee 2009; V. Smith, November 22, 2007 in a personal communication). Second, some elements of the evaluative method (e.g., the number of participants needed for a practice to be considered an EBP when using SSED) have not been empirically validated. Third, although the preliminary assessments of reliability and validity were positive (see Chap. 3), these assessments were conducted on a small sample by individuals closely connected with the development of the method. Validation of its application in real-world settings remains to be seen. Fourth, the evaluative method contains no method for assessing publication bias (Borenstein et al. 2009). Although the inclusion of an instrument capable of synthesizing research across multiple research methodologies is likely to lessen the impact of publication bias when compared to other methods of determining EBP, the threat of publication bias remains and should be acknowledged. Finally, as with any review, application of the evaluative method provides a picture of the research that was reviewed in that instance. Different reviews occurring at different times with different inclusion criteria are likely to produce conflicting results.

REFERENCES

Borenstein, M., Hedges, L. V., Higgins, J. P. T., & Rothstein, H. R. (2009). *Introduction to meta-analysis*. West Sussex: Wiley.

Children's Services Evidence-Based Practice Advisory Committee. (2009). *Interventions for autism spectrum disorders: State of the evidence*. Portland.

De Los Reyes, A., & Kazdin, A. E. (2008). When the evidence says, "yes, no, and maybe so": Attending to and interpreting inconsistent findings among evidence-based interventions. *Current Directions in Psychological Science, 17*, 47–51.

Doehring, P., Reichow, B., & Volkmar, F. R. (2007). Is it evidenced-based? How to evaluate claims of effectiveness for autism. Paper presented at the International Association for Positive Behavior Support Conference, March, Boston, MA.

Filipek, P. A., Accardo, P. J., Ashwal, S., Baranek, G. T., Cook, E. H., Jr., et al. (2000). Practice parameter: Screening and diagnosis of autism. *Neurology, 55*, 468–479.

Gast, D. L., & Spriggs, A. D. (2010). Visual analysis of graphic data. In D. L. Gast (Ed.), *Single subject research in behavioral methodology* (pp. 199–233). New York: Routledge.

Gersten, R., Fuchs, L. S., Coyne, M., Greenwood, C., & Innocenti, M. S. (2005). Quality indicators for group experimental and quasi-experimental research in special education. *Exceptional Children, 71*, 149–164.

Hawley, K. M., & Weisz, J. R. (2002). Increasing the relevance of evidence-based treatments review to practitioners and consumers. *Clinical Psychology: Science and Practice, 9*, 225–230.

Horner, R. H., Carr, E. G., Halle, J., McGee, G., Odom, S., & Wolery, M. (2005). The use of single subject research to identify evidence-based practice in special education. *Exceptional Children, 71*, 165–179.

Kratochwill, T. R., & Stoiber, K. C. (2002). Evidence-based interventions in school psychology: Conceptual foundations of the procedural and coding manual of Division 16 and the Society for the Study of School Psychology task force. *School Psychology Quarterly, 17*, 341–389.

Lilienfied, S. O. (2005). Scientifically unsupported and supported interventions for childhood psychopathology: A summary. *Pediatrics, 115*, 761–764.

Lonigan, C. J., Elbert, J. C., & Johnson, S. B. (1998). Empirically supported psychosocial interventions for children: An overview. *Journal of Clinical Child Psychology, 27*, 138–145.

Lord, C., Wagner, A., Rogers, S., Szatmari, P., Aman, M., et al. (2005). Challenges in evaluating psychosocial interventions for autistic spectrum disorders. *Journal of Autism and Developmental Disorders, 35*, 695–711.

National Autism Center. (2009). *National standards report*. Randolph: National Autism Center.

Reichow, B., & Volkmar, F. R. (in press) Introduction to evidence-based practices in autism. In B. Reichow, P. Doehring, D. V. Cicchetti, & F. R. Volkmar (Eds.). *Evidence-based practices and treatments for children with autism*. New York, NY: Springer.

Reichow, B., & Wolery, M. (2009). Comprehensive synthesis of early intensive behavioral interventions for young children with autism based on the UCLA Young Autism Project model. *Journal of Autism and Developmental Disorders, 39*, 23–41.

Reichow, B., Barton, E. E., Volkmar, F. R., & Cicchetti, D. V. (2007). The status of research on interventions for young children with autism spectrum disorders. Poster presented at the International Meeting for Autism Research, May, Seattle, WA.

Reichow, B., Volkmar, F. R., & Cicchetti, D. V. (2008). Development of an evaluative method for determining the strength of research evidence in autism. *Journal of Autism and Developmental Disorders, 38*, 1311–1319.

Rogers, S. J., & Vismara, L. A. (2008). Evidence-based comprehensive treatments for early autism. *Journal of Clinical Child and Adolescent Psychology, 37*, 8–38.

Straus, S. E., Richardson, W. S., Glasziou, P., & Haynes, R. B. (2005). *Evidence-based medicine: How to practice and teach EBM* (3rd ed.). Edinburgh: Elsevier.

APPENDIX A: RATING FORM FOR STUDIES USING GROUP RESEARCH DESIGN STUDIES

Study	Essential Quality Indicators						Desirable Quality Indicators						
	PART	IV	CC	DV	LRQ	STAT	RA	IOA	BR	FID	ATR	G/M	ES	SV

APPENDIX B: RATING FORM FOR STUDIES USING SINGLE SUBJECT EXPERIMENTAL DESIGNS

Study	Essential Quality Indicators						Desirable Quality Indicators					
	PART	DV	IV	BSLN	VIS ANAL	EXP CON	IOA	KAP	BR	FID	G/M	SV

Appendix C: EBP Status Worksheet

Study	Research method	Rigor rating	Successful N

Number of group *studies* with strong rigor ratings   = Group_S

Number of group *studies* with adequate rigor ratings   = Group_A

Number of *participants* from SSED studies with strong rigor ratings   = SSED_S

Number of *participants* from SSED studies with adequate rigor ratings   = SSED_A

Formula for determining EBP status

$$(\text{Group}_S * 30) + (\text{Group}_A * 15) + (\text{SSED}_S * 4) + (\text{SSED}_A * 2) = Z$$

Points (Z)	0	10	20	30	31	40	50	59	60+
EBP status	Not an EBP				Probable EBP				Established EBP

On the Reliability and Accuracy of the Evaluative Method for Identifying Evidence-Based Practices in Autism

Domenic V. Cicchetti

ABBREVIATIONS

EBP	Evidence-based practice
K	Kappa
PC	Proportion of chance agreement
PNA	Predicted negative accuracy
PO	Proportion of observed agreement
POneg	Proportion of observed negative agreement
POpos	Proportion of observed positive agreement
PPA	Predicted positive accuracy
QI–	Quality indicator absent
QI+	Quality indicator present
Se	Sensitivity
Sp	Specificity
SSED	Single subject experimental design

INTRODUCTION

The editors of this book recently described the development and application of an "evaluative method" for assessing evidence-based practices (EBP) in Autism (Reichow et al. 2008). The major results of this investigation, which were presented at the International Meeting for Autism Research (Reichow et al. 2007) indicated that the method produced highly reliable and valid results, whether deriving from an assessment of primary or secondary quality indicators from published peer-reviewed, group research reports or from published and peer-reviewed, single subject experimental design (SSED) reports. The levels of inter-examiner agreement, ranged between 85%, with a Kappa or chance-corrected

B. Reichow et al. (eds.), *Evidence-Based Practices and Treatments for Children with Autism*, DOI 10.1007/978-1-4419-6975-0_3, © Springer Science+Business Media, LLC 2011

level of 0.69 (Cohen 1960), and 96%, with a Kappa value of 0.93. By applying the criteria of Cicchetti (2001) and Cicchetti et al. (1995), the levels of reliability ranged between good (85%, with a Kappa value of 0.69) and excellent (96%, with a Kappa value equal to 0.93).

The two-fold purpose of this chapter is to discuss some biostatistical issues that need to be understood in the separate but conceptually related contexts of: some paradoxes that can occur in the application of the Kappa statistic and how they can be understood in the context of future reliability studies of the evaluative method for assessing EBP in autism; an elucidation of the most potent method for determining the validity or accuracy of rater assessments of EBP in autism; and the introduction of a new validity index that can be applied to the EBP evaluative method for research in autism, as well as more generally in biobehavioral research.

THE KAPPA STATISTIC DEFINED

When two raters, or clinical examiners, evaluate EBP in autism, the reliability research design for a given quality indicator can be depicted, as shown in Table 3.1.

The proportion of cases for which the two examiners agree that the studies contain evidence of the quality indicator is symbolized by the letter A and those for which they agree that the quality indicator is absent is symbolized by the letter D. To determine the level of overall chance-corrected inter-examiner agreement, the proportion of observed agreement (PO) is $(A+D)$, the proportion of chance agreement (PC) is $[(E_1F_1)+(E_2F_2)]$, and the maximum amount of chance-corrected agreement that is possible is $(1-PC)$. Kappa (K) is then defined as (Cohen 1960; Fleiss et al. 1969):

$$K = (PO - PC)/(1 - PC)$$

TABLE 3.1   Reliability research design for assessing evidence-based practice (EBP) in Autism[1]

	Rater 2		
Rater 1	Meets EBP Criterion	Fails EBP Criterion	Total
Meets EBP Criterion	A (E^1F^1)	B (E^2F^1)	F^1
Fails EBP Criterion	C (E^1F^2)	D (E^2F^2)	F^2
Total	E^1	E^2	1.00

Note[1]: The letters A and D refer, respectively, to the proportions of cases for which the two examiners agree either that the studies meet the EBP criterion (as symbolized by the letter A); or fail EBP criterion (symbolized by the letter D)

Kappa is constructed such that when rater agreement is no better than chance PO = PC, thereby resulting in a Kappa value of 0; when PO > PC, the usual case, then Kappa assumes a positive value; finally, when inter-rater agreement is at a level below chance expectation – a very unusual occurrence – then PC > PO, and Kappa assumes a negative value. The level of statistical significance of Kappa is determined by dividing the value of Kappa by its standard error and interpreting the result as a Z score, with the standard relationship between Z and statistical significance, or probability level (p), given as shown in Table 3.2.

Because a very low level of Kappa (e.g., as low as 0.10) is statistically significant at the 0.05 level, or beyond, based upon a sufficiently large enough sample size, biostatistical guidelines have been published to determine levels of Kappa that might be considered of practical or clinical significance. Conceptually similar Kappa guidelines have been provided by Landis and Koch (1977):

<0.00 Poor
0.00–0.20 Slight

0.21–0.40 Fair
0.41–0.60 Moderate
0.61–0.80 Substantial
0.81–1.00 Almost Perfect

by Fleiss (1981) and Fleiss et al. (2003):

<0.40 Poor
0.40–0.74 Fair to Good
≥0.75 Excellent

and by Cicchetti and Sparrow (1981) and Cicchetti (1994):

<0.40 Poor
0.40–0.59 Fair
0.60–0.74 Good
≥0.75 Excellent

When an investigator obtains a good to excellent level of agreement between any pair of raters or judges (say, 80–≥90%), the usual expectation is that the level of Kappa or chance-corrected agreement should correspondingly be good to excellent, as was shown for the Evaluative Method. As the next section indicates, this is not always true. It is possible to have a high level of agreement (say, 85%) associated with an unexpectedly low level of Kappa (say, <0.40 or poor, by the guidelines). This seemingly anomalous phenomenon has been identified as a "Kappa paradox" by Cicchetti (1988), Cicchetti and Feinstein (1990), and Feinstein and Cicchetti (1990).

TABLE 3.2   Level of statistical significance for Kappa

Z of Kappa	p of Kappa
< 1.65	not significant (ns)
1.65	.10
1.96	.05
2.24	.025
2.58	.01
2.81	.005
3.29	.001

KAPPA PARADOXES

We now show that when both PO and K are at a high level of rater agreement (e.g., PO = 0.85 and K = 0.60) then the agreement in both positive (POpos) and negative (POneg) cases is correspondingly high. In distinct contrast, when PO is high (e.g., 0.85) but K is very low (i.e., < 0.40), it signals a large discrepancy between inter-rater agreement on positive (POpos) and negative (POneg) cases.

Table 3.3 shows some reliability research results deriving from a hypothetical research investigation in which 100 group studies are assessed as to whether they demonstrated evidence of the primary quality indicators.

Using the formulae given in Table 3.1, it is readily seen that:

$$PO = (0.40 + 0.45) = 0.85$$
$$PC = (0.2254 + 0.2754) = 0.5008$$
$$K = (0.8500 - 0.5008) / (1 - 0.5008)$$
$$= 0.3492 / 0.4992 = 0.70.$$

This is a clear example of a reliability estimate in which the level of PO, at 85%,

TABLE 3.3   Illustrating data for calculating Kappa for assessing evidence-based practice (EBP) primary quality indicators deriving from 100 hypothetical group design studies

Rater 1	Rater 2		
	QI+	QI–	Totals
QI+	0.40(0.2254)	0.09(0.2646)	0.49
QI–	0.06(0.2346)	0.45(0.2754)	0.51
Totals	0.46	0.54	1.0

Unbracketed values refer to the proportions of cases EBP raters either agree or disagree. Bracketed values refer to the corresponding proportions of cases in which the two raters can be expected to agree by chance alone

is good (Cicchetti et al. 1995) and the level of Kappa, at 0.70, is also good (Cicchetti 1994). These results are virtually interchangeable with the aforementioned PO (also 0.85) and the K values (at 0.69) for primary quality indicators obtained when assessing EBP in autism based upon SSED; or for secondary quality indicators based upon group design research reports (Reichow et al. 2008).

Next, we show that when both PO and K have good inter-rater agreement, the POpos and POneg values are close to the PO value of 0.85. First, we calculate the rater agreement on positive cases, those in which a quality indicator is present (QI+), by the formula:

$$POpos = \frac{A}{(E_1 + F_1)/2} \qquad (3.1)$$

Analogously, the rater agreement on negative cases, those in which a quality indicator is absent (QI–), by the formula:

$$POneg = \frac{D}{(E_2 + F_2)/2} \qquad (3.2)$$

If we apply Formula (3.1) and Formula (3.2) to the data in Table 3.3, we obtain the following values:

$$POpos = \frac{0.40}{(0.49 + 0.46)/2} = \frac{0.40}{0.475} = 0.84$$

$$POneg = \frac{0.45}{(0.51 + 0.54)/2} = \frac{0.45}{0.525} = 0.86$$

It can be seen that the POpos and POneg values are both high and comparable to PO=0.85.

Let us now consider a hypothetical example in which PO is also 0.85, representing good agreement, but the corresponding level of Kappa is only 0.32 (poor). The hypothetical data upon which this result is based are shown in Table 3.4.

In distinct contrast to the previous case, it is shown that when PO is high but Kappa is low, then the relative values of POpos and POneg, are quite discrepant, relative to the PO of 0.85:

TABLE 3.4 Hypothetical data producing a Kappa paradox in the assessment of evidence-based practice (EBP) quality indicators derived from 100 hypothetical group design studies

	Rater 2		
Rater 1	QI+	QI–	Totals
QI+	0.05(0.015)	0.10(0.135)	0.15
QI–	0.05(0.085)	0.80(0.765)	0.85
Totals	0.10	0.90	1.0

Unbracketed values refer to the proportions of cases upon which the two EBP raters either agree or disagree. Bracketed values refer to the corresponding proportions of cases in which the two raters can be expected to agree or disagree by chance alone

$$POpos = \frac{0.05}{(0.15 + 0.10)/2} = \frac{0.05}{0.125} = 0.40$$

$$POneg = \frac{0.80}{(0.85 + 0.90)/2} = \frac{0.80}{0.875} = 0.9143$$

Note that PO (usually defined as A + D) can, using formulae (3.1) and (3.2), be defined as the weighted average of POpos and POneg:

$$PO = (0.9143 \times 0.875) + (0.40 \times 0.125)$$
$$= (0.80 + 0.05) = 0.85.$$

The question is, how can these two contrasting Kappa values (0.70 and 0.32) both associated with a PO of 0.85, be understood in a larger biostatistical and clinical framework? In order to accomplish this, one must determine where in the possible series of combinations that form a PO of 0.85 these two examples occur. As shown by the hypothetical data spread in Table 3.5, there are 43 such possibilities.

The best possible value of Kappa (Cases 1 and 2) is 0.70, with both POpos and POneg also at exactly 0.85. Case 3 is depicted in Table 3.3, with POpos and POneg at 0.84 and 0.86, respectively. Note that as

TABLE 3.5 Rank ordering of all values of Kappa, POpos and POneg when PO=0.85

Case	Pos	Neg	Kappa	POpos	POneg
1	0.42	0.43	0.70	0.85	0.85
2	0.41	0.44	0.70	0.85	0.85
3	0.40	0.45	0.70	0.84	0.86
4	0.39	0.46	0.70	0.84	0.86
5	0.38	0.47	0.70	0.84	0.86
6	0.37	0.48	0.70	0.83	0.86
7	0.36	0.49	0.70	0.83	0.87
8	0.35	0.50	0.69	0.82	0.87
9	0.34	0.51	0.69	0.82	0.87
10	0.33	0.52	0.69	0.81	0.87
11	0.32	0.53	0.69	0.81	0.88
12	0.31	0.54	0.68	0.81	0.88
13	0.30	0.55	0.68	0.80	0.88
14	0.29	0.56	0.68	0.79	0.88
15	0.28	0.57	0.67	0.79	0.88
16	0.27	0.58	0.67	0.78	0.89
17	0.26	0.59	0.66	0.66	0.89
18	0.25	0.60	0.66	0.77	0.89
19	0.24	0.61	0.65	0.76	0.89
20	0.23	0.62	0.65	0.75	0.89
21	0.22	0.63	0.64	0.75	0.89
22	0.21	0.64	0.63	0.74	0.90
23	0.20	0.65	0.62	0.73	0.90
24	0.19	0.66	0.62	0.72	0.90
25	0.18	0.67	0.61	0.71	0.90
26	0.17	0.68	0.60	0.69	0.90
27	0.16	0.69	0.58	0.69	0.90
28	0.15	0.70	0.57	0.67	0.90
29	0.14	0.71	0.56	0.65	0.90
30	0.13	0.72	0.54	0.63	0.91
31	0.12	0.73	0.52	0.62	0.91
32	0.11	0.74	0.50	0.59	0.91
33	0.10	0.75	0.48	0.57	0.91
34	0.09	0.76	0.46	0.55	0.91
35	0.08	0.77	0.43	0.52	0.91
36	0.07	0.78	0.40	0.48	0.91
37	0.06	0.79	0.36	0.44	0.91
38	0.05	0.80	0.32	0.40	0.91
39	0.04	0.81	0.26	0.35	0.92
40	0.03	0.82	0.20	0.29	0.92
41	0.02	0.83	0.16	0.21	0.92
42	0.01	0.84	0.04	0.12	0.92
43	0.00	0.85	–0.08	0.00	0.92

the discrepancy in size between POpos and POneg increases, the value of Kappa decreases. The inter-rater reliability data in Table 3.4 is shown in Table 3.5 as Case 38, with the Kappa value of 0.32 occurring when POpos is 0.40 and POneg is 0.91. Table 3.5 indicates that only five combinations produce lower Kappa values than this. More generally, these data indicate that high PO and low Kappa (a seeming paradox) occurs when POpos and POneg are widely discrepant with respect to the value of PO.

Another feature of the data spread in Table 3.5 is that it shows at a glance when either POpos or POneg reaches a value that represents poor reliability, that is <0.70, by the criteria set out by Cicchetti et al. (1995), in which 0.90–1.00 is excellent, 0.80–0.89 is good, 0.70–0.79 is fair, and < 0.70 is poor. It is noteworthy that this phenomenon begins at Case 26, in which POpos falls below 0.70 while POneg is at 0.90.

An essential question that is raised here is whether this information, gleaned from data on all possible hypothetical statistically controlled cases can be of utility in the field. Put another way, are the principles derived from this work of value in a research investigation in which quality indicators are evaluated for evidence of EBP in autism? This question was investigated by examining seven additional EBP autism studies reported at the International Association for Positive Behavior Support (Doehring et al. 2007). The data shown in Table 3.6 were derived from four SSED reports and three group design research reports and focused upon whether primary or secondary quality indicators were demonstrated in published and peer-reviewed autism intervention studies, as described in Reichow et al. (2008).

As with the hypothetical inter-rater reliability results presented in the Table 3.5, the data are ordered from the highest to the lowest Kappa values. It is very noteworthy that the same general phenomenon occurs in this uncontrolled field study as

TABLE 3.6   Rank ordering of varying values of PO, Kappa, and POpos and POneg by set of quality indicators across seven research studies assessing evidence-based practice (EBP) in autism

Study type:	Set of QIs	PO	Kappa	POpos	POneg
1. Group	Primary	1.00(E)	1.00(E)	1.00(E)	1.00(E)
2. SSED	Secondary	0.96(E)	0.90(E)	0.97(E)	0.93(E)
3. SSED	Primary	0.89(G)	0.77(E)	0.86(G)	0.90(E)
4. Group	Secondary	0.88(G)	0.75(E)	0.86(G)	0.90(E)
5. SSED	Primary	0.88(G)	0.71(E)	0.80(G)	0.91(E)
6. SSED	Secondary	0.88(G)	0.68(G)	0.90(E)	0.77(F)
7. Group	Primary	0.84(G)	0.65(G)	0.76(F)	0.88(G)

E excellent, *G* good, and *F* fair levels of interrater agreement by the criteria of Cicchetti (2001); and Cicchetti et al. (1995)

in the hypothetical data under statistically controlled conditions: as Kappa decreases, the absolute difference between POpos and POneg increases. Moreover, the values of POpos and POneg become more and more dissimilar from the value of PO.

Perhaps the best way to avoid both Kappa paradoxes and disparities in POpos and POneg values is the time-honored way, namely, to train the raters adequately, as was accomplished by Reichow et al. (2008). Note that the reliability results presented in Table 3.6, while showing disparities between POpos and POneg do not meet the criterion for a Kappa paradox (high PO but low, or poor, Kappa values). The obvious implication here is that the raters were trained adequately to apply the evaluative method in a highly reliable manner. In the next section, the issue of the validity of the evaluative method is discussed.

ASSESSING THE VALIDITY OF THE EVALUATIVE METHOD FOR PROVIDING EVIDENCE OF EBP IN AUTISM

Several sources of validity of the evaluative method were discussed by Reichow et al. (2008):

- Content validity, as it was made manifest through the operalization of the criteria needed to evaluate research study results for EBP in autism
- Concurrent validity, established by equating their definition of EBP with others that have been defined in the literature (Kratochwill and Stoiber 2002; Lonigan et al. 1998; Lord et al. 2001; Odom et al. 2005)
- Predictive validity, based upon the accuracy of evidence for EBP in autism, as established by agreement with an experienced rater on the basis of the application of extant validity indices that are applied in both medicine and biobehavioral clinical research endeavors

Of course, the gold standard for evaluating a physician's preliminary diagnosis in medicine is one that can be confirmed in the clinical laboratory. However, when this is not the case, and in the words of the late Joseph Fleiss (1975: 651):

In the absence of a laboratory or other test that might provide a standard against which to assess the correctness of the judgment, one must rely on the degree of agreement between different judges for information about error.

Indeed this is true in medical, psychiatric, neuropsychological and other areas of research, including the diagnosis of autism itself (Klin et al. 2000). Many diagnoses depend exclusively on an experienced clinician's best judgment, used as a "gold standard" best estimate. How this important aspect of validity is achieved is now addressed.

This section discusses the accuracy indices that are utilized in the predictive model. The four relevant validity indices are: sensitivity (Se); specificity (Sp); predicted positive accuracy (PPA); and predicted negative accuracy (PNA). The 2×2 contingency table and the formulae for defining each of four indices are shown in Table 3.7.

Using the notation presented in Table 3.7, the indices are defined, as follows:

- Sensitivity (Se) is defined as the proportion of confirmed positive cases, (QI+), based upon the best clinician diagnosis (Rater 2) that also test as positive by Rater 1:

$$Se = A / (A + C); \qquad (3.3)$$

- Specificity (Sp) refers to the proportion of confirmed QI– cases that both raters test as negative:

$$Sp = D / (B + D); \qquad (3.4)$$

- Predicted positive accuracy (PPA) is defined as the proportion of cases tested positive by Rater 1, that are confirmed as positive cases by Rater 2, defined as:

$$PPA = A / (A + B); \qquad (3.5)$$

- Predicted negative accuracy (PNA) is defined as the proportion of cases tested negative (QI–) by Rater 1, that are confirmed as negative by Rater 2:

$$PNA = D / (C + D). \qquad (3.6)$$

In the next section, these four validity indices are discussed using a hypothetical example in which an EBP rater has been trained by an experienced EBP specialist using the evaluative method. The data are given in Table 3.8.

Applying the formulae presented in Table 3.7 to the hypothetical data spread in Table 3.8, the indices are calculated as shown:

$$
\begin{aligned}
Se &= 0.42 / 0.50 = 0.84; \\
Sp &= 0.43 / 0.50 = 0.86; \\
PPA &= 0.42 / 0.49 = 0.8571; \\
PNA &= 0.43 / 0.51 = 0.8431.
\end{aligned}
$$

TABLE 3.7 Predictive validity research design for assessing evidence-based practice (EBP) in autism

	Rater 2		
Rater 1	QI+	QI–	Totals
QI+	A	B	(A+B)
QI–	C	D	(C+D)
Totals	(A+C)	(B+D)	1.0

The letters A and D refer, respectively, to the proportions of cases for which the two examiners agree either that the studies in which an EBP Quality Indicator is present (as symbolized by the letter A) or the EBP Quality Indicator is absent (symbolized by the letter D). Sensitivity = A / (A+C); specificity = D/ (B+D); predicted positive accuracy = A / (A+B); and predicted negative accuracy = D / (C+D)

TABLE 3.8 Hypothetical Data from 100 hypothetical single subject experimental design reports for assessing the predictive validity of the evaluative method

	Rater 2		
Rater 1	QI+	QI–	Totals
QI+	0.42(0.245)	0.07(0.245)	0.49
QI–	0.08(0.255)	0.043(0.255)	0.51
Totals	0.50	0.50	1.0

Unbracketed values refer to the proportions of cases upon which the two evidence-based practice (EBP) raters either agree or disagree. Bracketed values refer to the corresponding proportions of cases in which the two raters can be expected to agree by chance alone

Applying the criteria of Cicchetti (2001) and Cicchetti et al. (1995), each of these four indices represents a good level of rater accuracy or validity of EBP in autism, using the evaluative method.

It is important to note that there is a clear, but little-known, relationship between reliability and validity, above and beyond the well-known fact that reliability sets a lower bound on validity. If a phenomenon is not at least appropriately reliable, it will certainly fail the test for validity or accuracy. However, it is also true that when experienced judges are used as the closest approximation to a gold standard, there is a simple mathematical relationship between reliability and accuracy (or validity) of judgment.

THE MATHEMATICAL RELATIONSHIP BETWEEN INTER-RATER RELIABILITY AND PREDICTIVE VALIDITY

As discovered by Kraemer (1982) and based upon the J statistic, developed by the late biostatistical biochemist Jack Youden (1950), there is a mathematical relationship between chance-corrected inter-rater agreement, in the form of Kappa, and the two most widely applied indices of predictive validity, Sensitivity (Se) and Specificity (Sp):

$$K_{Youden} = (Se + Sp) - 1 \qquad (3.7)$$

This relationship holds under the condition, that both the test rater (Rater 1) and the confirmatory rater (Rater 2) make assignments to QI+ and QI– cases that are identical or nearly identical (e.g., they both assess 55% of the group studies in autism as QI+ and the remaining 45% as QI–).

Obviously there will be variability around this criterion and the next section determines how much deviation can occur

from strictly identical assignments while the relationship between Kappa and Se and Sp continues to hold.

Using the data from Table 3.8, we assume that Rater 1 has been extensively trained in the application of the EBP evaluative method and that Rater 2 is a very experienced EBP clinical examiner used as the best estimate gold standard. Recall that we calculated Se to be 0.42/0.50=0.84 and Sp to be 0.43/0.50=0.86. Calculating Kappa in the usual way (Cohen 1960), we obtain:

$$PO = 0.85;$$
$$PC = (0.245 + 0.255) = 0.50;$$
$$K_{Cohen} = (0.85 - 0.50)/0.50 = 0.70.$$

Using Youden's formula for Kappa (3.7), we obtain the following result:

$$\begin{aligned} K_{Youden} &= (Se + Sp) - 1 \\ &= (0.84 + 0.86) - 1 \\ &= 1.70 - 1 \\ &= 0.70 \end{aligned}$$

which is equal to Cohen's (1960) Kappa value, as previously calculated.

Now, while this relationship between Youden's statistic and the Cohen K statistic is noteworthy, it will be remembered that there are two further components of the Se–Sp model, namely, predicted positive accuracy (PPA) and Predicted Negative Accuracy. It is seen from the previous section that PPA=0.8571 and PNA=0.8431.

If we now replace Se and Sp in Formula (3.7) by PPA and PNA, respectively, then we can test whether the new Formula (3.8) bears the same relationship to Kappa:

$$Kappa = (PPA + PNA) - 1 \qquad (3.8)$$

Using the values of PPA and PNA, we obtain the following:

$$\begin{aligned} Kappa &= (0.8571 + 0.8431) - 1 \\ &= 1.7002 - 1 = 0.70, \end{aligned}$$

identical to both the Cohen and the Youden values.

Incorporating the information from both formulae (3.7) and (3.8) into a single formula, this time using all four indices of diagnostic agreement, we obtain the Dom-Index:

$$\text{Kappa}_{\text{Dom - Index}} = $$

$$\left(\begin{array}{c} (Se + Sp) - 1 \\ + (PPA + PNA) - 1 \end{array} \right) / 2 \quad (3.9)$$

COMPARING THE YOUDEN AND DOM-INDEX VALUES OF KAPPA TO COHEN'S KAPPA

In this section, again using Rater 2 as the gold standard, we pose and answer the question of how closely the Youden and Dom-Index interpretations of K hold to Cohen when the assignments of QI+ and QI– vary between essentially no difference (Rater 2 assigns QI+ to 50% of the studies and Rater 1 assigns QI+ to 49% of the studies) to a discrepancy of 15% (Rater 2 evaluates 57% of the studies as QI+ as compared to 42%

evaluated as QI+ by Rater 1). The results are shown in Table 3.9.

As shown in the last three columns, the $K_{\text{Dom-Index}}$ results are exactly the same as the K_{Youden} results. More importantly, the $\text{Kappa}_{\text{Cohen}}$ values, $\text{Kappa}_{\text{Youden}}$ values, and $\text{Kappa}_{\text{Dom-Index}}$ values all fall within a narrow range (0.70–0.74) of good levels of chance-corrected inter-rater agreement. This said, it is also important to emphasize that, even when Kappa values are essentially interchangeable, this in no way assures the accuracy of human judgments, when experienced raters are used as a proxy for gold-standard diagnoses. This is because the Se, Sp, PPA, and PNA validity indices can vary considerably with respect to each other, even when Kappa values vary only slightly or not at all.

Once again, we ask whether these hypothetical data can be of use in the field, where the controls that were put in place for the hypothetical data in Table 3.10 are not possible. We utilize the data in the contingency tables from which the data appearing in Table 3.6 were derived. These actual data appear in Table 3.10, where we portray Rater 2, again, as the gold-standard rater.

TABLE 3.9 Hypothetical data showing the relationship between Kappa (Cohen), Kappa (Youden) and Kappa Dom-Index with PO held constant at 0.85

Rater QI+							Kappa values		
Assign-ments	(+/−)	(−/+)	Se	Sp	PPA	PNA	(Cohen)	(Youden)	Dom-Index
1. 0.50–0.49	0.07	0.08	0.84	0.86	0.86	0.84	0.70	0.70	0.70
2. 0.51–0.48	0.06	0.09	0.82	0.88	0.88	0.83	0.70	0.70	0.70
3. 0.52–0.47	0.05	0.10	0.81	0.90	0.89	0.81	0.70	0.70	0.71
4. 0.53–0.46	0.04	0.11	0.79	0.91	0.91	0.80	0.70	0.71	0.71
5. 0.54–0.45	0.03	0.12	0.78	0.93	0.93	0.78	0.70	0.71	0.71
6. 0.55–0.44	0.02	0.13	0.76	0.96	0.95	0.77	0.70	0.72	0.72
7. 0.56–0.43	0.01	0.14	0.75	0.98	0.98	0.75	0.70	0.73	0.73
8. 0.57–0.42	0.00	0.15	0.74	1.00	1.00	0.74	0.71	0.74	0.74

TABLE 3.10   Rank ordering of the varying values of evidence-based practice (EBP) Quality Indicator Present (QI+) Rater Assignments and Corresponding PO, Kappa, and POpos and POneg Across Data from the Seven Research Studies Assessing EBP in Autism, given in Table 5

Rater QI+						Kappa values		
Study	Assignments	Se	Sp	PPA	PNA	(Cohen)	(Youden)	Dom-Index
1.	0.67–0.67	1.00	1.00	1.00	1.00	1.00	1.00	1.00
2.	0.71–0.67	1.00	0.88	0.94	1.00	0.90	0.88	0.91
3.	0.48–0.43	0.81	0.95	0.92	0.87	0.77	0.76	0.77
4.	0.50–0.375	0.75	1.00	1.00	0.80	0.75	0.75	0.775
5.	0.375–0.25	0.67	1.00	1.00	0.83	0.71	0.67	0.75
6.	0.71–0.70	0.90	0.79	0.91	0.76	0.68	0.68	0.68
7.	0.34–0.31	0.80	0.86	0.73	0.90	0.65	0.66	0.65

For Se, Sp, PPA, and PNA values: >0.90 = excellent; 0.80–0.89 = good; 0.70–0.79 = fair, and < 0.70 = poor level of accuracy (Cicchetti 2001, 1994; Cicchetti & Sparrow 1981; and Cicchetti et al. 1995); and for Kappa values: < 0.40 = poor; 0.40–0.59 = fair; 0.60–0.74 = good; and ≥ 0.75 = excellent

In Table 3.10, the discrepancy in rater assignments to QI + range from 0% (0.67 from both Rater 1 and Rater 2 in Study 1) and 12.5% (0.375 and 0.25 in Study 5). As was true for the hypothetical data, both the Youden and Dom-Index versions of Kappa hold up remarkably well. If we view the results from the hypothetical and field sources, together, we can conclude that the estimates of Cohen's Kappa are quite closely approximated by both the Youden and Dom-Index versions, both for hypothetical data and for data deriving from the field of EBP evaluative method research. The results are novel in the sense that they demonstrate quite unequivocally, that the previously implied stringent requirement that both rater assignments need to be the same or very similar in order for these approximations to hold is not true. As we have seen, even with marked differences in QI + assignments, the relationships hold. Finally, it appears that the newly constructed Dom-Index has added value in that, unlike the Youden approximation, it incorporates all four of the necessary components of diagnostic accuracy: sensitivity, specificity, predicted positive accuracy and predicted negative accuracy.

CONCLUSION

The purpose of the current chapter was to discuss some biostatistical issues that need to be understood: paradoxes that can occur in application of the Kappa statistic, namely, high inter-rater agreement that nonetheless results in poor and unacceptable levels of Kappa, in the form of chance-corrected agreement; how these paradoxes occur, how they may be identified, and most importantly, how they may be avoided; more broadly, how these fundamental psychometric issues can be understood in the context of future reliability studies of the evaluative method for assessing EBP in autism; an elucidation of the most potent method for determining the validity or accuracy of rater assessments of EBP in autism, using expert examiners as gold standards; and introducing a new validation index (the Dom-Index) that has been applied, for the first time, to the EBP Evaluative Method and is mathematically related to the Kappa statistic. In this fundamental sense, the Dom-Index, because it is defined in terms of all of the four validity indices (Se, Sp, PPA, and PNA), serves to help bridge the gap between reliable and valid assessments. In this general sense, the new index also has application more broadly in the field of biobehavioral research.

REFERENCES

Cicchetti, D. V. (1988). When diagnostic agreement is high, but reliability is low: Some paradoxes occurring in joint independent neuropsychology assessments. *Journal of Clinical and Experimental Neuropsychology, 10*, 605–622.

Cicchetti, D. V. (1994). Guidelines, criteria, and rules of thumb for evaluating normed and standardized assessment instruments in psychology. *Psychological Assessment, 6*, 284–290.

Cicchetti, D. V. (2001). The precision of reliability and validity estimates re-visited: Distinguishing between clinical and statistical significance of sample size requirements. *Journal of Clinical and Experimental Neuropsychology, 23*, 695–700.

Cicchetti, D. V., & Feinstein, A. R. (1990). High agreement but low Kappa: II. Resolving the paradoxes. *Journal of Clinical Epidemiology, 43*, 551–568.

Cicchetti, D. V., & Sparrow, S. S. (1981). Developing criteria for establishing interrater reliability of specific items: Applications to assessment of adaptive behavior. *American Journal of Mental Deficiency, 86*, 127–137.

Cicchetti, D. V., Volkmar, F., Klin, A., & Showalter, D. (1995). Diagnosing autism using ICD-10 criteria: A comparison of neural networks and standard multivariate procedures. *Child Neuropsychology, 1*, 26–37.

Cohen, J. (1960). A coefficient of agreement for nominal scales. *Educational and Psychological Measurement, 23*, 37–46.

Doehring, P., Reichow, B., & Volkmar, F. R. (2007). Is it evidenced-based? How to evaluate claims of effectiveness for autism. Paper presented at the International Association for Positive Behavior Support Conference, March, Boston, MA.

Feinstein, A. R., & Cicchetti, D. V. (1990). High agreement but low Kappa: I the problem of two paradoxes. *Journal of Clinical Epidemiology, 43*, 543–549.

Fleiss, J. L., Cohen, J., & Everitt, B. S. (1969). Large sample standard errors of kappa and weighted kappa. *Psychological Bulletin, 72(5).* 323–327.

Fleiss, J. L. (1975). Measuring agreement between two judges on the presence or absence of a trait. *Biometrics, 31*, 651–659.

Fleiss, J. L. (1981). *Statistical methods for rates and proportions* (2nd ed.). New York: Wiley.

Fleiss, J. L., Levin, B., & Paik, M. C. (2003). *Statistical methods for rates and proportions* (3rd ed.). New York: Wiley.

Klin, A., Lang, J., Cicchetti, D. V., & Volkmar, F. (2000). Inter-rater reliability of clinical diagnosis and DSM-IV criteria for autistic disorder: Results of the DSM-IV autism field trial. *Journal of Autism and Developmental Disorders, 30*, 163–167.

Kraemer, H. C. (1982). Estimating false alarms and missed events from interobserver agreement: Comment on Kaye. *Psychological Bulletin, 92*, 749–754.

Kratochwill, T. R., & Stoiber, K. C. (2002). Evidence-based interventions in school psychology: Conceptual foundations of the procedural and coding manual of Division 16 and the Society for the Study of School Psychology task force. *School Psychology Quarterly, 17*, 341–389.

Landis, J. R., & Koch, G. G. (1977). The measure of observer agreement for categorical data. *Biometrics, 3*, 159–174.

Lonigan, C. J., Elbert, J. C., & Johnson, S. B. (1998). Empirically supported psychosocial interventions for children: An overview. *Journal of Clinical Child Psychology, 27*, 138–145.

Lord, C., Bristol-Power, M., Filipek, P. A., Gallagher, J. J., Harris, S. L., et al. (2001). *Educating children with autism*. Washington, DC: National Academy.

Odom, S. L., Brantlinger, E., Gersten, R., Horner, R. H., Thompson, B., & Harris, K. R. (2005). Research in special education: Scientific methods and evidence-based practices. *Exceptional Children, 71*, 137–148.

Reichow, B., Barton, E. E., Volkmar, F. R., & Cicchetti, D. V. (2007). The status of research on interventions for young children with autism spectrum disorders. Poster presented at the International Meeting for Autism Research, May, Seattle, WA.

Reichow, B., Volkmar, F. R., & Cicchetti, D. V. (2008). Development of an evaluative method for determining the strength of research evidence in autism. *Journal of Autism and Developmental Disorders, 38*, 1311–1319.

Youden, W. J. (1950). Index for rating diagnostic tests. *Cancer, 3*, 32–35.

Treatment Reviews

Evidence-Based Treatment of Behavioral Excesses and Deficits for Individuals with Autism Spectrum Disorders

Michael D. Powers, Mark J. Palmieri, Kristen S. D'Eramo, and Kristen M. Powers

ABBREVIATIONS

ADHD	Attention deficit hyperactivity disorder
ASDs	Autism spectrum disorders
DRA	Differential reinforcement of alternative behavior
FCT	Functional communication training
High-p	High-probability request
Low-p	Low-probability request
NCR	Noncontingent reinforcement
SIB	Self-injurious behavior
SSED	Single subject experimental design

INTRODUCTION

The practice of evidence-based treatment of challenging behavior in autism has been heavily influenced by the application of principles and practices based on the experimental analysis of behavior, and particularly applied behavior analysis, to deficits or excesses in the behavioral repertoire of individuals with autism, Asperger Syndrome, and related pervasive developmental disorders. Indeed, for over 50 years, the learning principles established by Skinner (1938, 1953) and others have guided both the assessment and intervention process,

B. Reichow et al. (eds.), *Evidence-Based Practices and Treatments for Children with Autism*, DOI 10.1007/978-1-4419-6975-0_4, © Springer Science+Business Media, LLC 2011

evolving systematically as new findings are published and replicated. From early work addressing self-injury and aggression in those with severe developmental disabilities (Lovaas and Simmons 1969) to the most contemporary efforts to modify behavior through the use of antecedent manipulations (Luiselli and Cameron 1998), procedures based on functional equivalence (Carr 1988), and others based on positive behavior supports (Bambara and Kern 2005), applied behavior analysis has distinguished itself by a rigorous approach to quantification of variables responsible for treatment success, by a reliance on functional analysis (Iwata et al. 1994) including the direct observation of both the molecular and molar nature of behavior (Powers 1988), and by the demand for generalization, maintenance, and replicability of treatment effects (Baer et al. 1968). In order to meet these standards, the field has relied primarily upon the use of single subject experimental designs (SSED), but has demonstrated magnitude of effect by the replicability of findings by different researchers and clinicians. As such, the process of determining which practices are "evidence-based" is better understood as the description of *which* specific intervention strategies have demonstrated efficacy for *which* behavioral challenges maintained by *which* variables, in *which* child or adult, *under what* conditions. Within this rubric, it quickly becomes evident that precise treatment is impossible without precise assessment. The strategy that resolves these predictive, formative, and summative evaluation concerns is termed "functional behavioral assessment," while the intervention process is described in various ways, including behavioral treatment, applied behavior analysis, positive behavior support, etc. For purposes of this chapter, we use the term *applied behavior analysis* to describe the process of understanding why challenging behavior occurs and what to do about it.

Challenging behavior takes many forms, operates differentially in many environments, and can change depending on external antecedent and consequent factors, biological and medical conditions, and genetic factors. For example, aggression may be directed to others in the form of biting, throwing objects, or menacing words. Self-injury may occur as a result of reduced or nonexistent stimulation in the environment or as a result of internal pain (e.g., otitis media). While an individual may possess the Methyl CpG binding protein 2 (MECP2) genotype for Rett Syndrome, the phenotypic expression of hand stereotypy may present as hands clasped to midline, as hair twirling at midline, or as clapping. Further, expression can vary by age and degree of the mutation. While what we see (the topography) is important in our understanding of a challenging behavior, how the behavior functions in the environment is of utmost importance in assessment and intervention. As a result, while we always describe the *form*, we must also always understand the *function*. Treatment based on anything less not only constitutes poor practice, but also increases risk to the individual with autism spectrum disorder (ASD) by reducing opportunities for habilitation.

Applied behavior analysis addresses in a cumulative fashion problems of behavioral excesses and deficits in those with autism spectrum disorders. The predominant use of single-case experimental designs (Kazdin 1982) permits careful control of assessment and treatment variables, insuring treatment integrity and reducing threats to internal validity. The generally small number of subjects in any single study is an appropriate concern, but is addressed by the replicability of findings across settings and populations. In a manner of speaking, outcome studies produced in this manner all represent evidence-based practice, as each study must demonstrate the relationship between dependent and independent variables with reliability. The cumulative effect of multiple investigations producing similar findings, with rigorous treatment integrity, represents the power of these research methods (Horner et al. 2005; Kurtz et al. 2003; Odom et al. 2003). The issue of generalizability of findings is somewhat more complicated, however. Rather than using large population samples with statistical analysis to determine intervention effects, applied behavior analysis emphasizes the aggregate of smaller samples. Treatment effects, and indeed the individual components of specific treatments that overall are effective, cannot easily be generalized until there is a sufficient body of research to support widespread use. In addition, while there are certainly many studies that examine individuals with ASD specifically, there is a reasonable argument that well-constructed studies of individuals with significant disabilities other than ASD will contribute to the corpus of practices ultimately determined to describe evidence-based practice. This is particularly feasible with procedures derived from applied behavior analysis because assessment and intervention components and specific procedures must be defined operationally, with measurement of outcome and interobserver agreement (reliability). The emphasis on determination of behavioral function as a predictor of treatment provides some generalizability of strategies and findings across populations. Of course, variables associated with the specific diagnostic condition affecting the client influence responding (Iwata et al. 1986; Linscheid 2006), and must be understood and incorporated into the functional analysis and intervention process. This latter issue is well-conceptualized in contemporary analysis and intervention of challenging behavior from a functional ecological perspective (Powers 2005).

The process of accumulating such data is not linear; sometimes a particularly important clinical issue receives a tremendous amount of attention in a relatively short period of time (e.g., the development of nonaversive interventions to treat challenging behavior in ASD or the objective investigation of facilitative communication). In other situations, important clinical issues remain grossly underaddressed in the treatment literature (e.g., the effect of oral-motor deficits in treatment of feeding problems in children with ASD). This leaves the practitioner with the choice of utilizing only those assessment and treatment procedures with robust and well-replicated findings or utilizing those procedures while simultaneously continuing to evaluate systematically other issues that may contribute to enhanced treatment outcomes. If the principles of investigation, analysis, and intervention that are part of applied behavior analysis are incorporated into the second choice, then the dynamic process of developing contributions to *improve* evidence-based practice is enhanced as well. For purposes of the present chapter, we discuss specific evidence-based intervention strategies that might be used across a variety of situations (e.g., noncontingent reinforcement) and also the application of those strategies as part of evidence-based procedural interventions (e.g., the treatment of sleep disorders in those with ASD).

EVIDENCE-BASED COMPONENTS OF INTERVENTION

Behavior analytic intervention procedures are more accurately represented as a group of strategies that have demonstrated empiric efficacy and that could potentially be applied to any number of situations in order to increase prosocial and adaptive behavior or to decrease challenging behavior. With foundations in the experimental analysis of behavior going back over

70 years (Skinner 1938), what has come to be described as applied behavior analysis slowly coalesced through the 1940s and 1950s with the application of operant principles to individuals with significant psychiatric and developmental disabilities (Fuller 1949; Bijou 1957; Ayllon and Michael 1959) until 1968, when the seminal paper describing and defining the field was published by Donald Baer, Montrose Wolf, and Todd Risley in the new *Journal of Applied Behavior Analysis*. With the combined opportunities presented by a clearly articulated set of criteria for evaluating research and practice and a dissemination vehicle (in the form of a new journal) devoted to the rigorous application of those criteria and standards, both the number of investigations and the quality of work done expanded markedly, from a single journal in 1968 to well over 25 today. As importantly, expansion into other, non-behavioral, peer-reviewed journals followed as the body of well-conceptualized and implemented research studies demonstrating significant changes in problems of learning and behavior with children and adults in applied settings increased. The net effect of these factors is that there has been a broader understanding and recognition in the professional community of the role, function, and contributions of applied behavior analysis in successfully assessing and treating significant problems in living and that these contributions alone or in combination with other procedures constitute best, and evidence-based, practice.

In this section, we describe several specific intervention procedures, based upon the principles of applied behavior analysis, that enjoy a robust, substantial, and well-validated research history. We have considered only procedures that have been demonstrated to be effective in achieving their target outcomes, have demonstrated internal and external validity and inter-observer agreement, and have been replicated across multiple research settings with individuals with autism and related developmental disabilities. As such, those procedures selected all meet the most rigorous standards of clinical efficacy. Our choices here are neither exhaustive nor exclusive, however; the constraints of the chapter dictate a sampling rather than a comprehensive overview. For the latter, we refer the reader to the outstanding volume by Cooper et al. (2007). What we do wish to convey, however, is the assertion that *specific* strategies and *combined* treatment procedures can be discussed when considering evidence-based practices in treating behavioral challenges in ASD. As will be evident in our discussion of more "manualized" treatment procedures to address problems (e.g., sleep disorders) later in this chapter, the specific strategies discussed below, and others, are often components of those treatment packages. What is essential to remember is that not all specific strategies belong in all treatment protocols. While this may seem self-evident, consider that a clinician may misuse a procedure (i.e., reinforcing escape-maintained behavior), inadvertently contribute to procedural drift and compromise treatment integrity, or use an incorrect or inconsistent measurement or evaluation strategy to quantify change. The misuse of the procedure or the choice of an incorrect evaluation strategy is more a reflection on the clinician's judgment than on the integrity of the treatment strategy itself. Therefore, before we commence with the description of representative exemplary strategies, we offer the following caution: Any evidence-based strategy can be used poorly by an otherwise competent clinician, leading to a less-than-successful outcome. A strategy that enjoys little or no empirical support can be used by a competent (if misinformed) clinician, leading to a less-than-successful outcome. In both cases, the individual with ASD loses. Due diligence is the responsibility of the clinician. This is the primary thrust of applied behavior analysis and, indeed, of this book.

Functional Behavior Assessment

Functional behavior assessment or analysis is the evidence-based foundation of all that follows in the treatment of challenging behavior in those with ASD. Its importance is underscored by the inclusion of this technique at the beginning of this chapter. Simply put, whether the behavior problem is described as self-injury, aggression, food refusal, sleep disorders, pica, or any of a number of other *forms* of behavior, an analysis of behavioral *function* is essential. The behavioral treatment of challenging behavior in autism spectrum disorders without a prior functional assessment should be questioned in all cases, as it increases the risk of negative effects of treatment and compromised outcomes.

Assessing behavior through data-based collection procedures is a necessary component of applied behavior analysis, facilitating the primary goal of establishing a reliable relationship between the treatment and behavior change. This concept forms the basis for the assessment of challenging behavior in applied behavior analysis. Functional analysis is the procedure by which environmental conditions are manipulated to reliably evoke a target behavior (Carr and Durand 1985; Cooper and Harding 1993; Iwata et al. 1990, 1994/1982, 1994b). Based upon the results of these assessments, maladaptive behavior is conceptualized as being motivated by a particular function, thus allowing appropriate interventions to be developed. An important component of functional analytic methodology is that behavior must be understood by its consequences within the environment and not solely by its topography or form (Cooper and Harding 1993). Further, the process of completing a functional analysis often requires attention to individual-specific variables that are systematically programmed for within a more traditional

analogue model (Carr et al. 1997; LaBelle and Charlop-Christy 2002). As the research base on various analogue functional analysis procedures expands, consistency among critical components often remains as the majority of functional analysis procedures currently used are based upon the seminal work of Iwata et al. (Herzinger and Campbell 2007).

Functional analysis methodology has been applied to a variety of treatment settings. The original research on these procedures was conducted in highly controlled treatment settings (Carr and Durand 1985; Cooper and Harding 1993; Iwata et al. 1994/1982, 1990). In these environments, experimenters have exposed participants to repeated treatment conditions in order to establish a reliable relationship between environmental contingencies and the occurrence of a target behavior (Carr and Durand 1985; Cooper and Harding 1993; Iwata et al. 1990, 1994/1982). Recently, research attention has shifted toward evaluating the use of functional analytic procedures in outpatient settings with less precise and sustained control (Asmus et al. 2002; Cihak et al. 2007; Cooper and Harding 1993; Sigafoos and Saggers 1995). This research has provided a great deal of support for brief functional analysis as a means of assessing challenging behavior (Cihak et al. 2007; Cooper et al. 1992; Derby et al. 1994). These assessments follow the same conceptual guides as does extended functional analysis; however, their structure and duration allows for them to be more successfully integrated into outpatient settings.

Empirical Foundations of Functional Analysis

While Carr (1977) established the conceptual foundation for functional analysis, the model for clinical practice is most closely associated with the work of Iwata et al. (1994/1982) and Carr and Durand (1985).

The methodology developed in these studies has since been widely examined and used extensively in the applied behavior analysis literature (Hanley et al. 2003).

The initial study by Iwata et al. (1994/1982) utilized four assessment conditions to evaluate self-injurious behavior in nine individuals diagnosed with developmental disability, ranging in age from 19 months to 17 years and 2 months. The conditions included in the functional analysis were social disapproval, academic demand, unstructured play, and alone. During the assessments, conditions lasted for 15 min and were randomly ordered for each participant. The functional analysis continued until stable levels of responding were observed in each condition or until 12 days of assessment were completed.

The social disapproval condition was designed to replicate contingencies for positive reinforcement in the form of attention for engaging in self-injury. The participant was instructed to play with toys while the experimenter worked. If the participant engaged in self-injury, the experimenter provided physical and vocal attention. The academic demand condition tested for the presence of negative reinforcement contingencies in the form of escape from work for engaging in self-injury. The experimenter ran academic programs appropriate to each participant's ability level. Social praise was delivered after each response whether or not the response was correct. If the participant engaged in self-injurious behavior, the experimenter turned away and terminated the learning trial. The alone condition was designed to assess for self-injurious behavior maintained by automatic reinforcement. The participant was left alone without access to attention or tangible items. The experimenter did not provide a consequence for an occurrence of self-injury. Finally, the unstructured play condition served as a control condition for the functional analysis. In this condition,

the experimenter provided noncontingent attention and gave no demands. Again, no consequence was provided contingent upon an occurrence of self-injury.

To address individual differences in the topography of self-injury, operational definitions were provided for the self-injury that each participant experienced. Interobserver agreement was calculated to ensure that all observers were able to reliably identify all the topographies of challenging behavior. The results of the Iwata et al. (1994/1982) study demonstrated that similar topographies of behavior can serve different functions. In their study, the level of responding varied from individual to individual across the assessment conditions. As a result of these data, Iwata et al. (1994/1982) supported functional analysis as a means of systematically evaluating the stimuli-maintaining behavior and, subsequently, the use of individualized assessment and intervention procedures for self-injurious behavior.

Carr and Durand (1985) confirmed the Iwata et al. (1994/1982) results, showing that similar forms of challenging behavior can be maintained by different contingencies in each individual. The study evaluated a number of topographies of challenging behavior experienced by four participants, aged 7–14 years, with either developmental disabilities or brain damage. The functional analysis conditions were designed to assess escape and attention motivations for each target behavior. The "easy 100" condition served as the control condition for the analysis. In this condition, the experimenter provided easy demands and attention during 100% of the condition's intervals. In the "easy 33" condition, the experimenter again utilized easy demands but only provided attention during 33% of the intervals. This condition was used to assess for an attention motivation for each target behavior. During the "difficult 100" condition, the participants were given challenging demands and attention during 100% of the condition's intervals. It was expected that this condition would assess for an escape function maintaining any target behavior.

Consequences were provided for all topographies of behavior in the same manner during each condition. All behavior except darting and responses that risked physical injury were placed on extinction (Carr and Durand 1985). If the participant darted from work and did not return in 10 s, she or he was physically guided back to the table. In cases where physical risk was a concern, the participant's hands were restrained for 5–10 s while the experimenter followed through with the work demands. The results of the functional analyses suggested that the various forms of challenging behavior of the participants were maintained by different environmental contingencies. The data from Carr and Durand (1985) supported those obtained by Iwata et al. (1994/1982), substantiating functional analysis as an efficient means for evaluating challenging behavior.

Carr and Durand (1985) further supported functional analysis as a means of assessing and treating challenging behavior by implementing functional communication training for each of the participants. The targets of the training were mands for attention and help, consistent with the attention and escape motivations for the forms of challenging behavior. By providing consistent reinforcement for appropriate requests for attention and help, all participants' challenging behavior decreased. Functionally equivalent interventions were thereby supported as the optimal treatment for challenging behavior.

Considerable research has been conducted on functional analysis methodology since the seminal studies by Carr and Durand (1985) and Iwata et al. (1994/1982). Systematic reviews of the literature on functional analysis have consistently supported the procedure's efficacy in identifying the function or functions of challenging behavior (Hanley et al. 2003; Herzinger and

Campbell 2007; Iwata et al. 1994b). Hanley et al. (2003) reviewed 575 functional analysis studies, 96% of which rendered usable outcomes. While the functional analysis procedures utilized in typical studies are rarely identical, the basic premise of controlled antecedents and consequences as defined by environmental manipulations has aided in the development of functionally equivalent interventions leading to a decrease in problem behavior and an increase in targeted replacement skills (Hanley et al. 2003; Iwata et al. 1994b). The clinical utility of these procedures has been consistently supported, even though they often require significant resources. In a review of 58 articles detailing 106 functional behavior assessment procedures, Herzinger and Campbell (2007) found that treatments derived from the completion of functional analysis procedures were more successful at treating challenging behavior than were those derived from behavioral assessment procedures that did not include systematic manipulations of environmental contingencies.

Hanley et al. (2003) reviewed the literature to identify trends for best practices in functional analysis methodology. Their review supported the use of functional analysis to study many topographies of challenging behavior in individuals with disabilities of varying severities. While functional analysis has been applied primarily to learners with pervasive developmental disorder or intellectual disabilities, it is important to note that a variety of other mental disorders and mild behavior problems have been included in analyses (Cooper et al. 1990; Doggett et al. 2001).

Critical Issues in the Development of Functional Analysis Conditions

The experimental conditions most prevalent in the literature are based upon those used by Iwata et al. (1994/1982). These conditions, social positive reinforcement (attention), social negative reinforcement (escape), automatic reinforcement (alone), and control, appear as they were described above. In addition, a "tangible" condition has been applied in a number of studies (Asmus et al. 2002; Fisher et al. 2000; Moore et al. 2002; Mueller et al. 2001; Shirley et al. 1999). In this condition, the individual is typically given access to a highly preferred item for 1 min at which point the experimenter removes the item and places it out of reach (Mueller et al. 2001). The participant is told that the target item is unavailable and directed toward low-preference items. Upon the occurrence of the target behavior, the experimenter grants access to the high preference item.

Session confounds. A number of concerns are common in developing the conditions for a functional analysis. These concerns primarily focus on the presence of confounds or the failure to identify essential variables for use in assessment conditions (Carr et al. 1997; Hanley et al. 2003; Moore et al. 2002; Shirley et al. 1999). Hanley, Iwata, and McCord note that the research on functional analysis has yet to render a unified set of rules for assessment implementation; however, components have been identified that can be considered evidence-based practices. This is made more complicated by the need for highly individualized procedures with analogue frameworks if the conditions are to reliably evoke the target response (Carr et al. 1997). Indeed, without appropriate informed analysis conditions using indirect methods (i.e., clinical interviews) analyses can fail to incorporate an essential, though idiosyncratic, stimulus. Included here are topics such as limiting assessment to a manageable number of responses, considering the influence of establishing operations on the contingencies active in each condition, relatively short sessions, brief designs that can be expanded on an individual basis, and programming for consequences (Hanley et al. 2003).

Concerns regarding session confounds were illustrated by Moore et al. (2002) regarding the influence that attention can play during a tangible condition. In their investigation, a functional analysis was conducted on a child's self-injurious behavior (SIB). The results of the analysis suggested that SIB was a multi-operant behavior maintained by positive reinforcement in the form of attention and access to preferred items (Moore et al. 2002). In a follow-up analysis, the level of attention provided during the tangible condition was evaluated. By reducing the amount of attention paired with the presentation of the tangible, the rate of SIB was decreased. Moore et al. (2002) suggested that the attention inadvertently delivered during the tangible condition was acting as a confound and evoking SIB. Weakening the contingency between the target behavior and access to attention (e.g., delivering attention noncontingently) may serve to control for the influence of confounds (Moore et al. 2002). If the contingent presentation of attention does confound the tangible condition, it stands to reason that all independent variables should be carefully controlled during the development of functional analysis sessions.

Another methodological concern was identified by Shirley et al. (1999) in a study on incidental maintenance in the tangible condition. A functional analysis conducted on an individual's hand mouthing suggested that the behavior was maintained by automatic reinforcement and access to tangible items. Observations of the behavior indicated that the preferred items used in the assessment were almost never provided as a natural consequence. Therefore, the functional analysis may have identified a tangible function that was not actually maintaining the challenging behavior, but could have if presented contingently. Shirley, Iwata, and Kahng suggest caution when using the results of a preference assessment without collecting some form of data on the natural environment.

Length of sessions. Session duration is an important topic in functional analysis methodology. A number of studies have demonstrated the use of functional analysis in less-controlled settings such as schools and outpatient clinics (Asmus et al. 2002; Cooper et al. 1992; Cooper and Harding 1993; Iwata et al. 2000; Moore et al. 2002; Umbreit 1995). To be applied within these settings, topics related to the efficient application of functional analysis procedures must be considered. A study by Wallace and Iwata (1999) considered the influence of session duration on determining function. A group of 46 individuals participated in functional analyses based on the model described by Iwata et al. (1994/1982). Tangible conditions were also run for those individuals whose indirect assessment suggested that access to tangible items might evoke the target behavior. The sessions were videotaped and three sets of data were prepared for each participant, by using the first 5, 10, and 15 min of the sessions. Trained independent raters evaluated data from each video. The results rendered strong agreement between the 15- and 10-min sessions and only three disagreements between 15- and 5-min sessions. As a result, shorter session duration was supported as a means for increasing the practical application of functional analysis methodology (Wallace and Iwata 1999).

Functional analysis in diverse treatment settings. The majority of research on functional analysis has been conducted in controlled settings where naturally occurring environmental events are much less likely to influence assessment conditions. One potential result of this structure is that the functional analysis may suggest a relationship that does not exist in the natural environment (Hanley et al. 2003) and may compromise the ecological validity of the findings. In addition, most individuals referred for treatment are not admitted directly to inpatient facilities; typically, intervention attempts on an outpatient basis constitute the first stage of treatment

(Cooper et al. 1990). By developing a model compatible with an outpatient treatment facility and using parents during a functional analysis, Cooper et al. (1990) were able to identify the functions maintaining different topographies of challenging behavior and develop successful treatment interventions.

A growing body of research has demonstrated the use of functional analysis procedures in a variety of treatment settings, such as outpatient clinics, schools, and homes (Asmus et al. 2002; Cooper and Harding 1993; Cooper et al. 1990; Doggett et al. 2001; Lohrmann-O'Rourke and Yurman 2001; Umbreit 1995). Often, these procedures incorporate parent or teacher training components (Lohrmann-O'Rourke and Yurman 2001) in an attempt to evoke the fewest changes possible to the natural environment. Such procedures have resulted in the completion of functional analyses within naturalistic settings which, potentially as a result of an improved quality of data collection and social validity, may then better inform treatment planning.

Hypothesis-driven condition selection. To help address the time-consuming nature of a full functional analysis, professionals in outpatient and classroom settings may use indirect and direct descriptive data collection methods as practical ways to gain information before constructing the assessment conditions (Asmus et al. 2002; Cooper and Harding 1993; Cooper et al. 1992; Herzinger and Campbell 2007). Asmus, Vollmer, and Borrero offer a model for progressing from initial background data collection procedures and through functional analysis at home and at school. In such models the indirect data collection procedures directly inform decision-making and analysis procedures. Once constructed, functional analysis conditions that are informed by many levels of information collection are typically more easily incorporated into naturalistic environments where trained teachers or parents run the assessment conditions

(Cooper and Harding 1993; Cooper et al. 1992; Lohrmann-O'Rourke and Yurman 2001). The benefits of this procedure may include ecological validity and an improved understanding of intervention methodology by the primary treatment staff.

Doggett et al. (2001) and Umbreit (1995) tested the application of functional analysis methodology in classroom environments. Their studies focused on developing a process in which the conceptual foundations of applied behavior analysis were incorporated with an efficient use of classroom resources. In a similar way to Cooper et al. (1992) and Cooper and Harding (1993), they stressed the importance of using indirect data collection procedures, as well as descriptive analyses and observations, to aid in the interpretation of functional analysis data.

In the Doggett et al. (2001) study, behavioral consultants assisted general education classroom teachers in conducting an entire functional assessment. The functional analysis component of the assessment was implemented during periods of general classroom instruction. Behavioral consultants trained and supervised the entire assessment procedure, ensuring that the teachers played a primary role in hypothesis development and data analysis. Similarly, in Umbreit (1995) a teacher was supported in the implementation of a functional analysis that proved successful in identifying a function of the student's challenging classroom behavior. The successful implementation of functional analysis in a typical classroom setting further demonstrates the technology's use outside of controlled inpatient clinics (Cooper and Harding 1993; Doggett et al. 2001; Umbreit 1995).

Brief Assessment Models

Modifications to extended functional analysis procedures have attempted to develop systematic models for the implementation of conditions in a variety of settings (Cooper et al. 1990; Harding et al. 1994; Northup et al. 1991). In addition to developing structured models, recent attempts have focused upon utilizing functional analysis in treatment settings with significant time constraints for evaluating each case (Northup et al. 1991; Derby et al. 1992, 1994). Subsequent studies have examined how these methods can then be applied to public settings (Cihak et al. 2007).

In some of the initial research in this area, Cooper et al. (1990) developed a functional analysis procedure that could be incorporated into an outpatient clinic designed to assess maladaptive behavior and develop treatment recommendations for families or treatment providers. In order to facilitate the rapid evaluation of many patients, Cooper et al. (1990) proposed a functional analysis procedure that could be conducted within a 90-min period. To implement the procedure, operational definitions were constructed for appropriate, inappropriate, and off-task forms of behavior for each participant. In this functional analysis model, parents conducted each assessment condition. As training, the parents received written directions that were prepared for each condition regarding the consequences for appropriate and inappropriate behavior as well as 5-min practice sessions to allow the parents to rehearse the conditions with the experimenter.

The functional analysis followed a three-phase design: baseline, initial assessment, and replication (Cooper et al. 1990). The replication consisted of the best and worst conditions conducted in series. In the baseline condition, the parent and child were left alone in a room to play with toys and interact freely. The "high-demand–parent-attention" condition consisted of challenging academic demands and parent attention for all appropriate behavior. Inappropriate behavior resulted in a redirection to the demand. In the "high-demand–parent-ignore" condition, the parents initially presented difficult demands and provided no attention for appropriate behavior. Off-task behavior resulted in a redirection to the task. The "low-demand–parent-attention" condition consisted of easy academic demands and parent attention for appropriate behavior. Similarly to the high-demand–parent-attention condition, the participants were redirected to work upon the occurrence of inappropriate behavior. Finally, the "low-demand–parent-ignore" condition utilized easy academic demands and provided no attention for appropriate behavior. Again, the participants were redirected to the demand when off-task behavior occurred. Immediately following the initial analysis, the conditions with the lowest and highest rates of inappropriate behavior were replicated.

Based upon the assessment data, treatment recommendations were constructed. Cooper et al. (1990) also conducted social validity and challenging behavior assessments on all participants' challenging behavior following the implementation of the treatment recommendations. The data indicated that the treatments derived from the functional analysis were considered appropriate by the parents and resulted in generally lower rates of forms of challenging behavior in the participants.

The Cooper et al. (1990) study was replicated by Cooper et al. (1992). The model applied to the initial study was modified slightly to include task preference as a possible contingency maintaining challenging behavior. In this study the researchers were able to conduct their brief functional analysis procedure in both a school and an outpatient clinic setting. By replicating their initial findings and extending the model to other treatment settings, Cooper et al. (1992) rendered support for the components of functional analysis to be efficiently incorporated into brief assessment protocols.

Harding et al. (1994) developed a 90-min functional analysis procedure for use in an outpatient setting. The model was designed to systematically evaluate the influence of antecedents and consequences on challenging behavior and to arrive at a recommendation for treatment interventions within a 90-min period. This assessment model was hierarchical in nature as each condition added a component to the previous condition's contingencies. The design included a baseline control condition followed by the systematic implementation of the condition hierarchy until improvements in appropriate behavior were noted. Upon the occurrence of improved rates of appropriate behavior, the previous condition was implemented in a reversal design with the successful condition.

Parents conducted each condition with the participants, following a brief training period including written directions describing the required contingencies. The "free play" condition served as the control for the study (Harding et al. 1994). The parents were instructed to play freely with their child without providing any demands. Further, Harding et al. utilized a second control condition in the study. The "general directions" conditions instructed parents to tell their child to begin working on a nonpreferred task and to ignore any appropriate behavior. Inappropriate behavior resulted in a prompt to return to work. The "specific directions" condition was identical to the previous condition except the parents provided a clear statement regarding the required demand. The next condition allowed the participants the opportunity to choose the task to be completed. The subsequent conditions incorporated differential reinforcement of appropriate behavior, differential reinforcement of communication, and access to a preferred task following the completion of the initial demand. Finally, punishment contingencies (time-out or guided compliance) were implemented based upon the hypotheses regarding the contingencies maintaining the participant's challenging behavior.

The Harding et al. (1994) study achieved improved rates of appropriate behavior in all seven participants. The conditions that evoked improved behavior varied by participant, as did the percentage increase in appropriate responding. Further, experimental control via brief reversals was demonstrated for six participants. All assessments were completed within the 90-min period and allowed for treatment recommendations to be provided to the parents (Harding et al. 1994). Follow-up reports from the parents regarding the implementation of the treatment suggestions indicated a high degree of satisfaction with the treatments derived from the analysis. The model proposed by Harding et al. further supports the use of brief assessment models.

Similar to Cooper et al. (1990) and Harding et al. (1994), Northup et al. (1991) developed a model for brief assessment that could be completed within 90 min and contained a contingency reversal phase. In addition, Northup et al. enhanced the brief analysis model by including the reinforcement of an alternative behavior. The initial analogue assessment conditions (alone, social attention, and escape) followed those outlined by Iwata et al. (1994/1982). In addition, a tangible condition was included where the participants were granted access to items contingent on an occurrence of the target behavior.

The contingency reversal phase began following the initial assessment. The condition producing the highest amount of the target behavior was repeated; however, in the contingency reversal, a functionally equivalent alternative behavior was identified and reinforced (e.g., providing access to a break, a tangible, or attention for communicating "please") (Northup et al. 1991). The reversal was achieved by reinstating the contingencies that evoked the highest levels of the target behavior. That is, the challenging behavior was again

reinforced and all appropriate behavior was ignored. Finally, the contingency reversal condition was repeated. Northup et al. 1991 both decreased inappropriate behavior during the contingency reversal and increased the target skills. These manipulations were then cited as indications of a potentially effective treatment derived from the analogue functional analysis.

The model proposed by Northup et al. (1991) was partially replicated by Derby et al. (1992). Derby et al. summarized the brief assessments conducted with 79 patients. These assessments, however, were conducted in an outpatient setting with the participant's parents acting as therapists. The target topographies of behavior were evoked by the assessments in 63% of the cases. Of those assessments, 74% identified the maintaining contingencies and 54% resulted in a decrease in the target behavior. Derby et al. suggested that the brief assessment model was limited to those patients that exhibit the target behavior at high rates. The inability of the assessment to reliably evoke all target behavior could be conceptualized as a limitation of the procedure. Cihak et al. (2007) adapted the models described by Northup et al. (1991) and Vollmer et al. (1993) to implement analyses in community settings. Their strategies provided information that appropriately informed treatment planning and allowed for an evaluation of those procedures likely to evoke therapeutic change and maximize teacher impressions of social validity.

Functional assessment procedures, including indirect data collection, descriptive analyses, and functional analyses, have been consistently supported within the literature as appropriate procedures for identifying the maintaining variables of challenging behavior. This information then informs treatment planning in a reliable fashion. There is increasing evidence that among the broad range of functional assessment procedures, functional analyses are more effective (Herzinger and Campbell 2007). The use of such procedures, however, remains complicated. This is perhaps most evident in public school settings which often find it difficult to achieve the training and time resources necessary for their implementation (Johnston and O'Neill 2001). As the already substantial empirical foundation for functional analysis methodology continues to expand to offer further iterations of procedures that include brief models, public settings,

and caregiver training, the discrepancy between procedures conducted in well-controlled, highly resourced, environments and public settings will continue to decrease.

Functional behavior assessment and functional analysis are well-documented and empirically supported procedures that remain essentially consistent with those described by Iwata et al. (1994/1982). From this substantial basic and applied research literature, a number of practice parameters emerge, which are presented in Table 4.1.

TABLE 4.1   Practice parameters for evidence-based functional behavior assessment for the treatment of problem behaviors in individuals with ASD

1. Each topography of behavior must be operationally defined so that all individuals responsible for participation in the functional analysis can reliably identify an instance of the challenging behavior. Further, functional assessment procedures must collect information on each topography of challenging behavior separately in order to avoid any inappropriate grouping of topographies into response classes. Such grouping requires reliable data indicating equality in maintaining variables.

2. In any functional analysis procedure, all conditions must be fully described with respect to environmental characteristics, antecedent manipulations, consequences to challenging behavior, stimuli to be included in the analysis, session duration, and data collection procedures. Further, while AB models of functional analysis have rendered meaningful findings, ABC models are considered more rigorous. Without a comprehensive description of each condition, implementation errors are likely, thereby nullifying the ability of the analysis to appropriately inform treatment planning.

3. Indirect data collection procedures should be undertaken to thoroughly inform the development of functional analysis conditions. These include procedures such as clinical interviews, rating scales, and archival reviews that are likely to render essential background information on the client. Also, descriptive assessment procedures (e.g., ABC) are often completed to better conceptualize the case and facilitate the development of hypotheses regarding the maintaining variables of the target behavior. These procedures become essential if the functional assessment process do not include an analogue analysis as they offer a useful alternative to achieve direct observation data collection.

4. Measures of procedural fidelity allow researchers and clinicians to verify the integrity of the data collection before making recommendations for treatment planning. Given the complexity of session implementation and data collection, it is essential that all procedures are reviewed consistently.

5. While no consistent standard exists for executing data analysis (e.g., statistical versus visual), it is essential that the functional analysis protocol clearly delineate those procedures to be used so that they may be objectively evaluated.

FUNCTIONAL COMMUNICATION TRAINING

Functional communication training (FCT) was initially described by Carr and Durand (1985) as a method of replacing aberrant behavior with an alternative communicative response that serves the same function as the problem behavior. FCT bears some similarity to differential reinforcement of alternative behavior (DRA) procedures as it teaches an alternative communicative response which elicits the reinforcer that previously maintained the challenging behavior. However, by placing the client in control of the schedule of reinforcement, the client can access a greater rate of reinforcement by manding (requesting) using the functionally equivalent alternative communicative response (Wacker et al. 1990). By allowing the client to achieve the reinforcer with greater efficiency by providing more consistent reinforcement and less delay in the period of time between the response by the client and the delivery of reinforcement (Carr 1988), the alternative communicative response becomes a reliable antecedent to diminish the problem behavior (Fisher et al. 1998).

Functional communication training has two main components: functional behavior assessment of the problem behavior in order to determine reinforcing stimuli that maintain the behavior and using those stimuli to understand and select an alternative communicative response to replace the problem behavior (Carr and Durand 1985). In practical terms, if a problem behavior has communicative intent, then it is reasonable to teach a communicative response that is more adaptive, efficient and functionally equivalent to the problem behavior to replace the aberrant response.

Numerous studies have supported the use of FCT with individuals with aggression (Durand et al. 1989), self-injury (Hanley et al. 2001), destructive behavior

(Wacker et al. 2008), stereotypies (Repp et al. 1988), and tantrums (Durand et al. 1989). For example, Carr and Durand (1985) reported the effects of FCT on four children with developmental disabilities exhibiting aggressive and disruptive behavior. After initially determining the function of behavior to provide access to positive or negative reinforcement for each specific child, each child was taught to solicit praise (positive reinforcement) or to request assistance for help with a difficult task (negative reinforcement). Episodes of aggressive and disruptive behavior decreased significantly in all cases and maintained over time. While in this study inappropriate behavior was ignored (placed on extinction), other researchers have followed the same FCT procedures but applied extinction with subsequent redirection to another activity contingent upon inappropriate behavior (Steege et al. 1989).

Wacker et al. (1990) conducted a component analysis of FCT across different forms of behavior (e.g., self-injury, stereotypy, and aggression) with differing functions (escape, access to tangible positive reinforcement, sensory consequences). Two components were studied in three individuals with developmental disabilities (one with autism): the effect on FCT if an intervention for inappropriate behavior following initial training was provided and the effect of the control over reinforcement exercised by the functional communicative response. Their results indicate that with the maintaining function quickly identified during assessment, the alternative communicative response was learned rapidly. While the FCT procedure alone reduced problem behavior, a more significant and sustained decrease was observed when an additional intervention for inappropriate behavior (e.g., graduated guidance, extinction) was applied following initial FCT training. Consistent with previous studies, treatment results were not contingent on specific behavior forms or functions.

Finally, the data clearly supported the assertion that client control over reinforcement is an important component of FCT.

An important concern in the use of FCT is whether the schedule of reinforcement necessary to establish the alternative behavior (typically a fixed ratio 1 schedule) can be modified ("thinned") after the behavior has been established, so as to approximate a more natural, community-referenced schedule of reinforcement. As a practical concern, it is important to know whether the new, functional communicative response will continue to be used and will maintain low rates of challenging behavior when reinforcement is not available for every correct alternative communicative response demonstrated by the client. Hanley et al. (2001) addressed this issue with three adults with profound intellectual disabilities whose self-injury and aggression was determined through functional analysis to be maintained by positive reinforcement. After teaching a functional communicative response to access positive reinforcement to each client, several different schedules of reinforcement were investigated for their impact on maintaining problem behavior at low rates and alternative functional communicative responses at treatment levels. Their results indicate that a multiple schedule reinforcement arrangement (whereby white and red cards, signaling reinforcement or extinction, respectively, were alternatively presented to the client) was superior to a reinforcer delay procedure, fixed interval schedules of reinforcement, and mixed schedule of reinforcement without signaling in maintaining targeted behaviors at initial treatment levels. These findings are important as they address the practical problem of thinning the schedule of reinforcement after acquisition of an alternative communicative response, while simultaneously keeping problem behavior at low rates. Further, they provide support for the use of prediction or

signaling reinforcement opportunities as a component of FCT with those with significant developmental disabilities.

In a further investigation of schedule thinning, Hagopian et al. (2005) demonstrated that FCT combined with extinction (i.e., removal of the reinforcing stimulus contingent upon the problem behavior) and access to competing stimuli was more successful than FCT with extinction alone in maintaining low rates of problem behavior once the reinforcement schedule was reduced. Three children with autism or pervasive developmental disorder with concurrent ADHD who demonstrated a range of significant behavioral challenges were participants. Following a functional analysis and subsequent determination of a functionally equivalent communicative response, a preference assessment to determine potential reinforcers was undertaken with caregivers. All children then participated in an assessment of competing stimuli, whereby items identified in the preference assessment as associated with the lowest rates of problem behavior were determined. These items were provided noncontingently and continuously during the FCT with extinction (of the problem behavior) and access to competing stimuli condition, while only FCT with extinction was provided in the comparison condition. It was hypothesized that access to competing stimuli would produce reinforcement for the child that effectively competed with the reinforcement maintaining the problem behavior, thereby reducing that behavior. Results for all three children confirm this, as rates of problem behavior decreased more substantially with the provision of competing stimuli and maintained during schedule thinning more successfully than when FCT with extinction alone was used. While conducted in an inpatient setting without probes to assess generalization to more natural rates of response and reinforcement in the community, the finding that the process of fading the reinforcement schedule following establishment of a viable functional communicative alternative can be enhanced is an important one.

In a large-scale investigation of 21 clients with developmental disabilities, Hagopian et al. (1998) evaluated the effectiveness of FCT on reducing aggression and self-injury when used alone or in conjunction with extinction, extinction plus fading, and with brief punishment (i.e., a 60-s chair time out, a 2-min room time out, or a 60-s basket hold). Their findings identify a 90% reduction in problem behavior from baseline in half of the cases when extinction procedures were incorporated and a 90% reduction in target behaviors in every case when punishment procedures were added. (The authors note that the punishment procedures described above were not added unless the FCT plus extinction procedure failed to produce significant reductions of the target behavior.) These results further define potential treatment progressions to be considered when FCT is implemented in combination with extinction procedures, but fail to produce reductions in behavior to acceptable levels. While the results are limited to those clients with severe developmental disabilities whose behavior is so severe as to require inpatient hospitalization, the strength of the findings across a large number of clients is especially noteworthy.

In a related evaluation of components necessary to enhance the efficacy of FCT, Steege et al. (1989) combined extinction plus redirection to treat a high rate of self-injury in two children with severe multiple disabilities. For the first child, baseline rates of self-injury were in excess of 90% of observation intervals. For the second, self-injury was observed in 45% and 68% of observed intervals across two separate tasks. Results for both children indicate rapid reduction in self-injury to near zero rates within 2–6 sessions of treatment, with maintenance at zero for 6 months for the first child and 15 months for the second. In addition to replicating the applicability of the initial procedure and demonstrating the maintenance of treatment effects, this study extends the importance of conducting formal preference assessments after completion of the functional analysis, in order to identify objectively those reinforcers that will be used in the training procedure.

The applicability of functional communication training to the treatment of challenging behavior is well-established in the literature. Researchers have expanded upon the original conceptualization proposed by Carr and Durand (1985) to define additional components to the treatment package that significantly increase efficacy of the procedure. Practice parameters for FCT are presented in Table 4.2.

NONCONTINGENT REINFORCEMENT

Noncontingent reinforcement (NCR) is a method of increasing access to reinforcing stimuli by providing these stimuli on a fixed-time or variable-time schedule, independent of a child's behavior (Vollmer et al. 1993). In contrast to contingent access to reinforcement, whereby a child gains access to the reinforcer only after demonstrating the desired behavior, NCR schedules reinforcing stimuli based on elapsed time. Following identification of the reinforcer maintaining a challenging behavior during functional analysis, that reinforcer is provided independent of the occurrence of the behavior. For example, where the functional analysis identifies that access to tangible positive reinforcement maintains problem behavior, access to reinforcing tangibles is provided on a fixed-time or variable-time schedule independent of the problem behavior's occurrence. This disrupts the response–reinforcer relationship. With the environment enhanced by

TABLE 4.2   Practice parameters for evidence-based functional communication training for the treatment of challenging behaviors in individuals with ASD

1. A functional analysis must be conducted in order to identify variables maintaining the problem behavior. Results of the functional analysis will directly guide selection of the functionally equivalent communicative alternative.

2. An alternative, functionally equivalent communicative response must be selected to be taught as a replacement for the problem behavior. This communicative response must match the maintaining variable identified in the functional analysis. That is, if the functional analysis indicated that the problem behavior was maintained by social attention, then use of the FCT response must access social attention (cf. Repp et al. 1988).

3. A communication modality must be selected for training the new response. Verbal responses, manual signs, picture exchanges and microswitch activation all have been used. The modality must be within the repertoire of the individual, or prerequisite skills must be evident that would permit rapid acquisition of the response modality.

4. A preference assessment should be conducted prior to training in order to establish potential reinforcers (cf. Steege et al. 1989).

5. Reinforcement schedules should be thinned after the FCT response is established, so that the period of time between a communicative response and the delivery of reinforcement is gradually increased (Hagopian et al. 1998; Hanley et al. 2001).

6. Consequent procedures for problem behaviors (e.g., extinction plus redirection) can be incorporated as necessary in order to achieve and maintain low and stable rates of problem behavior (Steege et al. 1989; Hagopian et al. 1998).

7. In order to reduce the potential for prompt dependency is important to gradually reduce verbal prompts during the implementation of FCT, once the response has been established (Cooper et al. 2007; Miltenberger et al. 1998).

reinforcing stimuli that are provided frequently and without any expectation by the child, the motivation to engage in the problem behavior is reduced. This effect is termed an *abolishing operation* (Michael 2004), a specific type of motivating operation that decreases the effectiveness of a known reinforcer (e.g., playing the Wii frequently may reduce the effectiveness of the Wii as a reinforcer). NCR has been demonstrated to be effective in the treatment of various forms of problem behavior including stereotypy (Britton et al. 2002), self-injury (Vollmer et al. 1993), disruptive behavior (Fisher et al. 1996), and aggression (Vollmer et al. 1997). It has also proven effective in treating challenging behavior maintained by automatic reinforcement (Roane et al. 2003), negative reinforcement or escape from demands (Kodak et al.

2003), positive reinforcement from social attention (Hanley et al. 1997; Kahng et al. 2000b), and tangible positive reinforcement (Marcus and Vollmer 1996).

The role of positive reinforcement in NCR with children with autism has been considered by several researchers. For example, Hagopian et al. (1994) investigated the role of NCR in the treatment of self-injury, aggressive and disruptive behavior maintained by social attention in 5-year-old female identical quadruplets diagnosed with pervasive developmental disorder and intellectual disability. In particular, these researchers were interested in whether dense or lean schedules of response-dependent attention had a significant differential effect on reduction of these challenging behaviors. A multi-element design with schedule fading and generalization phases (across therapists and settings) was used. During the lean NCR treatment condition, a child received one 10 s period of social attention every 5 min. In the dense condition, the child received six 10 s periods of social attention each minute (essentially, a continuous reinforcement schedule). Results for all four children were dramatic under the dense NCR condition, with 90% reduction from baseline rates of aggressive, self-injurious, or disruptive behavior. Under the lean schedule condition, three of the four children demonstrated a decrease from baseline rates (ranging from 65% to 77%), while the fourth, most impaired, sibling increased slightly. With the subsequent implementation of a systematic fading procedure from dense-to-lean schedules, all four siblings were able to establish low rates of problem behavior consistent with initial reductions during the first NCR phase, and to generalize them across therapists, with maintenance at 1- and 2-month observations. The authors note that the discrepant range of sessions required for fading for each sibling (i.e., 16, 27, 29, 34) highlights the importance of having specific response criteria for fading sessions, such that as behavior rate increases with the introduction of a leaner schedule, there is a systematic means of moving back a step to re-establish low rates of behavior before moving forward with the fading procedure. They further suggest that a dense schedule may be the most effective in establishing low rates of behavior when using NCR, with systematic thinning of the schedule as behavior rates continue to decline.

Wilder et al. (2005) noted that noncontingent positive reinforcement in the form of continued access to a preferred movie was successful in increasing food acceptance and also reducing escape-motivated, self-injurious behavior in a girl with autism. Ingvarsson et al. (2008) extended these findings in their investigation of the role of NCR in the treatment of aggressive and disruptive behavior in an 8-year-old girl, where the problem behaviors were maintained by both escape from demands and access to edibles. In addition, these authors evaluated the effect of the density of reinforcer delivery on the effectiveness of NCR and the effect of NCR on compliance. Results indicated that both lean and dense schedules of reinforcement were equally successful in producing significant reduction, to near zero rates, in challenging behavior and that these effects were achieved through the delivery of edibles during the NCR phase without necessity of escape extinction as a treatment component in the demand context. Noncontingent delivery of edibles also increased compliance from less than 20% during baseline to approximately 80% following use of NCR, with no significant difference between lean and dense schedules of reinforcement. Together these three studies offer support for the role of NCR in the treatment of self-injurious, aggressive and disruptive behavior, and additional support for the efficiency of using relatively lean schedules of reinforcement in the NCR procedure.

The relationship between variable- and fixed-time schedules of reinforcement and treatment effectiveness has also been investigated by several authors. Britton et al. (2000) used NCR on a fixed-time schedule plus extinction (of the target) and schedule thinning to successfully treat various aberrant behaviors in three individuals with severe developmental disabilities, including one with autism. Following demonstration of the effectiveness of NCR across a multiple baseline design for all clients, systematic schedule thinning problem behaviors were maintained at near zero rates when NCR was provided on a fixed 5-min schedule. Fisher et al. (2004) compared the effect of NCR plus extinction on a fixed schedule to extinction alone in treating the severe self-injurious, aggressive, and destructive behavior in four individuals (aged 5, 7, 9, and 33) with significant intellectual disability. Their results indicate clear differences between treatment sessions that provided NCR in the form of social attention or tangibles from those where extinction alone was used. Van Camp et al. (2000) compared the effects of fixed-time and variable-time schedules of reinforcer delivery during NCR on the aggressive and self-injurious behavior of two students with severe-to-profound intellectual disability. Results showed that problem behavior in one individual decreased from a baseline of approximately four episodes per minute to near zero by the 40th session, and for the second individual behavior decreased from about 1.5 episodes per minute during baseline to zero by the 50th session. Both schedules were similar in their effectiveness, providing support for the use of variable-time schedules as

the clinical situation dictates. Carr et al. (2009) conducted a comprehensive review of research on NCR to treat challenging behavior of individuals with developmental disabilities and concluded that, overall, fixed-time schedules of reinforcer delivery with extinction and schedule thinning were superior to both fixed-time and variable-time schedules with extinction, with the former being identified as well-established as an evidence-based treatment and the latter two as probably efficacious.

The efficacy of noncontingent reinforcement procedures for the treatment of a wide range of behavioral topographies and functions has been well established in the literature. Operational components that significantly increase the effectiveness of NCR are shown in Table 4.3.

TABLE 4.3   Practice parameters for noncontingent reinforcement for the treatment of problem behaviors in individuals with ASD

---

1. A functional analysis must first be conducted in order to determine the positive, negative, or automatic reinforcers maintaining problem behavior (Iwata et al. 1994/1982; Hanley et al. 2003).

2. A reinforce preference assessment should be completed, and repeated throughout treatment as necessary, in order to determine those stimuli to be used during the NCR intervention (DeLeon et al. 2000).

3. Noncontingent reinforcement must be presented more frequently than the baseline schedule of reinforcement (Ringdahl et al. 2001; Kahng et al. 2000a, b).

4. Fixed-time reinforcement schedules combined with extinction and schedule thinning procedures are the most effective, but fixed-time schedules incorporating extinction and variable-time schedules incorporating extinction are also effective, even as they have a slightly less-conclusive research foundation (Carr et al. 2009).

5. Adventitious reinforcement can be problematic, and chance pairings of the NCR delivery of reinforcement and the problem behavior should be monitored so that the problem behavior does not increase (Hagopian et al. 1994; Vollmer et al. 1997).

6. Terminal criteria should be established for NCR (Kahng et al. 2000a, b; Cooper et al. 2007). That is, the amount of time to increase between presentation of stimuli during NCR should be scheduled (schedule thinning) should be accompanied by establishing the final duration of the NCR schedule. Kahng and colleagues (2000) observed that 5 min has become something of a convention in behavior analytic literature, and this duration remains effective. The degree to which this duration effectively matches natural schedules of reinforcement in an individuals' typical environment, and the extent to which behavior gains can be maintained with treatment integrity, remains an area for further investigation.

BEHAVIORAL MOMENTUM (HIGH-PROBABILITY OR HIGH-P COMMAND SEQUENCE)

Behavioral momentum is the metaphor used to describe the tendency for a behavior that has historically been maintained through specific schedules of reinforcement to persist even after reinforcement conditions change (Mace et al. 1988). The term, borrowed from the infrahuman experimental literature (Nevin 1996), applies to the application of a high-probability (high-p) command sequence immediately preceding a low-probability command. By providing requests or commands that have a high probability of reinforcement, the client achieves a "momentum" that increases the likelihood of responding correctly and being reinforced for a request that previously had a low probability of correct responding. While the terms "behavioral momentum" (Mace et al. 1988) and "interspersed requests" (Horner et al. 1991) have been used to describe this phenomenon, the process is most accurately described as the *high-p request sequence* (Cooper et al. 2007).

High-p request sequences have been used to increase task completion (Horner et al. 1991; Mace and Belfiore 1990), to increase appropriate behavior during transition from recess to instructional group time (Singer et al. 1987), to increase social initiations and responding (Davis et al. 1994), to increase compliance with self-care routines (Mace et al. 1988) and compliance with simple requests (Zuluaga and Normand 2008), to increase generalized responding (Davis et al. 1992), to increase compliance with a self-medication regimen (Harchik and Putzier 1990), to reduce self-injury (Horner et al. 1991; Zarcone et al. 1994), to teach object labels (Volkert et al. 2008), and to decrease stereotypy (Mace and Belfiore 1990). Since the seminal and elegant series of studies presented by Mace et al. (1988), researchers have, for the most part, sought to better understand the specific conditions under which the high-p sequence is most successful and whether it is most effective in combination with other strategies (e.g., with escape extinction) when treating problem behavior maintained by specific functional consequences (e.g., escape-maintained self-injury).

Several researchers have demonstrated the effectiveness of the high-p request sequence in the treatment of compliance with individuals with autism and related severe developmental disabilities. For example, Wilder et al. (2007) evaluated the effectiveness of noncontingent reinforcement, the high-p request sequence, and a verbal warning on increasing compliance in three children, one of whom had Fragile-X syndrome. The high-p sequence was effective only for the child with Fragile-X, while the other two children (both with typical development) required the addition of an extinction component in order to generate stable compliant responding. Zuluaga and Normand (2008) assessed the effects of providing reinforcement or no reinforcement for compliance to high-p instructions on compliance to low-p instructional requests with two children (aged 4 and 5) with developmental disabilities. Programmed reinforcement for the high-p requests increased compliance significantly in the low-p requests, compared to non-reinforcement for high-p requests. These authors also conducted a preference assessment prior to beginning intervention and used the results of those assessments to select reinforcers for the high-p sequences, suggesting the importance of a preference assessment in the high-p request protocol. Bullock and Normand (2006) also evaluated the effect of the high-p sequence with reinforcers informed by a preference assessment on increasing compliance to low-p requests in two young children (both typical). These authors compared the effectiveness of the high-p sequence with fixed-time interval reinforcement for compliance with low-p requests, the latter maintained by escape from demands (negative reinforcement). Both strategies worked equally well. The authors suggest that the effectiveness of escape as a reinforcer may have been reduced because the preferred items offered as reinforcement constituted an abolishing operation, an observation consistent with findings by others (Lalli et al. 1999).

Ducharme and Worling (1994) evaluated the effect of stimulus fading in maintaining the durability of responding to low-p compliance requests in two children (aged 5 and 15) with developmental disabilities and mild-to-severe intellectual challenges. Using a multiple baseline design across subjects, the authors found that systematically fading high-p requests and increasing the latency between the high-p and low-p requests was more effective than an abrupt change in the high-p sequence, and that the stimulus fading procedure maintained treatment levels of compliance after 16 weeks. As importantly, these procedures were implemented successfully by parents. In a preliminary study to evaluate components of successful high-p interventions, Kennedy et al. (1995) investigated the effect of interspersed high-p requests with and without neutral social comments that did not require a response from the client on noncompliant behavior in two individuals aged 18 and 19 with severe developmental disabilities. Their results suggested that compliance was increased when low-p requests were preceded by high-p requests accompanied by social comments. Mace et al. (1988) found that neutral comments delivered prior to high-p requests had no effect on compliance, but the current findings raise the interesting question as to whether reinforcing stimuli presented noncontingently before a *low-p* request would contribute to a decrease in noncompliant behavior.

Task avoidance is a commonly observed behavior problem in individuals with autism, typically maintained by negative reinforcement. Mace et al. (1988) presented a series of five studies evaluating the effect of the high-p response sequence on reducing task avoidance and decreasing response latency in four adults with severe developmental disabilities, all with intellectual disability. These authors noted not only that task avoidance and response latency were reduced significantly, but also that duration to task completion was also reduced.

The use of the high-p request sequence to promote task participation and skill acquisition with individuals with autism and other developmental disabilities has also been discussed by several authors. Davis et al. (1994) extended the earlier work of Mace and others and used a high-p sequence to increase social initiations and social interactions in three young children diagnosed with autism and intellectual disabilities. They found that child responsiveness to low-p requests for social exchanges was increased when preceded by high-p requests and that there was an increase in generalized unprompted initiations and interactions in nontraining settings. Results were maintained after all prompts were removed.

Volkert et al. (2008) taught object labels to six children, five of whom were diagnosed with autism. A comparison of similar and dissimilar interspersed tasks yielded no difference in acquisition of labels, but the quality of reinforcers offered had a positive effect on acquisition rates. These authors speculated that praise may not be as potent a reinforcer for children with autism as for those with other developmental disabilities, an observation made earlier by Mace and Belfiore (1990). However, in an extension of earlier work, Mace et al. (1997) reported on the effectiveness of the high-p sequence in reducing aggression and increasing compliance in two adolescents with autism and "autistic features," and determined that reinforcer quality increased behavioral momentum and likely contributed to the reduction of problem behavior. Given the seminal work of Klin et al. (2009) describing the atypical gaze patterns in those with autism compared to individuals with other or no disabilities, it is likely that the salience of a variety of socially-mediated reinforcers (including praise, positive affect, etc.) differs with various populations. While the application of this particular consideration to the use of the high-p sequence with those with autism remains to be investigated, it is certainly reasonable to conduct preparatory preference assessments with this distinction in mind.

Aggressive, disruptive, and self-injurious behaviors are among the most insidious problems encountered by parents and professionals, and these challenges can restrict learning as well as integration opportunities of those with autism in very significant ways (Matson and LoVullo 2008). In an early study, Horner et al. (1991) reported on the effectiveness of interspersed high-p requests on the successful completion of low-p requests, and on the aggression and self-injury that accompanied low-p requests in three adolescents with severe intellectual disabilities. Not only did interspersal of high-p requests increase compliance to low-p requests, but self-injury and aggression also reduced significantly. Horner, Day, and their colleagues suggested that the response class of "instruction following" was reinforced, leading to an increase in instructional responses and a concomitant decrease in problem behaviors. In a related study, Zarcone et al. (1993) addressed escape-maintained self-injury, in the form of headbanging on hard surfaces, in a 33-year-old man with profound intellectual disability. While the application of the high-p sequence alone was unsuccessful in reducing self-injury, a high-p sequence combined with escape extinction led to significant reductions in the problem

behavior and also increased compliance to low-p requests. These results suggest that for escape-maintained problem behavior, a high-p sequence alone may be insufficient to override the negative reinforcing value of terminating instruction. Zarcone et al. (1994) replicated and extended these findings with two adult men with profound intellectual disabilities who were institutionalized. For these individuals, escape-maintained self-injury took the form of hand-biting, headbanging, face-slapping, and finger-biting. The high-p sequence alone was again ineffective but when escape from the demand was on extinction and self-injury could not successfully terminate the demand (the men were redirected back to the task to completion upon episodes of self-injury), self-injury decreased to near zero levels, from an average of approximately four per minute, and compliance increased from less than 20% to approximately 80% to over 90% for low-p and high-p requests, respectively. These findings confirm the importance of escape extinction as a component to a high-p request sequence when noncompliance is accompanied by self-injury.

While self-injury and related aggressive and disruptive behaviors constitute important problems for those with autism, stereotypy is also frequently observed. Mace and Belfiore (1990) investigated the use of a high-p sequence to reduce escape-maintained stereotypy (repetitive touching of others with the hands or feet) in a 38-year-old woman with severe developmental disabilities. These authors found that high-p requests that were functionally incompatible with stereotypy (household tasks) reduced and then maintained low rates of stereotypy, while also increasing compliance to tasks. As the client increased her engagement with high-p tasks and was reinforced at high rates, subsequent refusal or avoidance of low-p requests would have effectively terminated reinforcement

opportunities. Mace and Belfiore speculate that "compliance to instructions" as
a response class served as an abolishing
operation, momentarily reducing the reinforcing value of escape.

The high-probability (high-p) request
sequence has demonstrated utility in the
treatment of a variety of behavior problems in those with severe developmental disabilities including autism. While a
substantial body of evidence exists establishing it as a highly effective antecedent
intervention with aggressive, disruptive,
noncompliant, and self-injurious behavior,
treatment efficacy for problem behavior
maintained by escape from demands has
also been established. The operational
dimensions and practice recommendations
shown in Table 4.4 should be considered in
implementation.

Behavioral Treatment of Sleep Problems in Individuals with Autism Spectrum Disorder

The previous section identified several
specific strategies that enjoy substantial
empirical support. Treatment in autism is
often based on multi-component interventions, however, incorporating two or more
procedures. In this section, we consider
the use of behavioral strategies to reduce
sleep disorders in children with autism.
While this particular area has not been as
extensively studied with those with autism
spectrum disorders, a significant research
literature exists documenting the effectiveness of various behavioral strategies

TABLE 4.4   Practice parameters for using the high-probability (high-p) request sequence to treat problem behaviors in individuals with ASD

1. The quality of reinforcers chosen is important, especially with escape-maintained behavior (Zarcone et al. 1994). To the extent that salient and powerful reinforcers follow compliance, the effectiveness of the high-p intervention is enhanced (Mace 1996).
2. High-p sequence requests must be within the repertoire of the client, and should be easily accessible, so that the opportunity for reinforcement is maintained a high levels during high-p presentations (Mace 1996).
3. Speed matters and the law of contiguity applies. Low-p requests should follow in quick succession from the reinforcer for a high-p request, and intervals between all requests should be short (Cooper et al. 2007; Davis and Reichle 1996).
4. Instructor error can take several forms. If used after the occurrence of a problem behavior reinforcement for the high-p request might strengthen the problem behavior. In addition, with escape-maintained behavior procedural drift may occur whereby the intervenor inadvertently begins to offer fewer low-p requests (as these elicit the problem behavior) and more high-p requests in order to avoid the challenging behavior (Cooper et al. 2007; Horner et al. 1991).
5. For escape-maintained behavior, escape extinction can increase the effectiveness and efficiency of a high-p request sequence. Where aggression or self-injury are present, response blocking and redirection to the low-p task to completion is an effective strategy (Zarcone et al. 1993, 1994).
6. Teaching compliance to instructional requests is an important objective in using a high-p request sequence, as it likely constitutes a response class with more generalized utility (Mace and Belfiore 1990; Horner et al. 1991).

with other populations of individuals with severe developmental disabilities and also with typically developing children. Individual components are described as *well-established, probably efficacious, or possibly efficacious* based upon the preponderance of empirical support and independent replicated findings available for review, as well as whether published research identified children with autism more specifically among those treated. As with individual procedures described earlier in this chapter, only published research that clearly operationalized target behaviors, demonstrated a functional relationship between the intervention and the rate of behavior change, and where a procedure was replicated across multiple settings or individuals was considered. While a concurrent review of assessment and treatment procedures for organically-based sleep disorders (e.g., obstructive sleep apnea) is beyond the scope of this chapter, excellent reviews of medication management are available elsewhere (Owens 2009).

Sleep problems are prevalent in those with identified autism spectrum disorder, with estimates ranging from 44% to 83% (Liu et al. 2006; McDougall et al. 2005; Patzold et al. 1998; Richdale and Prior 1995; Paavonen et al. 2008; Wiggs and Stores 1996), far exceeding the estimates for typically developing young children. The types of sleep disorder found among children with autism are generally not unique to ASD, but are more frequent and severe than in the general population and also when compared to children with other disabilities. While some studies of parents of individuals with ASD (Schreck and Mulick 2000) report similar quantitative sleep dimensions (e.g., the number of hours spent sleeping), other studies of parents identify significant discrepancies in the duration and quality of sleep (Honomichl et al. 2002). Parents also typically report that their children have sleep problems more frequently, including significant sleep onset and maintenance problems (Malow and McGrew 2008), irregular sleep–wake patterns, early waking, and poor sleep routines (Patzold et al. 1998; Mindell et al. 2006; Quine 2001; Schreck and Mulick 2000; Honomichl et al. 2002). Sleep problems have also been shown to be related to problems with daytime behavioral functioning in children with autism spectrum disorders (Malow et al. 2006; Schreck et al. 2004) and to sleep problems in the parents of children with autism (Lopez-Wagner et al. 2008).

While there is a substantial literature investigating treatment of sleep problems with typically developing children (Mindell et al. 2006), the research literature on sleep problems experienced by those with autism spectrum disorders is quite small, comprising perhaps less than 20 well-designed studies. In their exhaustive review of the literature on behavioral treatment of sleep problems in typically developing children, Mindell, Kuhn, and their colleagues reviewed 52 treatment studies and concluded that 94% of studies reported successful outcomes, with over 80% maintenance of gains at 3 and 6 months. Extinction procedures (without modifications) and parent education procedures had the strongest support in the literature reviewed. In contrast, a review of behavioral treatment of sleep problems in children with autism spectrum disorders by Schreck (2001) identified only six studies emphasizing strategies based on the principles of applied behavior analysis. A later review by Kodak and Piazza (2008) similarly reports a small number of studies.

Common sleep problems of childhood have been comprehensively described (Owens 2009) and can be divided into four basic etiologic categories: insufficient sleep for basic biologic needs (e.g., behavioral insomnia and lifestyle sleep restrictions); fragmented or disrupted sleep caused by conditions that result in prolonged or frequent arousal (e.g., obstructive sleep apnea and periodic limb movement disorder);

excessive daytime sleepiness (e.g., narco-lepsy); and circadian rhythm disorders, whereby sleep is structurally normal but occurs at undesirable times (e.g., delayed sleep phase disorders). While sleep disorders can be split, for practical purposes, into those that are medically or organically and those that are behaviorally based, these two considerations frequently co-exist, are influenced by psychosocial and environmental factors, and must be comprehensively assessed prior to development of a treatment plan. Malow and McGrew (2008) discuss the evaluation and treatment of sleep disturbances in autism and recommend that, following determination and treatment of any potential underlying organic cause for the sleep problem (e.g., obstructive sleep disorder or circadian rhythm disorder), behavioral treatments should be the first-line interventions. Their conceptualization of treatment is consistent with earlier recommendations (Wiggs and France 2000) which drew the distinction between the treatment of sleep *disorders* and sleep *architecture*, noting that while behavioral interventions often appropriately addressed the former, attention to the latter (which includes a wide range of organic or medical conditions) is essential.

In discussing the research on treatment of sleep disturbances in autism we would reiterate the recommendation of Malow and McGrew (2008) that a thorough review of physical systems be undertaken prior to initiating behavioral treatment. This is important for several reasons, including the possibility to an organic basis may contribute to symptoms and behavior presentation. For example, Malow et al. (2006) documented the effect of adenotonsillectomy on behavioral symptomatology of a 5-year-old girl with autism spectrum disorder with obstructive sleep apnea, reporting significant improvements in alertness, emotional reactivity, and social communication and decreases in tactile sensitivity

and repetitive behavior. It is reasonable to consider that reduced upper airway size or muscle tone (as may be observed in children with craniofacial syndromes or Down syndrome, respectively) may also be contributory factors that must be accounted for in the treatment planning process.

In this section, we consider various behavioral interventions that have been used to treat a number of sleep problems in children with autism. There are several caveats, however. As noted earlier, the literature on intervention with children diagnosed with autism spectrum disorders is quite small. A somewhat broader literature evaluating and treating those with other developmental disabilities contributes more conclusively to our understanding of treatment efficacy, particularly where specific evidence-based strategies are applied (e.g., extinction procedures). As such, while we note studies that included people with a diagnosis in the autism spectrum in our review, we believe that it is appropriate to also consider the results of treatment with individuals with different but related neurodevelopmental disorders (e.g., Fragile-X Syndrome or severe intellectual disability) in any evaluation of treatment efficacy.

Extinction and its variants (e.g., graduated and non-graduated extinction procedures) have been studied extensively in typical children (Bramble 1997; Mindell et al. 2006) with consistent success, justifying use as an evidence-based procedure in those without developmental disabilities. Extinction has also been the subject of research in those with autism and related neurodevelopmental disorders. Non-graduated extinction represents a traditional extinction process, whereby the maintaining variable is systematically withheld contingent upon the problem behavior. Thus, in the case of a child who tantrums for social attention by an adult after being put to bed, removal of the social attention constitutes non-graduated extinction. In an early study with a 3-year-old with autism,

Wolf et al. (1964) used such an extinction procedure that also included a structured bedtime routine and a consequent procedure (door closed to the bedroom contingent upon tantrum behavior). Consistent with the experimental literature on extinction the child responded with an extinction burst, but then a dramatic decrease in problem behavior, with near zero rates after day 6. Weiskop et al. (2001) and Weiskop et al. (2005) also investigated the effect of non-graduated extinction on children with autism. Weiskop et al. (2001) reported on the use of positive routines, reinforcement for appropriate bedtime behavior, and extinction in reducing co-sleeping and remaining in bed throughout the night with a 5-year-old with autism. These authors found that positive routines and reinforcement were insufficient to reduce sleep problems, but with the addition of extinction procedures the child was able to fall asleep on his own and remain asleep in his bed throughout the night within 6 days. Results maintained at 3- and 12-month follow-ups. Weiskop et al. (2005) extended these findings by evaluating the effects of bedtime routines, positive reinforcement and extinction to reduce sleep problems in six children with autism and seven children with Fragile-X syndrome, all of whom ranged in age from 1+11 to 7+11 years, using a multiple-baseline-across-participants design. Functional assessment identified positive reinforcement or social attention as the variable maintaining problem behaviors, which included pre-sleep disturbances, waking during the night, falling asleep alone, and requiring a parent to sleep with the child. Consistent with results in their previous investigation, Weiskop et al. (2005) found that improvements in behavior were significant within 2–3 days post-intervention, but only with the introduction of non-graduated extinction procedures. The effect of extinction on early morning waking and rocking was also evaluated, but findings indicated that these behaviors were unresponsive to the treatment procedures (suggesting that different maintaining variables were responsible for these two behaviors). Results maintained at 3- and 12-month follow-ups for 75% of participants with autism and 80% of children with Fragile-X syndrome.

In a related study with three children with intellectual disability, Thackeray and Richdale (2002) evaluated the effect of reinforcement, parent education in sleep hygiene, positive bedtime routines, and non-graduated extinction on falling asleep without a parent present, co-sleeping, and night waking. Extinction procedures were clearly most effective, reducing episodes of disruptive behavior to zero levels quickly for two of the three children, with the third child averaging slightly less than one episode per night after 4 weeks of treatment. The treatment rates maintained at 3-month follow-up for the two children who were most successful initially, while the third child experienced a slight increase then a subsequent decrease at follow-up. Didden et al. (1998) also investigated the effect of extinction on reducing various sleep problems including crying and disruptive behavior during bedtimes in six children with a range of severe physical or intellectual disabilities. Functional assessment identified positive reinforcement in the form of parental attention as the maintaining variable in four children, with anxiety following a traumatic event hypothesized for the fifth child, and an organic cause (a possible seizure disorder) responsible for the sixth child. Treatment procedures included non-graduated extinction for the four whose behavior was maintained by attention or positive reinforcement, while a stimulus fading procedure with differential reinforcement was introduced for the fifth child. The sixth child was subsequently diagnosed with, and treated for, a seizure disorder during baseline. Following stabilization of the seizure disorder non-graduated extinction was used. All children exposed to the extinction procedure showed significant reductions of nighttime disruptive behavior, with two children achieving zero rates between 20 and 30 days, three showing a much reduced but more variable response rate (in all cases with decreases of at least 50%). The child diagnosed with a seizure disorder experienced a decrease in disruptive behavior following psychopharmacologic intervention, but no additional effect with the use of extinction. Finally, when the stimulus fading with differential reinforcement procedure was implemented with the sixth child, he successfully completed all steps in the procedure by the 24th night and was able to sleep alone in his bed throughout the night without disruptive behavior. With the exception of the child with a seizure disorder, all participants maintained appropriate behavior at 3-month follow-up.

Graduated extinction has also been used to treat sleep problems. This variant involves putting a child to bed and following a gradual extinction routine systematically. For example, contingent upon the disruptive behavior a parent might ignore the behavior for a pre-set interval (e.g., 5 min) initially. If the problem behavior continues at that interval juncture the parent would enter the room and neutrally re-settle the child, providing as little attention as possible. Intervals are then systematically increased over time, for example from 5, to 10, to 15 min before re-entering the room. Adams and Rickert (1989) evaluated the effects of using positive routines and graduated extinction on 36 young typically developing children who exhibited tantrums at bedtime. Children were assigned to one of three groups: positive routines, graduated extinction, and a control group. Positive routines and extinction were significantly more effective than a no treatment control condition, with the more rapid decrease in tantrums evident after implementation in those children assigned to the positive routine group. By follow-up, these differences

between positive routines and extinction groups had evaporated. Those in the control group showed little change. Reid et al. (1999) also investigated the effect of nongraduated extinction, graduated extinction, and no treatment (a wait-list control group) on decreasing bedtime behavior problems (i.e., extensive time to settle into sleep or night waking requiring co-sleeping by a parent, for at least four nights per week) with 49 typically developing children. Their results are consistent with those of Adams and Rickert (1989), confirming that both types of extinction procedure were effective in quickly reducing bedtime behavior problems, with results maintaining at a 2-month follow-up.

In the only study evaluating the use of graduated extinction to reduce night waking and bedtime disturbances with children with autism and other neurodevelopmental disorders, Durand et al. (1996) used a multiple-baseline design to assess the effects of treatment procedures. Both graduated extinction and development of consistent bedtime routines were included. For the two children with intellectual disability secondary to identified chromosomal abnormalities the treatment procedure successfully reduced night waking by at least half of baseline rates, maintaining at follow-up. Bedtime behavioral disturbances were targeted in the two children with autism, including property destruction, tantrumming, screaming, and self-injury. Graduated extinction for the first child involved increasing increments 3 min initially, then 2 min each night on subsequent evenings. For the second child, a wait time of 5 min was initially selected, followed by 5-min increases on subsequent nights. Following implementation of the treatment procedure, behavior occurrences decreased in one child from a baseline of 100% to a mean of 22.3% of nights per week and in the other child from a mean of 65.1% per week to 22.3% per week. While preliminary and in need of replication, these results are a promising extension of the well-established efficacy of graduated extinction in typically developing children.

Extinction involves the removal of the reinforcing stimulus contingent upon the problem behavior and, as such, can generate characteristic immediate increases in problem behavior after initial implementation of the procedure. This temporary increase in the behavior (typically referred to as an extinction burst) can be difficult for parents to confront, sometimes compromising treatment integrity. Alternatives to the use of extinction procedures designed to alter sleep onset patterns have been investigated, including sleep restriction procedures and bedtime scheduling. Durand and Christodulu (2004) evaluated the effectiveness of sleep restriction procedures on reducing night waking and bedtime problem behavior with two 4-year-old children, one with autism and one with developmental delays. While sleep restriction strategies have been reported previously for use with older patients (Lichstein and Morin 2000) and with typical children (Spielman et al. 1987), use of these procedures to treat children with autism and related developmental disabilities has been underrepresented. The two children in this study displayed a range of bedtime disruptions including tantrums, delayed onset of sleep unless accompanied by a parent, and night waking culminating in co-sleeping. Assessment included completion of several sleep problem questionnaires, as well as a sleep diary identifying sleep schedule, night waking, behavior problems experienced, frequency and duration of naps, etc.

Durand and Christodulu (2004) provide a detailed description of this procedure. Sleep restriction procedures involved limiting the child's time in bed to 90% of the total time the child slept each night, derived from the data in the sleep diary. The sleep schedule was then reduced by altering either the child's bedtime or time awakened in the morning. If bedtime alterations were made and the child remained awake when taken to bed, she was removed and allowed to engage in a relaxing activity until she appeared tired. Elimination or significant reductions in bedtime problem behavior over the course of 1 week led to an increase in bedtime by 15 min. For example, for the child with autism in this study baseline hours slept per night averaged 8.75 h. Her sleep restriction schedule duration was set at 7 h per night, with bedtime moved to midnight with awakening at 7 a.m. Bedtime was then systematically faded back to a more typical hour as she progressed. Results indicate that while bedtime disturbances were not evident in the child with autism during baseline (due to the use of melatonin throughout baseline), when melatonin was discontinued following introduction of the sleep restriction schedule, behavior problems remained at low levels. For this child, night waking also decreased significantly from a mean of 7.17 per week to 1.4 per week. For the second child, bedtime problems occurred nightly, but after intervention reduced to an average of .25 per week. Duration of these problems decreased from 1.05 h per week to .01 h per week. Finally, night waking decreased from an average of 2.55 per week to 1.38 per week, with duration dropping to .07 h per week from a baseline of .14 h per week. Parent satisfaction measures were consistent with these treatment successes.

In a related study Christodulu and Durand (2004) again investigated sleep restriction but also incorporated positive routines into the intervention package. Consistent with earlier reports, positive routines included a series of relaxing activities followed consistently that presumably would help the child transition more successfully into sleep (e.g., reading a story, taking a bath). Four children participated, two of whom were diagnosed with an autism spectrum disorder. Several dependent measures were investigated across a multiple-baseline design, including number of bedtime disturbances, number of nighttime awakenings, total sleep time, and parent satisfaction. Results indicate that all children experienced fewer bedtime disturbances from baseline to intervention, with three of the four demonstrating a significant reduction in nighttime awakenings. Sleep restriction and positive routines was more effective in 75% of the children, including both diagnosed with an autism spectrum disorder. Three of the four children also experienced a decrease in total sleep time (including both of those with autism), while the fourth child showed no change from baseline. All results maintained at 40- and 42-week follow-up. All parents reported greater satisfaction with their child's sleep habits following intervention.

Bedtime scheduling has also been used to eliminate sleep difficulties in children with developmental disabilities. Bedtime scheduling involves creating an established time and routine for bedtime, scheduling naps as appropriate daily, and having a set wake-up time in the morning. The key element in this intervention strategy is consistency and the provision of a series of stimulus cues that predict upcoming steps in the schedule. In an early study with typical infants and young children, Rickert and Johnson (1988) compared extinction and bedtime scheduling in the treatment of night waking and crying in 33 young typically developing children (mean age 20 months), randomly assigned to one of three groups: scheduled awakenings, systematic ignoring, or control. Scheduled awakenings involved waking the child at times during the evening preceding when the child normally would have awakened the parents. During this awakening interval, the parent would engage in whatever activity would have occurred if the child had awakened them (e.g., soothe or feed the child). The child would then be returned to bed. Their results indicate that while systematic ignoring was more effective than scheduled awakenings during the first week of treatment, both procedures were equally effective subsequently, and both were more effective in reducing night waking and tantrums than no treatment controls. Results maintained at follow-up at 3 and 6 weeks post-treatment. The response effort differs in some ways for these two procedures: in one case the parent must commit to allowing the child to "cry it out", while in the other case the parent must commit to waking the child from a sleep state. As importantly, the social invalidity of the extinction procedure for some parents may preclude their being able to implement the strategy successfully. Rickert and Johnson's findings suggest that viable alternatives exist with typically developing toddlers.

In an extension of these findings, Durand (2002) treated three children with autism who experienced chronic night terrors with a scheduled awakening procedure. Parents were initially instructed to keep detailed sleep records, identifying the time and duration of their child's night terrors. Scheduled awakenings consisted of waking the child 30 min prior to the time that night terrors typically occurred, in an effort to interrupt Stage 3 and 4 non-REM sleep (when sleep terrors are most likely to occur), and then allow the child to fall back to sleep. This was to be done nightly until seven nights with no sleep terrors was achieved, at which time parents were instructed to skip one scheduled awakening each week, adding one skipped night per week as long as night terrors remained at zero. If an episode occurred, the parents were instructed to return to the nightly schedule and begin the schedule anew. Results indicate that all children reduced their weekly number of night terrors significantly from baseline (a mean of 7 for child one, 3 for child two, and 2.5 per week for child three) to less than .1 per week after implementation of the procedure. The mean number of weeks needed to achieve treatment criterion and discontinue the scheduled awakenings was 5.7. All children maintained at zero night terrors at 12-month follow-up.

Piazza and Fisher (1991) investigated the effect of faded bedtimes on the disruptive behavior of two children, one with ADHD and one with tuberous sclerosis. Bedtime fading involves setting a bedtime when the child is likely to fall asleep and then gradually moving this earlier to a more acceptable and developmentally normal bedtime as the child demonstrates rapid sleep onset. Both children showed significant improvement in targeted responses following treatment, both in the increase of percentage of appropriate sleep time or onset and also a reduction in inappropriate sleep. While not specifically discussed by the authors, it is possible that the fading procedure served as a motivating operation for sleep onset, enhancing its efficacy and stability. Piazza et al. (1997) extended this work to 14 children with developmental disabilities, five of whom had an autism spectrum diagnosis, all exhibiting delayed sleep onset, night waking, or early waking. Bedtime scheduling was compared with a faded bedtime with response cost procedure. The response cost procedure added in this study involved removing the child from bed if sleep onset had not occurred within 15 min of the prescribed time and keeping the child awake for 1 h before returning to bed. Bedtime scheduling involved having the child go to bed and awaken at the same time each morning. Results indicate that bedtime fading, both with and without response cost, was successful in reducing all sleep problems and superior to bedtime scheduling. Two of three children with an autism spectrum disorder enrolled in the bedtime fading with response cost procedure successfully eliminated sleep concerns. Of the two children with autism spectrum disorders in the bedtime scheduling group, one showed minor improvements in sleep onset and a somewhat less successful response to reducing night waking. The other child showed no difference from baseline in either early waking or night waking. These results lend support for the use of bedtime fading with or without response cost over the use of bedtime scheduling alone to treat sleep problems in children with autism spectrum disorders.

The incorporation of bedtime routines into treatment protocols is typical in studies of sleep problems in autism. For example, Durand et al. (1996), Christodulu and Durand (2004), and Adams and Rickert (1989) all incorporated a specific schedule of predictable activities to be accomplished as part of the bedtime ritual into their intervention protocols. While only one study specifically evaluated the effectiveness of predictable routines (Christodulu and Durand 2004) in the treatment of bedtime problems in children with autism, these authors found that routines alone were not as successful as routines combined with another procedure, in their case, sleep restriction. Milan et al. (1981) compared enforced bedtimes (essentially escape extinction), following a "natural sleep baseline" (allowing the child to fall asleep on his or her own and subsequently placing the child in bed asleep), with the use of positive routines (essentially a set of predictable pre-retirement bedtime steps that are chained together and then systematically faded) to treat the behavior problems of three children with significant bedtime disruptions and developmental disabilities (but not autism). Results supported the efficacy of positive routines over escape extinction (i.e., enforced bedtimes) in reducing behavioral episodes associated with a required bedtime that is not preceded by a routine schedule.

One study reporting the effect of what is essentially a stimulus fading procedure is reported in the literature. Howlin (1984) discusses the effect of gradually moving the parent of a 6-year-old with autism away from the child, who had become accustomed to his mother remaining with him to support sleep onset. The mother was proximally faded over time, from the child's bed, to an air mattress, to outside the child's door, and finally to the mother's room. While the child successfully learned to initiate sleep onset independently, periodic behavior problems associated with bedtime remained at follow-up. While the use of stimulus fading procedures has intuitive appeal and is likely incorporated into components of behavioral treatment protocols on a regular basis, it remains to be demonstrated whether this strategy is efficacious alone, or only in combination with other strategies.

While the literature on the behavioral treatment of sleep problems in those with autism spectrum disorders has been relatively sparse, there are several important implications for treatment derived from those that do exist. Moreover, given the structural nature of treatment of sleep and bedtime behavior problems in those with neurodevelopmental disorders, it appears imprudent to ignore the research addressing these problems in children with other significant developmental disabilities simply because the study sample does not include individuals with autism. As such, in proposing the following guidelines, we emphasize evidence-based procedures derived from the literature on autism, while also incorporating support from the treatment literature for children with other severe developmental disabilities Table 4.5.

TABLE 4.5   Practice parameters for the treatment of sleep problems for children with ASD

1. The use of non-graduated extinction procedures enjoys considerable empirical support in treatment literature, and should be considered an *established evidence-based procedure.*

2. Non-graduated extinction procedures appear to be most efficient and effective when combined with differential reinforcement strategies. This conclusion is consistent with the use of attention extinction and escape extinction for other behavior problems encountered by individuals with ASD.

3. Graduated extinction appears to be effective in many cases, but does not enjoy the level of replication as the more traditional procedure. The use of graduated extinction can be considered as *probably efficacious,* for sleep problems maintained by positive reinforcement in the form of social attention. It remains to be demonstrated whether empirical support exists for sleep problems maintained by positive reinforcement in the form of tangibles.

4. The use of bedtime routines (including positive routines) and bedtime scheduling have demonstrated efficacy, but in a smaller number of studies and with a smaller number of individual cases. Nonetheless, these procedures are often part of the intervention package crafted to respond to the individual needs of the child with autism and related disorders. As such, while they should be deemed *probably efficacious* there is a sufficient basis to consider including them in an individually-tailored treatment plan if the assessment data so dictate.

5. Sleep restriction procedures show promise, especially when combined with other procedures such as positive routines. At this time, however, there does not exist a sufficient empirical basis for widespread use of this strategy as an evidence-based procedure, and sleep restriction should more appropriately be considered *possibly efficacious* in reducing night waking and bedtime behavior problems.

6. Parent education in sleep hygiene and in the implementation of treatment procedures is an almost ubiquitous component of intervention, but the extent to which it has been formally evaluated is surprising small. With an understanding that data do not exist to conclusively include this procedure as an evidence-based procedure, successful implementation by parents of treatment procedures is well documented in other domains of need within autism and in other areas of child development. As such, it is at once appropriate to highlight the need for more substantial research in this area, but also to suggest that parent education and training should be incorporated into treatment protocols, minimally for purposes of supporting generalization and maintenance of gains achieved in more highly-controlled intervention settings.

7. The use of stimulus fading deserves greater research efforts, but our current understanding of the conditions of its use, and its comparative value in the treatment armamentarium remains to be determined with respect to the treatment of sleep problems for children with ASD.

Other Evidence-Based Practices for Treating Problem Behavior in Individuals with Autism Spectrum Disorders

While the task of providing a comprehensive review of all evidence-based procedures for assessing and treating problem behavior in autism is clearly well beyond the scope of this chapter, we would highlight several particular strategies that enjoy a very well-established empirical foundation in general, but also specifically with respect to those with autism spectrum disorders. Each should be defined as an evidence-based practice, subject to appropriate use determined by a comprehensive assessment, including functional assessment or analysis. Positive reinforcement and related differential reinforcement variant (Cooper et al. 2007), negative reinforcement (Iwata 1987), extinction, including escape extinction, attention extinction, and sensory extinction (Lerman and Iwata 1996), generalization and maintenance procedures (Horner et al. 1988), treatment of feeding problems (Ledford and Gast 2006; Kodak and Piazza 2008), treatment of enuresis (Houts 2003), treatment of self-injury (Rojahn et al. 2009; Matson and LoVullo 2008), and the treatment of pica (McAdam et al. 2004) have all been addressed comprehensively in the literature, with clearly articulated practice parameters. The interested reader is encouraged to consult these resources as necessary and appropriate.

Conclusion

In this chapter, we have reviewed a subset of assessment and treatment strategies which, used individually or in combination, constitute effective and evidence-based practices for treating problem behavior in those with autism spectrum disorders. While we necessarily cannot be comprehensive in reviewing all effective practices, we have attempted to review several noteworthy procedures in depth, offering suggestions for practice parameters as the evidence dictates. As we noted at the beginning of this chapter, data-driven decision-making is the foundation of effective intervention. With careful attention to treatment integrity, client assets, needs, and characteristics, and the social and environmental context upon which we layer intervention, we increase exponentially the likelihood of successful outcomes. In the final analysis, however, two points matter most. The practice of reducing or eliminating problem behavior must be reconceptualized as the practice of teaching replacement behaviors that are at once adaptive, prosocial, functionally equivalent, and socially valid. The second point allows us to come full circle and remember our roots: To paraphrase Skinner, the learner is always right. If an individual with an autism spectrum disorder is not learning a skill or behavior that we seek to develop, then we are not learning from them and we are not modifying our instructional tactics to their needs effectively. That due diligence is both the clinician's mandate and the clinician's responsibility.

References

Adams, L. A., & Rickert, V. I. (1989). Reducing bedtime tantrums: Comparison between positive routines and graduated extinction. *Pediatrics, 84*, 756–759.

Asmus, J. M., Vollmer, T. R., & Borrero, J. C. (2002). Functional behavioral assessment: A school-based model. *Education and Treatment of Children, 25*, 67–90.

Ayllon, T., & Michael, J. (1959). The psychiatric nurse as a behavioral engineer. *Journal of the Experimental Analysis of Behavior, 2,* 323–334.

Baer, D. M., Wolf, M. M., & Risley, T. R. (1968). Some current dimensions of applied behavior analysis. *Journal of Applied Behavior Analysis, 1,* 91–97.

Bambara, L. M., & Kern, L. (2005). *Individualized supports for students with problem behaviors: Designing positive behavior plans.* New York: Guilford Press.

Bijou, S. W. (1957). Patterns of reinforcement and resistance to extinction in young children. *Child Development, 28,* 47–54.

Bramble, D. (1997). Rapid-acting treatment for a common sleep problem. *Developmental Medicine and Child Neurology, 39,* 543–547.

Britton, L. M., Carr, J. E., Kellum, K. K., Dozier, C. L., & Weil, T. M. (2000). A variation of noncontingent reinforcement in the treatment of aberrant behavior. *Research in Developmental Disabilities, 21,* 425–435.

Britton, L. N., Carr, J. E., Landaburu, H. J., & Romick, K. S. (2002). The efficacy of noncontingent reinforcement as treatment for automatically reinforced stereotypy. *Behavioral Interventions, 17,* 93–103.

Bullock, C., & Normand, M. P. (2006). The effects of a high-probability instruction sequence and response-independent reinforce delivery on child compliance. *Journal of Applied Behavior Analysis, 39,* 495–499.

Carr, E. G. (1977). The motivation of self-injurious behavior: A review of some hypotheses. *Psychological Bulletin, 84,* 800–816.

Carr, E. G. (1988). Functional equivalence as a mechanism of response generalization. In R. Horner, R. Koegel, & G. Dunlap (Eds.), *Generalization and maintenance: Life-style changes in applied settings* (pp. 221–241). Baltimore: Paul Brookes.

Carr, E. G., & Durand, M. V. (1985). Reducing behavior problems through functional communication training. *Journal of Applied Behavior Analysis, 18,* 111–126.

Carr, E. G., Yarbrough, S. C., & Langdon, N. A. (1997). Effects of idiosyncratic stimulus variables on functional analysis outcomes. *Journal of Applied Behavior Analysis, 30,* 673–686.

Carr, J. E., Severtson, J. M., & Lepper, T. L. (2009). Noncontingent reinforcement is an empirically supported treatment for problem behavior exhibited by individuals with developmental disabilities. *Research in Developmental Disabilities, 30,* 44–57.

Christodulu, K. V., & Durand, V. M. (2004). Reducing bedtime disturbance and night waking using positive bedtime routines and sleep restriction. *Focus on Autism and Other Developmental Disabilities, 19,* 130–139.

Cihak, D., Alberto, P. A., & Fredrick, L. D. (2007). Use of brief functional analysis and intervention evaluation in public settings. *Journal of Positive Behavior Interventions, 9,* 80–93.

Cooper, L. J., & Harding, J. (1993). Extending functional analysis procedures to outpatient and classroom settings for children with mild disabilities. In J. Reichle & D. P. Wacker (Eds.), *Communicative alternatives to challenging behavior: Integrating functional assessment and intervention strategies* (Communication and Language Series, Vol. 3, pp. 41–62). Baltimore: Paul Brookes.

Cooper, L. J., Wacker, D. P., Sasso, G. M., Reimers, T. M., & Donn, L. K. (1990). Using parents as therapists to evaluate appropriate behavior of their children: Application to a tertiary diagnostic clinic. *Journal of Applied Behavior Analysis, 23,* 285–296.

Cooper, L. J., Wacker, D. P., Thursby, D., Plagmann, L. A., Harding, J., Millard, T., et al. (1992). Analysis of the effects of task preferences, task demands, and adult attention on child behavior in outpatient and classroom settings. *Journal of Applied Behavior Analysis, 25,* 823–840.

Cooper, J. O., Heron, T. E., & Heward, W. L. (2007). *Applied behavior analysis* (2nd ed.). Upper Saddle River, NJ: Prentice Hall.

Davis, C. A., & Reichle, J. (1996). Variant and invariant high-probability requests: Increasing appropriate behavior in children with emotional-behavioral disorders. *Journal of Applied Behavior Analysis, 29,* 471–482.

Davis, C. A., Brady, M. P., Hamilton, R., McEvoy, M. A., & Williams, R. E. (1994). Effects of high-probability requests on social interactions of young children with severe disabilities. *Journal of Applied Behavior Analysis, 27,* 619–637.

Davis, C. A., Brady, M. P., Williams, R. E., & Hamilton, R. (1992). Effects of high-probability requests on the acquisition and generalization of responses to requests in young children with behavior disorders. *Journal of Applied Behavior Analysis, 25,* 905–916

DeLeon, I. G., Anders, B. M., Rodriguez-Catter, V., & Neider, P. L. (2000). The effects of noncontingent access to single-versus multiple-stimulus sets on self-injurious behavior. *Journal of Applied Behavior Analysis, 33,* 623–626.

Derby, K. M., Wacker, D. P., Sasso, G., Steege, M., Northup, J., et al. (1992). Brief functional assessment techniques to evaluate aberrant behavior in an outpatient setting: A summary of 79 cases. *Journal of Applied Behavior Analysis, 25*, 713–721.

Derby, K. M., Wacker, D. P., Peck, S., Sasso, G., DeRaad, A., et al. (1994). Functional analysis of separate topographies of aberrant behavior. *Journal of Applied Behavior Analysis, 27*, 267–278.

Didden, R., Curfs, L. M. G., Sikkema, S. P. E., & de Moor, J. (1998). Functional assessment and treatment of sleeping problems with developmentally disabled children: Six case studies. *Journal of Behavior Therapy and Experimental Psychiatry, 29*, 85–97.

Doggett, R. A., Edwards, R. P., Moore, J. W., Tingstrom, D. H., & Wilczynski, S. M. (2001). An approach to functional assessment in general education classroom settings. *School Psychology Review, 30*, 313–328.

Ducharme, J. M., & Worling, D. E. (1994). Behavioral momentum and stimulus fading in the acquisition and maintenance of child compliance in the home. *Journal of Applied Behavior Analysis, 27*, 639–647.

Durand, V. M. (2002). Treating sleep terrors in children with autism. *Journal of Positive Behavioral Interventions, 4*, 66–72.

Durand, V. M., & Christodulu, K. V. (2004). Description of a sleep-restriction program to reduce bedtime disturbances and night waking. *Journal of Positive Behavior Interventions, 6*, 83–91.

Durand, V. M., Crimmins, D., Caulfield, M., & Taylor, J. (1989). Reinforcer assessment I: Using problem behavior to select reinforcers. *Journal of the Association for Persons with Severe Handicaps, 14*, 113–126.

Durand, V. M., Gernert-Dott, P., & Mapstone, E. (1996). Treatment of sleep disorders in children with developmental disabilities. *Journal of the Association for Persons with Severe Handicaps, 21*, 114–122.

Fisher, W. W., Ninnes, H. A., Piazza, C. C., & Owen-DeSchryver, J. S. (1996). On the reinforcing effects of the content of verbal attention. *Journal of Applied Behavior Analysis, 29*, 235–238.

Fisher, W. W., Kuhn, D. E., & Thompson, R. H. (1998). Establishing discriminative control of responding using functional and alternative reinforcers during functional communication training. *Journal of Applied Behavior Analysis, 31*, 543–560.

Fisher, W. W., O'Connor, J. T., Kurtz, P. F., DeLeon, I. G., & Gotjen, D. L. (2000). The effects of noncontingent delivery of high and low-preference stimuli on attention-maintained destructive behavior. *Journal of Applied Behavior Analysis, 33*, 79–83.

Fisher, W. W., DeLeon, I. G., Rodriguez-Catter, V., & Keeny, K. M. (2004). Enhancing the effects of extinction on attention-maintained behavior through noncontingent delivery of attention on stimuli identified via a competing stimulus assessment. *Journal of Applied Behavior Analysis, 37*, 171–184.

Fuller, P. R. (1949). Operant conditioning of a vegetative organism. *The American Journal of Psychology, 62*, 587–590.

Hagopian, L. P., Fisher, W. W., & Legacy, S. M. (1994). Schedule effects of noncontingent reinforcement on attention-maintained destructive behavior in identical quadruplets. *Journal of Applied Behavior Analysis, 27*, 317–325.

Hagopian, L. P., Fisher, W. W., Sullivan, M. T., Acquisto, J., & LeBlanc, L. A. (1998). Effectiveness of functional communication training with and without extinction and punishment: A summary of 21 inpatient cases. *Journal of Applied Behavior Analysis, 31*, 211–235.

Hagopian, L. P., Contrucci-Kuhn, S. A., Long, E. S., & Rush, K. S. (2005). Schedule thinning following communication training: Using competing stimuli to enhance tolerance to decrements in reinforce density. *Journal of Applied Behavior Analysis, 38*, 177–193.

Hanley, G. P., Piazza, C. C., & Fisher, W. W. (1997). Noncontingent presentation of attention and alternative stimuli in the treatment of attention-maintained destructive behavior. *Journal of Applied Behavior Analysis, 30*, 229–237.

Hanley, G. P., Iwata, B. A., & Thompson, R. H. (2001). Reinforcement schedule thinning following treatment with functional communication training. *Journal of Applied Behavior Analysis, 34*, 17–38.

Hanley, G. P., Iwata, B. A., & McCord, B. E. (2003). Functional analysis of problem behavior: A review. *Journal of Applied Behavior Analysis, 36*, 147–185.

Harchik, A., & Putzier, V. (1990). The use of high-probability requests to increase compliance with instructions to take medication. *Journal of the Association for Persons with Severe Handicaps, 15*, 40–43.

Harding, J., Wacker, D. P., Cooper, L. J., Millard, T., & Jensen-Kovalan, P. (1994). Brief hierarchical assessment of potential treatment components with children in an outpatient clinic. *Journal of Applied Behavior Analysis, 27*, 291–300.

Herzinger, C. V., & Campbell, J. M. (2007). Comparing functional assessment methodologies: A quantitative synthesis. *Journal of Autism and Developmental Disorders, 37*, 1430–1445.

Honomichl, R. D., Goodlin-Jones, B. L., Burnham, M., Gaylord, E., & Anders, T. F. (2002).

Sleep patterns of children with pervasive developmental disorders. *Journal of Autism and Developmental Disorders, 32,* 553–561.

Horner, R. H., Dunlap, G., & Koegel, R. L. (1988). *Generalization and maintenance: Lifestyle changes in applied settings.* Baltimore: Paul Brookes.

Horner, R. H., Day, H. M., Sprague, J. R., O'Brien, M., & Heathfield, L. T. (1991). Interspersed requests: A nonaversive procedure for reducing aggression and self-injury during instruction. *Journal of Applied Behavior Analysis, 24,* 265–278.

Horner, R. H., Carr, E. G., Halle, J., McGee, G., Odom, S., & Wolery, M. (2005). The use of single subject research to identify evidence-based practice in special education. *Exceptional Children, 71,* 165–179.

Houts, A. C. (2003). Behavioral treatment for enuresis. In A. E. Kazdin & J. R. Weisz (Eds.), *Evidence-based psychotherapies for children and adolescents* (pp. 389–406). New York: Guilford.

Howlin, P. (1984). A brief report on the elimination of long-term sleeping problems in a six-year-old autistic boy. *Behavioural Psychotherapy, 12,* 257–260.

Ingvarsson, E. T., Kahng, S., & Hausman, N. L. (2008). Some effects of noncontingent positive reinforcement on multiply controlled problem behavior and compliance in a demand context. *Journal of Applied Behavior Analysis, 41,* 435–440.

Iwata, B. A. (1987). Negative reinforcement in applied behavior analysis: An emerging technology. *Journal of Applied Behavior Analysis, 20,* 361–378.

Iwata, B. A., Pace, G. M., Willis, K. D., Gamache, T. B., & Hyman, S. L. (1986). Operant studies of self-injurious hand-biting in the Rett syndrome. *American Journal of Medical Genetics, 24,* 157–166.

Iwata, B. A., Pace, G. M., Kalsher, M. J., Cowdery, G. E., & Cataldo, M. F. (1990). Experimental analysis and extinction of self-injurious escape behavior. *Journal of Applied Behavior Analysis, 23,* 11–27.

Iwata, B. A., Dorsey, M. F., Slifer, K. J., Bauman, K. E., & Richman, G. S. (1994). Toward a functional analysis of self-injury. *Journal of Applied Behavior Analysis, 27,* 197–209. Reprinted from *Analysis and Intervention in Developmental Disabilities* (1982), 2:3–20.

Iwata, B. A., Pace, G. M., Dorsey, M. F., Zarcone, J. R., Vollmer, T. R., & Smith, R. G. (1994b). The functions of self-injurious behavior: An experimental-epidemiological analysis. *Journal of Applied Behavior Analysis, 27,* 215–240.

Iwata, B. A., Wallace, M. D., Kahng, S., Lindberg, J. S., Roscoe, E. M., Conners, J., et al. (2000).

Skill acquisition in the implementation of functional analysis methodology. *Journal of Applied Behavior Analysis, 33,* 181–194.

Johnston, S. S., & O'Neill, R. E. (2001). Searching for effectiveness and efficiency in conducting functional assessments: A review and proposed process for teachers and other practitioners. *Focus on Autism and Other Developmental Disabilities, 16,* 205–214.

Kahng, S. W., Iwata, B. A., DeLeon, I. G., & Wallace, M. D. (2000a). A comparison of procedures for programming noncontingent reinforcement schedules. *Journal of Applied Behavior Analysis, 33,* 223–231.

Kahng, S. W., Iwata, B. A., Thompson, R. H., & Hanley, G. P. (2000b). A method for identifying satiation versus extinction effects under noncontingent reinforcement schedules. *Journal of Applied Behavior Analysis, 33,* 419–432.

Kazdin, A. E. (1982). *Single-case research designs: Methods for clinical and applied settings.* Boston: Allyn & Bacon.

Kennedy, C. H., Itkonen, T., & Lindquist, K. (1995). Comparing interspersed requests and social comments as antecedents for increasing student compliance. *Journal of Applied Behavior Analysis, 28,* 97–98.

Klin, A., Lin, D. J., Gorrindo, P., Ramsay, G., & Jones, W. (2009). Two-year-olds with autism fail to orient towards human biological motion but attend instead to non-social, physical contingencies. *Nature, 459,* 257–261.

Kodak, T., & Piazza, C. C. (2008). Assessment and behavioral treatment of feeding and sleep disorders in children with autism spectrum disorders. *Child and Adolescent Psychiatric Clinics of North America, 17,* 887–905.

Kodak, T., Miltenberger, R. G., & Romaniuk, C. (2003). The effect of differential negative reinforcement of other behavior and noncontingent escape on compliance. *Journal of Applied Behavior Analysis, 36,* 379–382.

Kurtz, P. F., Chin, M. D., Huete, J. M., Tarbox, R., O'Connor, J. T., Paclawsky, T. R., et al. (2003). Functional analysis and treatment of self-injurious behavior in young children: A summary of 30 cases. *Journal of Applied Behavior Analysis, 36,* 205–219.

LaBelle, C. A., & Charlop-Christy, M. (2002). Individualizing functional analysis to assess multiple and changing functions of severe behavior problems in children with autism. *Journal of Positive Behavior Interventions, 4,* 231–241.

Lalli, J. S., Vollmer, T. R., Progar, P. R., Wright, C. A., Borrero, J., et al. (1999). Competition between positive and negative reinforcement

90   M.D. POWERS ET AL.

in the treatment of escape behavior. *Journal of Applied Behavior Analysis, 32,* 285–296.

Ledford, J. R., & Gast, D. L. (2006). Feeding problems in children with autism spectrum disorders: A review. *Focus on Autism and other Developmental Disabilities, 21,* 153–166.

Lerman, D. C., & Iwata, B. A. (1996). Developing a technology for the use of operant extinction in clinical settings: An examination of basic and applied research. *Journal of Applied Behavior Analysis, 29,* 345–382.

Lichstein, K. L., & Morin, C. M. (Eds.). (2000). *Treatment of late-life insomnia.* Thousand Oaks, CA: Sage.

Linscheid, T. R. (2006). Behavioral treatments for pediatric feeding disorders. *Behavior Modification, 30,* 6–23.

Liu, X., Hubbard, J. A., Fabes, R. A., & Adams, J. B. (2006). Sleep disturbances and correlates of children with autism spectrum disorders. *Child Psychiatry and Human Development, 37,* 179–191.

Lohrmann-O'Rourke, S., & Yurman, B. (2001). Naturalistic assessment of and intervention for mouthing behaviors influenced by establishing operations. *Journal of Positive Behavior Interventions, 3,* 19–27.

Lopez-Wagner, M. C., Hoffman, C. D., Sweeney, D. P., & Gilliam, J. E. (2008). Sleep problems of parents of typically developing children and parents of children with autism. *The Journal of Genetic Psychology, 169,* 245–259.

Lovaas, I., & Simmons, J. Q. (1969). Manipulation of self-destruction in three retarded children. *Journal of Applied Behavior Analysis, 2,* 143–157.

Luiselli, J. K., & Cameron, M. J. (1998). *Antecedent Control: Innovative approaches to behavioral support.* Baltimore: Paul Brookes.

Mace, F. C. (1996). In pursuit of general behavioral relations. *Journal of Applied Behavior Analysis, 29,* 557–563.

Mace, F. C., & Belfiore, P. (1990). Behavioral momentum in the treatment of escape-motivated stereotypy. *Journal of Applied Behavior Analysis, 23,* 507–514.

Mace, F. C., Hock, H. L., Lalli, J. S., West, B. J., Belfiore, P., et al. (1988). Behavioral momentum in the treatment of noncompliance. *Journal of Applied Behavior Analysis, 21,* 123–141.

Mace, F. C., Mauro, B. C., Boyajian, A. E., & Eckert, T. L. (1997). Effects of reinforcer quality on behavioral momentum: Coordinated applied and basic research. *Journal of Applied Behavior Analysis, 30,* 1–20.

Malow, B. A., & McGrew, S. G. (2008). Sleep disturbances and autism. *Sleep Medicine Clinics, 3,* 479–488.

Malow, B. A., Marzec, M. L., McGrew, S. G., Wang, L., Henderson, L., et al. (2006a). Characterizing sleep in children with autism spectrum disorders: A multidimensional approach. *Sleep, 29,* 1563–1571.

Malow, B. A., McGrew, S. G., Harvey, M., Henderson, L. M., & Stone, W. L. (2006b). Impact of treating sleep apnea in a child with autism spectrum disorder. *Pediatric Neurology, 34*(4), 325–8.

Marcus, B. A., & Vollmer, T. R. (1996). Combining noncontingent reinforcement and differential reinforcement schedules as treatment for aberrant behavior. *Journal of Applied Behavior Analysis, 29,* 43–51.

Matson, J. L., & LoVullo, S. V. (2008). A review of behavioral treatments of self-injurious behaviors in persons with autism spectrum disorders. *Behavior Modification, 32,* 61–76.

McAdam, D. B., Sherman, J. A., Sheldon, J. B., & Napolitano, D. A. (2004). Behavioral intervention to reduce pica of persons with developmental disabilities. *Behavior Modification, 28,* 45–72.

McDougall, A., Kerr, A. M., & Espie, C. A. (2005). Sleep disturbance in children with Rett Syndrome. *Journal of Applied Research in Intellectual Disabilities, 18,* 201–215.

Michael, J. (2004). *Concepts and principles of behavior analysis* (revisedth ed.). Kalamazoo, MI: Society for the Advancement of Behavior Analysis.

Milan, M. A., Mitchell, Z. P., Berger, M. I., & Pierson, D. F. (1981). Positive routines: A rapid alternative to extinction for the elimination of bedtime tantrum behavior. *Child Behavior Therapy, 3,* 13–24.

Miltenberger, R. G., Fuqua, R. W., & Woods, D. W. (1998). Applying behavior analysis to clinical problems: Review and analysis of habit reversal. *Journal of Applied Behavior Analysis, 31,* 447–469.

Mindell, J. A., Kuhn, B., Lewin, D. S., Meltzer, L. J., & Sadeh, A. (2006). Behavioral treatment of bedtime problems and night waking in infants and young children. *Sleep, 29,* 1263–1276.

Moore, J. W., Edwards, R. P., Sterling-Turner, H. E., Riley, J., DuBard, M., & McGeorge, A. (2002a). Teacher acquisition of functional analysis methodology. *Journal of Applied Behavior Analysis, 35,* 73–77.

Moore, J. W., Mueller, M. M., Dubard, D., Roberts, D. S., & Sterling-Turner, H. E. (2002b). The influence of therapist attention on self-injury during a tangible condition. *Journal of Applied Behavior Analysis, 35,* 283–286.

Mueller, M. M., Wilczynski, S. M., Moore, J. W., Fusilier, I., & Trahant, D. (2001). Antecedent manipulations in a tangible condition: Effects of stimulus preference on aggression. *Journal of Applied Behavior Analysis, 34*, 237–240.

Nevin, J. A. (1996). The momentum of compliance. *Journal of Applied Behavior Analysis, 29*, 535–547.

Northup, J., Wacker, D., Sasso, G., Steege, M., Cigrand, K., et al. (1991). A brief functional analysis of aggressive and alternative behavior in an outclinic setting. *Journal of Applied Behavior Analysis, 24*, 509–522.

Odom, S., Brown, W., Frey, T., Karasu, N., Smith-Cantor, L., & Strain, P. (2003). Evidence-based practice for young children with autism: Contributions of single subject research. *Focus on Autism and Other Developmental Disabilities, 10*, 166–175.

Owens, J. A. (2009). Sleep and sleep disorders in children. In W. Carey, A. C. Crocker, E. Elias, H. Feldman, & W. L. Coleman (Eds.), *Developmental-behavioral pediatrics* (4th ed. - text revision). Philadelphia: W. B. Saunders.

Paavonen, E. J., Vehkalahti, K., Vanhala, R., von Wendt, L., Niemenen-von Wendt, T., & Aronen, E. T. (2008). Sleep in children with Asperger syndrome. *Journal of Autism and Developmental Disorders, 38*, 41–51.

Patzold, L. M., Richdale, A. L., & Tonge, B. J. (1998). An investigation into the sleep characteristics of children with autism and Asperger's disorder. *Journal of Paediatrics and Child Health, 34*, 528–533.

Piazza, C. C., & Fisher, W. W. (1991). Bedtime fading in the treatment of pediatric insomnia. *Journal of Behavior Therapy and Experimental Psychiatry, 22*, 53–56.

Piazza, C. C., Fisher, W. W., & Scherer, M. (1997). Treatment of multiple sleep problems in children with developmental disabilities: Faded bedtime with response cost versus bedtime scheduling. *Developmental Medicine and Child Neurology, 39*, 414–418.

Powers, M. D. (1988). Behavioral assessment of autism. In E. Schopler & G. B. Mesibov (Eds.), *Diagnosis and assessment of autism* (pp. 139–165). New York: Plenum.

Powers, M. D. (2005). Behavioral assessment of individuals with autism: A functional ecological approach. In F. Volkmar, A. Klin, R. Paul, & D. Cohen (Eds.), *Handbook of autism and pervasive developmental disorders* (3rd ed., pp. 817–830). Hoboken, NJ: Wiley.

Quine, L. (2001). Sleep problems in primary school children: Comparison between mainstream and special school children. *Child: Care, Health and Development, 27*, 201–221.

Reid, M. J., Walter, A. L., & O'Leary, S. G. (1999). Treatment of young children's bedtime refusal and nighttime waking: A comparison of standard and graduated ignoring procedures. *Journal of Abnormal Child Psychology, 27*, 5–16.

Repp, A., Felce, D., & Barton, L. (1988). Basing the treatment of stereotypic and self-injurious behaviors on hypotheses of their causes. *Journal of Applied Behavior Analysis, 21*, 281–289.

Richdale, A. L., & Prior, M. R. (1995). The sleep/wake rhythm in children with autism. *European Journal of Child and Adolescent Psychiatry., 4*, 175–186.

Rickert, V. I., & Johnson, C. M. (1988). Reducing nocturnal awakening and crying episodes in infants and young children: A comparison between scheduled awakenings and systematic ignoring. *Pediatrics, 81*, 203–212.

Ringdahl, J. E., Vollmer, T. R., Borrero, J. C., & Connell, J. E. (2001). Fixed-time schedule effects as a function of baseline reinforcement rate. *Journal of Applied Behavior Analysis, 34*, 1–15.

Roane, H. S., Kelly, M. L., & Fisher, W. W. (2003). The effects of noncontingent access to food on the rate of object mouthing across three settings. *Journal of Applied Behavior Analysis, 36*, 579–582.

Rojahn, J., Schroeder, S. R., & Hoch, T. A. (2009). *Self-injurious behavior in intellectual disabilities.* New York: Elsevier.

Schreck, K. A. (2001). Behavioral treatments for sleep problems in autism: Empirically supported or just universally accepted? *Behavioral Interventions, 16*, 265–278.

Schreck, K. A., & Mulick, J. A. (2000). Parental report of sleep problems in children with autism. *Journal of Autism and Developmental Disorders, 30*, 127–135.

Schreck, K. A., Mulick, J. A., & Smith, A. F. (2004). Sleep problems as possible predictors of intensified symptoms of autism. *Research in Developmental Disabilities, 25*, 57–66.

Shirley, M. J., Iwata, B. A., & Kahng, S. (1999). False-positive maintenance of self-injurious behavior by access to tangible reinforcers. *Journal of Applied Behavior Analysis, 32*, 201–204.

Sigafoos, J., & Saggers, E. (1995). A discrete-trial approach to the functional analysis of aggressive behaviour in two boys with autism. *Australia and New Zealand Journal of Developmental Disabilities, 20*, 287–297.

Singer, G., Singer, J., & Horner, R. H. (1987). Using pretask requests to increase the probability of compliance for students with severe disabilities. *Journal of the Association for Persons with Severe Handicaps, 12*, 287–291.

Skinner, B. F. (1938). *The Behavior of Organisms.* New York: Appleton-Century-Crofts.

Skinner, B. F. (1953). *Science and Human Behavior.* New York: MacMillan.

Spielman, A. J., Caruso, L. S., & Glovinsky, P. B. (1987). A behavioral perspective on insomnia. *The Psychiatric Clinics of North America, 10,* 541–553.

Steege, M., Wacker, D., Berg, W., Cigrand, K., & Cooper, L. (1989). The use of behavioral assessment to prescribe and evaluate treatments for severely handicapped children. *Journal of Applied Behavior Analysis, 22,* 23–33.

Thackeray, E., & Richdale, A. (2002). The behavioural treatment of sleep difficulties in children with intellectual disability. *Behavioral Interventions, 17,* 211–231.

Umbreit, J. (1995). Functional assessment and intervention in a regular classroom setting for the disruptive behavior of a student with attention deficit hyperactivity disorder. *Behavioral Disorders, 20,* 267–278.

Van Camp, C. M., Lerman, D. C., Kelley, M. E., Contrucci, S. A., & Vorndran, C. M. (2000). Variable-time reinforcement schedules in the treatment of socially-maintained problem behavior. *Journal of Applied Behavior Analysis, 33,* 545–557.

Volkert, V. M., Lerman, D. C., Trosclair, N., Addison, L., & Kodak, T. (2008). An exploratory analysis of task-interspersal procedures while teaching object labels to children with autism. *Journal of Applied Behavior Analysis, 41,* 335–350.

Vollmer, T. R., Iwata, B. A., Zarcone, J. R., Smith, R. G., & Mazaleski, J. L. (1993). The role of attention in the treatment of attention-maintained self-injurious behavior: Noncontingent reinforcement and differential reinforcement of other behavior. *Journal of Applied Behavior Analysis, 26,* 9–21.

Vollmer, T. R., Ringdahl, J. E., Roane, H. S., & Marcus, B. A. (1997). Negative side effects of noncontingent reinforcement. *Journal of Applied Behavior Analysis, 30,* 161–164.

Wacker, D., Steege, M., Northrup, J., Sasso, G., Berg, W., et al. (1990). A component analysis of functional communication training across three response topographies of severe behavior problems. *Journal of Applied Behavior Analysis, 23,* 417–429.

Wacker, D. P., Harding, J. W., & Berg, W. K. (2008). Evaluation of mand-reinforcer relations following long-term functional communication training. *Journal of Speech Language Pathology and Applied Behavior Analysis, 24–31,* 25–35. doi:10:1901/japplied behavior analysis.2008.-25.

Wallace, M. D., & Iwata, B. A. (1999). Effects of session durations on functional analysis outcomes. *Journal of Applied Behavior Analysis, 32,* 175–183.

Weiskop, S., Matthews, J., & Richdale, A. (2001). Treatment of sleep problems in a 5-year-old boy with autism using behavioural principles. *Autism, 5*(2), 209–221.

Weiskop, S., Richdale, A., & Matthews, J. (2005). Behavioural treatment to reduce sleep problems in children with autism or Fragile-X syndrome. *Developmental Medicine and Child Neurology, 47,* 94–104.

Wiggs, L., & France, K. (2000). Behavioural treatments for sleep problems in children and adolescents with physical illness, psychological problems or intellectual disabilities. *Sleep Medicine Reviews, 4,* 299–314.

Wiggs, L., & Stores, G. (1996). Severe sleep disturbances and daytime challenging behavior in children with severe learning disabilities. *Journal of Intellectual Disability Research, 40,* 518–528.

Wilder, D. A., Normand, M., & Atwell, J. (2005). Noncontingent reinforcement as treatment for food refusal and associated self-injury. *Journal of Applied Behavior Analysis, 38,* 549–553.

Wilder, D. A., Zonneveld, K., Harris, C., Marcus, A., & Reagan, R. (2007). Further analysis of antecedent interventions on preschooler's compliance. *Journal of Applied Behavior Analysis, 40,* 535–539.

Wolf, M. M., Risley, T. R., & Mees, H. (1964). Application of operant conditioning procedures to the behavior problems of an autistic child. *Behaviour Research and Therapy, 1,* 305–312.

Zarcone, J. L., Iwata, B. A., Hughes, C. E., & Vollmer, T. R. (1993). Momentum versus extinction effects in the treatment of self-injurious escape behavior. *Journal of Applied Behavior Analysis, 26,* 135–136.

Zarcone, J. L., Iwata, B. A., Mazaleski, J. L., & Smith, R. G. (1994). Momentum and extinction effects on self-injurious escape behavior and noncompliance. *Journal of Applied Behavior Analysis, 27,* 649–658.

Zuluaga, C. A., & Normand, M. P. (2008). An evaluation of the high-probability instruction sequence with and without programmed reinforcement for compliance with high-probability instructions. *Journal of Applied Behavior Analysis, 41,* 453–457.

Evidence-Based Treatments in Communication for Children with Autism Spectrum Disorders

Patricia A. Prelock, Rhea Paul, and Elizabeth M. Allen

ABBREVIATIONS

ADHD	Attention deficit hyperactivity disorder
ASDs	Autism spectrum disorders
CBT	Cognitive behavioral therapy
CGI	Clinical global improvement
DSM-IV	Diagnostic and Statistical Manual of Mental Disorders 4th edition
NIMH	National Institutes of Mental Health
OCD	Obsessive–compulsive disorder
ODD	Oppositional defiant disorder
PCIT	Parent–child interaction therapy
RCT	Randomized control trial
RUPP	Research Units on Pediatric Psychopharmacology
SSED	Single subject experimental design

INTRODUCTION

This chapter considers treatments that aim to enhance the ability of children with autism spectrum disorders (ASD) to communicate and use language. Since disorders of communication constitute one of the core symptom areas in ASD and represent an aspect of function in which all children on this spectrum experience significant disability, virtually every child on the autism spectrum will require some form of communicative intervention. Moreover, communication is vital for learning and establishing connections with others, so that deficits in communication skill not only characterize the syndrome, but set limits on opportunities for play, socialization, academic achievement, and integration. Thus, interventions aimed at improving communication in ASD are crucial to success both in school programs and

B. Reichow et al. (eds.), *Evidence-Based Practices and Treatments for Children with Autism*,
DOI 10.1007/978-1-4419-6975-0_5, © Springer Science+Business Media, LLC 2011

functional, real-world adaptation. In considering interventions to improve communication and the evidence that supports them, we focus on three broad developmental periods:

1. The *prelinguistic communication* phase, which refers to that period in typical development from eight to 12–18 months, when children begin communicating intentionally, at first using means other than words
2. The *early language* phase, which spans the period between 12–18 and 24–36 months in typical development, during which children begin saying single words and combining them into simple multiword utterances
3. The *basic-to-advanced language* phase, which refers to the preschool and school-aged periods in typical development when children progress from early multi-word combinations through the acquisition of full sentences and the ability to use language to accomplish a variety of social goals and express a range of abstract ideas

In each section, we briefly outline the typical milestones of communicative development, discuss the ways in which children with autism differ from the typical picture, and review a selected set of interventions for which empirical evidence of efficacy is available.

PRELINGUISTIC COMMUNICATION

Prelinguistic Development in Typical Children

A typical infant shows interactive behaviors from the first days of life, including responding to the mother's voice; synchronizing patterns of gaze, movements, and facial expressions of affect; and participating in vocal turn-taking (Fernald 1983). Although infants engage in numerous social interactions during this time, the first 8 months of life are typically referred to as the *preintentional* phase of communication, because the child has not yet developed the ability to retain goals in mind and pursue them through action. Although adults often treat the behavior of preintentional children as if it were communicative, serving as one of the avenues by which children learn to communicate, it is not until the end of their first year that intentional communication of the typical child begins to appear. These early communication intentions are, at first, expressed with simple gestures, such as reaching to indicate a request or pushing away to indicate rejection. Later, children acquire more conventional gestures such as pointing to request, or shaking the head to mean "no." These expressions are highly coordinated with the infant's gaze, either toward the adult or between the adult and an object of interest. Gradually, these expressions become accompanied, and eventually replaced, by vocalization and speech (Acredolo and Goodwyn 1988; Bloom 1993). They continue to be tightly coupled with gaze. Early intentional behaviors have been found to express three basic communicative functions: the *regulation* of others' behavior by requesting or rejecting objects and actions, calling attention to objects or events and commenting on their appearance to establish *joint attention*, and calling attention to self for the purpose of *social interaction* (Bates 1976; Carpenter et al. 1998). Research suggests that joint attention is particularly important to the development of communication (Charman 2003; Mundy et al. 1990; Wetherby and Prizant 1992; Wetherby et al. 1998, 2000). It requires an ability to coordinate visual attention to an external object or activity with another person to demonstrate mutual interest and social engagement (Carpenter and Tomasello 2000; Mundy and Stella 2000) and has been shown to predict language development (Charman et al. 2003; Dawson et al. 2004; Mundy et al. 1990; Sigman and Ruskin 1999).

Prelinguistic Communication in ASD

Although one of the nearly universal features of children with ASD (with the exception of those with Asperger syndrome) is a significant delay in the acquisition of first words and word combinations, recent research has shown that delays in the development of preverbal communication occur even earlier, in the first and second years of life. At the prelinguistic level of communication, children diagnosed with ASD show:

- A depressed rate of preverbal communicative acts (Wetherby et al. 1998)
- Delayed development of pointing and other conventional gestures, both in terms of use and responsiveness (Dawson et al. 1998)
- Unconventional means of communicating, such as pulling a person by the hand instead of pointing or looking (Stone et al. 1997)
- Reduced responsiveness to speech and to hearing their name called (Osterling and Dawson 1994; Paul et al. 2007a)
- A restricted range of communicative behaviors, limited primarily to regulatory functions (getting people to do or not do things), with very limited use of communication for social interaction or to comment or establish joint attention (Mundy and Stella 2000)
- Lack of coordination among gaze, gestures, and vocalizations (Stone et al. 1997)
- Atypical preverbal vocalizations (Sheinkopf et al. 2000)
- Deficits in pretend and imaginative play (Rogers et al. 2005)
- A limited ability to imitate others' actions and vocalizations (Volkmar et al. 1997)

The consequence of this collection of preverbal behavior patterns is that children with ASD fail not only to begin talking at the normal time, but do not compensate for their lack of speech by attempting to communicate in other ways, as children with other language delays generally do (Stone et al. 1997; Thal 1991). Moreover, children with ASD not only fail to express communicative acts, they have difficulty in responding to speech and gestures and in following others' attempts to establish joint attention (Yoder and McDuffie 2006). This is likely to be a result of their failure to have acquired, during the preverbal period of development, the basic concept of reciprocal, intentional interpersonal communication as a means to attain objects, activities, and pleasurable interaction with others. Thus, as we shall see, interventions to improve communication in children with ASD who function at prelinguistic levels vary according to whether they aim primarily to elicit speech or to lay a foundation for language in the acquisition of earlier-emerging behaviors using gestures, gaze, and vocalizations to increase the frequency and range of expression of early communicative functions.

Interventions at the Prelinguistic Level

Although the prelinguistic period ends by the first birthday in typical development, for children with ASD, it can last much longer. Some children with ASD persist in preverbal communication well into the preschool years; for others, spoken language may fail to emerge at all (Tager-Flusberg et al. 2005). This scenario suggests that prelinguistic children with ASD require communication interventions that address several different targets. First, for young children who do not speak, it is important to provide treatment that attempts to elicit vocal production, vocal imitation, and eventually speech, since this is the most universal means of communication and enables the greatest degree of integration into mainstream environments and activities. In addition, however, interventions that focus on developing other skills known to be related to language development can help to establish a broader foundation for the acquisition of conventional communication skills. Research suggests that behaviors most likely to serve this function are *imitation* (McDuffie et al. 2005; Rogers et al. 2003; Sigman and Ruskin 1999; Smith et al. 2007), *play* (Yoder 2006; Paul et al. 2008; Smith et al. 2007), and *joint attention* (Charman 2003; Dawson et al. 2004; Mundy et al. 1990; Paul et al. 2008; Smith et al. 2007). Finally, because some preverbal children establish unusual, hard-to-interpret ways to communicate their wants and needs or use maladaptive behaviors to communicate intent (Paul and Sutherland 2005; Prelock 2006), it is also important to provide alternate means for preverbal children to express themselves in more acceptable ways, either until they acquire spoken language or as an alternative modality if spoken language does not emerge. Thus, a preverbal child with ASD may benefit from one, or two, or all three of these kinds of intervention. A communication intervention program for a child at this level does not necessarily mean choosing one method to the exclusion of others. A carefully implemented combination of approaches, with each method provided by a therapist who is well-trained in that intervention approach (National Research Council 2001; Reichow et al. 2009) may be considered. In reviewing evidence-based intervention approaches for children at this level, then, we attempted to identify interventions that would target each of the three areas of prelinguistic communication development.

Five intervention approaches are discussed in this context. The first, discrete trial intervention, is aimed specifically at increasing vocal imitation and eliciting speech. Three others – joint attention training (Kasari et al. 2006, 2008), More Than Words (Sussman 1999) and milieu communication training (Kaiser and Hester 1994; Warren and Yoder 1998; Yoder and Warren 2002) – are designed to support joint attention, play and imitation as foundations for the emergence of language. The fifth intervention, Picture Exchange Communication System (Bondy and Frost 1998), provides an alternate means of communication.

Discrete trial intervention. One of the first attempts at systematic education for children with ASD was an early intensive behavioral intervention, referred to as the Young Autism Program, developed by (Lovaas 1987). This program relied primarily on a discrete trial intervention (DTI) method. DTI entails dividing the target skill into a hierarchy of components and training each component individually, using highly structured, drill-like procedures and rewarding correct responses with positive reinforcement. Intensive training utilizes one-to-one sessions employing shaping, prompting, prompt fading, and reinforcement strategies. Trials continue until the child produces the target response with minimal prompting; at which point the next step in the hierarchy of behaviors is presented and trained.

A relatively large literature (reviewed by Reichow and Wolery (2009)) based primarily on single subject experimental designs (SSED) and small sample studies has demonstrated the efficacy of these approaches in eliciting vocal imitation (Ross and Greer 2003) and speech (Jones et al. 2006; Tsiouri and Greer 2003; Yoder and Layton 1988) from nonverbal children. In their meta-analysis of studies using programs based on the Lovaas method, Reichow and Wolery (2009) conclude that, for the six studies reporting sufficient data to be evaluated, early intensive behavioral intervention has been effective in improving both expressive and receptive language for children with ASD, with effect sizes calculated for each of the six studies ranging from small to very large. Table 5.1 provides a summary of studies implementing discrete trial intervention to facilitate speech and language in children with ASD.

Because discrete trial approaches rely heavily on teacher direction, prompted responses, and contrived forms of reinforcement, they have an inherent weakness: they often lead to a passive style of communication, in which children respond to prompts to communicate but do not initiate communication or transfer the behaviors acquired to situations outside the teaching context (Paul and Sutherland 2005; Stokes 1977). These difficulties in generalizing and maintaining behaviors taught through DTI approaches, along with changes in theoretical views of language learning that emphasize the central role of social exchanges in the acquisition of language, have led away from reliance on DTI as a primary means of teaching early communication skills to children with ASD. Nonetheless, DTI approaches have demonstrated effectiveness (Eikeseth et al., 2007) and, in combination with some of the other, more naturalistic methods discussed below, they merit consideration as a component of a comprehensive program for preverbal children.

Joint attention training. As discussed above, children on the autism spectrum generally communicate primarily to regulate others' behavior, rather than to achieve social interaction or joint attention (Mundy and Burnette 2005; Wetherby 1986). They are less likely to point or show objects, to make gaze shifts back and forth between a person and an interesting object or event, and have difficulty following a "line of regard" (i.e., understanding the direction of another person's gaze). Deficits in the capacity for establishing joint attention highlight the lack of communication for social purposes described for children

with ASD (Wetherby et al. 2000). Further, failure to develop joint attention has been linked to limitations in play, language acquisition, and in the development of peer relationships. Considering the critical role of joint attention in making early social and symbolic connections, it is often described as a priority treatment goal (Prelock 2006) or a pivotal skill (Koegel and Koegel 2006) for children with ASD.

Several treatment studies examining the effectiveness of joint attention training have been carried out since 2002. Some of these studies have relied on parents as intervention agents for their children with ASD, following the logic that parents spend the most time with the child and thus will have the greatest number of opportunities to provide instruction. Other studies have targeted direct work by clinicians and special educators with children with ASD. Notably, the research in joint attention training has utilized strong experimental designs, including both randomized control trials and multiple baseline SSED. As presented in Table 5.2, the effects of joint attention training have been powerful for increasing verbalization (Drew et al. 2002), facilitating reciprocal social interaction (Aldred et al. 2004), and increasing response to and initiation of joint attention that generalized to other contexts (Jones et al. 2006; Kasari et al. 2006, 2008; Schertz and Odom 2007; Whalen and Shreibman 2003) in young children with ASD, from 2 to 5 years of age.

More Than Words. Several studies have examined parents' abilities to support the communication and social responsiveness of their children with ASD. Aldred et al. (2004) found that parents respond sensitively to their children with ASD and interpret their actions as meaningful. Delaney and Kaiser (2001) describe parents as able to support the communication and responsiveness of their children. Mahoney and Perales (2003) report that parents use responsive interactions to enhance the social–emotional functioning of their children. Further, parents

TABLE 5.1 Studies designed to improve speech and language in individuals with ASD using discrete trial intervention

Research design (SSED or group)	Study	Participants	Outcome
Multiple group comparison	Lovaas (1987)	59 children with autism under the age of 46 months:	• *Experimental group*: 40 h of 1-on-1; *Control group* 1: received less than 10 h per week of 1-on-1; *Control group* 2: no intervention • Experimental group was significantly higher on level of academic placement than the control groups (there were no pre-treatment differences between groups and there were no differences between the control groups at follow-up). • Experimental group demonstrated significantly greater gains in IQ scores compared to the control groups. • Mental age and IQ scores remained the same between intake and follow-up in the control groups. • Prorated mental age was significantly related to outcome in both the Experimental Group and Control Group 1. • Abnormal speech was significantly related to outcome in Control Group 1.
Group pretest–posttest design; SSED multiple-baseline designs	Ander-son et al. (1987)	14 children with autism or autistic-like symptoms, 18 to 64 months old upon entry into the study	• There were statistically significant gains in receptive and expressive language performance at both one-year and 2-year follow-ups (based on performance on *Symbolic Play Test*, *Peabody Picture Vocabulary Test Form L*, *Preschool Language Scale*, *Sequenced Inventory of Communicative Development*). • After 1 year, 12 children demonstrated gains in all three domains (social/self-help, pre-academic, communication – based on the *Uniform Performance Assessment System*); the most significant gains occurred in the social/self-help domain with some children functioning at or near age level; the smallest gains occurred in the communication domain, with all children continuing to perform well below age level. • Two children demonstrated little or no change; both children had entry level mental-age, social-age, and language-age scores below 12 months. • One of 11 children in school settings upon entry to the program was in a socially integrated school placement; after 1 year in the study, 23% (out of 13 enrolled in school settings) were integrated at least 2 h a week. • Gains on specific behaviors did not occur until the intervention was systematically introduced.

Design	Study	Sample	Results
Group compari-son (follow-up to Lovaas 1987)	McEachin et al. (1993)	38 children with autism with a mean age of 11.5 years (range: 6–19 years), from the experimen-tal group of Lovaas (1987) and control group 1	• Participants in the experimental group maintained level of intellectual functioning since previous assessment at a mean age of 7 years (mean IQ was significantly higher than that of the control group). • Experimental group demonstrated significantly higher level of functioning *than the control group on adaptive behavior* (Vineland) and personality (*Personality Inventory for Children*). • Nine participants in the experimental group who had been classified as "best outcome" by Lovaas consistently demonstrated average intelligence and average levels of adaptive func-tioning (measured by *Weschler's Intelligence Scale for Children, Revised; Vineland; Personality Inventory for Children, Clinical Rating Scale* addressing friendships, family relations, school and community activities).
Control group comparison study (not random assignment)	Birnbrauer and Leach (1993)	14 children (10 boys, four girls) ages 22–47 months diagnosed with PDD, PDD-NOS, or autistic disorder	• Two of nine children in the intervention group demonstrated a higher than normal develop-mental rate on language development (based on *Receptive Expressive Emergent Language* and *Reynell* scores). • Four of nine children in the intervention group were considered high achieving (achieving IQ scores on at least one scale >80 and demonstrating substantial gains in language and adaptive behavior) and the other five were considered moderate–low achieving. • One out of five children in the control group was considered to be high achieving although language development was not accelerated beyond expected normal rate.
Group compari-son study (group assignment based on therapist avail-ability and treat-ment eligibility)	Smith et al. (1997)	21 children (19 boys, two girls), 46 months of age or younger with PDD and men-tal retardation	• Mean IQ of the experimental group increased at follow-up; mean IQ of the comparison group decreased at follow-up; the difference in IQ at follow-up was statistically significant (it was not at intake). • No child spoke in words at intake; 10 of 11 children in the experimental group spoke in words at follow-up to label objects and express words (two of which were using phrases), which was a significant difference from intake; two of 10 children in the comparison group spoke in words at follow-up. • Large variability in individual differences in the experimental group at follow-up; less variability in the comparison group.

(Continued)

TABLE 5.1 (Continued)

Research design (SSED or group)	Study	Participants	Outcome
Control group comparison study (control group pairwise matched)	Sheinkopf and Siegel (1998)	22 children, ages 23–47 months, with autism or PDD-NOS	• Experimental group had significantly higher IQ scores at follow-up compared to the control group (no difference pre-treatment). • All children in the experimental group had IQ scores above 65 at follow-up, versus six of the 11 in the control group. • Number of positive symptoms in the experimental group declined from pre-treatment to post-treatment, but did not reach significance. • Experimental group received significantly lower severity ratings on a four-point scale at post-treatment compared to the control group. • All participants still met diagnostic criteria for autism/PDD-NOS at follow-up.
Correlational study	Weiss (1999)	20 children (19 boys, one girl), ages 20–65 months, with autism or PDD-NOS receiving intensive behavior analytic intervention at home for 40 h a week	• Prior to intervention, all children scored in the severely autistic range on the *Childhood Autism Rating Scale* (*CARS*); following 2 years of intervention, nine scored in the non-autistic range, four had mild manifestations of autism noted, four were in the mild–moderate range, and three scored in the severe range. • There was variability in acquisition rates among participants. • Scores on second administration of CARS were predicted by Verbal Imitation, Receptive Commands, and Object Manipulation.
RCT group study (matched pair, random assignment procedure)	Smith et al. (2000b)	28 children (23 boys, five girls) between the ages of 18 and 42 months with autism (*N* = 14) or PDD-NOS (*N* = 14)	• There were no statistically significant between-group differences at intake. • Intensive treatment group made significantly greater gains in language development compared to the parent training group, as measured by the total score on the *Reynell Developmental Language Scales* (there were no significant differences between groups on the Comprehension or Expressive subscales). • Four children in the intensive treatment group achieved maximum scores on the Comprehension and Expressive Language subscales at follow-up (no children in the parent training group did so). • Intensive treatment group had significantly less restrictive school placements than the parent training group. • Children with PDD-NOS in the intensive training group obtained higher scores than children with autism at follow-up testing but no significant differences were found. • Two children in the intensive treatment group met criteria for "best outcome" (McEachin et al. 1993) and two met the placement criterion with IQ scores just below the cutoff; all four of these children scored in the average range on all tests (except for one child for whom clinically significant behavior problems were noted on the *Child Behavior Checklist*); only one child from the parent training group scored in the average range on a test at follow-up.

SSED multiple baseline across participants (with random assignment to a baseline lasting 1, 3, or 5 months)	Smith et al. (2000a)	Six boys with autism or PDD-NOS who were between the ages of 31 and 45 months at intake	• Following treatment implementation (in a period of 5 months), five of the six children substantially increased correct responding to receptive actions, nonverbal imitation, and verbal imitation; two of the children also increased correct responding to expressive labeling (to a maximum of 30% correct following 5 months of treatment). • At follow-up after 2–3 years, two of the children demonstrated increases >10 on *Reynell and Vineland*; one child demonstrated a decline; two children's scores remained stable; one child's scores were mixed.
Longitudinal study over 12 months and cross-sectional with respect to time into treatment	Bibby et al. (2001)	66 children (11 girls, 55 boys) with autism, autistic spectrum disorder or PDD; mean age of 45 months (SD = 11.2 months) at onset of treatment	• Group mean IQ did not change across 31.6 months of intervention. • Mean mental age increased significantly, but the mean increase was 16.8 months over 31.6 months of intervention. • Significant increase in *Vineland Adaptive Behavior* scores from early in treatment to follow-up. • Pathology scores dropped significantly following intervention. • Speech ratings, made by researchers based on parent interviews, increased following intervention: 37 children had no recognizable words at the beginning of treatment compared to five children following treatment. • Mean outcome IQ for children over 72 months old was significantly less than that of the children in Lovaas (1987); there was no significant difference between their mean and the means for control groups. • No "best outcomes" following treatment for children over 72 months (i.e., no "educationally normal functioning children"). • Four children under 72 months of age at the 6–9-month follow-up approximated "best outcome" (IQ>85 and succeeding in regular schools with no or minimal adult support). • For children who received intervention for 12 months, mean Vineland scores in Communication increased significantly; progress demonstrated on Reynell Comprehension and Expression subscales, but less than typically expected in 12 months, except fore five children who gained >12 months on both scales; two demonstrated regression on both Reynell scales. • Pre-treatment IQ was significantly positively correlated with IQ at Time 1 and Time 2. • Children who began treatment before 43 months of age demonstrated greater gains in IQ from intervention.

(Continued)

TABLE 5.1 (Continued)

Research design (SSED or group)	Study	Participants	Outcome
Outcome survey (retrospective case review and parent questionnaire)	Boyd and Corley (2001)	22 children (16 boys, six girls) with a primary diagnosis of autism ($n = 19$) or PDD-NOS ($n = 3$) younger than 4 years old at onset of intervention (mean: 41 months, range: 29–48 months)	• No child achieved recovery based on Lovaas' (1987) criteria (with normal intelligence and in regular education without a 1:1 aide). • Measures of behavior indicated a mean that was very close to the threshold of "very serious behavior problems" and it was no different than a mean for children with similar diagnoses not receiving the intervention. • Language, compliance, and pre-academic skills were reported most often by parents as showing improvement although nearly half of the children were non-verbal following the intervention.
Comparison group study (assignment based on availability of supervisors)	Eikeseth et al. (2002)	25 children (17 boys, eight girls) with autism, aged 4 to 7 years old	• Participants in the behavioral and eclectic treatment groups received an average of 28.52 h of 1:1 treatment per week. • Behavioral group demonstrated significantly greater gains on IQ, language (based on performance on all scales of the *Reynell* or the *WPPSI-R*), and adaptive behavior (*Vineland Communication and Composite scores*). • Children in the behavioral group were more likely to have IQs in the average range at follow-up. • Intake IQ of the behavioral group was strongly correlated with follow-up IQ and language, and change in language.
Group RCT (clinic-directed EIBI of 38.6 h/week or parent-directed of 31.7 h/week)	Sallows and Graupner (2005)	24 children (19 boys, five girls) with autism and a mean age of 33–34 months at intake	• No significant differences between groups at pre- or post-test. • When groups were combined, significant increases were seen on Full Scale IQ, Verbal IQ, Performance IQ, receptive language, *Vineland Communication and Socialization*, and *ADI-R Social Skills and Communication*. • "Rapid learners" demonstrated significant gains in all areas measured, with all scores reaching the average range over 4 years; only one of these children continued to demonstrate a delay in language. • 12 "moderate learners" showed increases in developmental age equivalents, but did not catch up to peers. • Teacher ratings of Communication and Socialization on the Vineland Classroom Edition were average for rapid learners; deficiencies were noted in both areas for moderate learners. • Eight of the 11 rapid learners scored in the nonautistic range on all three scales of the ADI (some had diagnoses removed). • Ability to imitate was highly correlated with performance on IQ, language, and social skills. • Language skill acquisition strongly related to Early Learning Measures (receptive language, nonverbal imitation, verbal imitation), *Vineland Daily Living Skills*, and ADI-Communication.

| Three-year prospective outcome group study, quasi-experimental design (groups based on parental preference for EIBI or local public school special education classes) | Cohen et al. (2006) | 42 children (4:1 male:female) with autism or PDD-NOS, aged 18–42 months at diagnosis and under 48 months at onset of intervention | • EIBI (in a community setting) group had significantly greater gains in IQ following intervention.
• EIBI group increased more in *Reynell* Receptive and Expressive language: receptive language approached significance, expressive language scores did not.
• EIBI group made significantly greater gains on *Vineland Composite* and Communication and Daily Living Skills subscales.
• At year three, 17 of the 21 EIBI participants were in regular education classrooms, compared to one out of 21 in the control group.
• Scores in IQ, *Vineland, Merrill-Palmer, and Reynell* Comprehension and Expression demonstrated similar patterns of gains across the 3 years. |
| Retrospective group comparison (10–20 h per week of 1:1 behavioral treatment vs. combination of two to three treatments for the "eclectic" group) | Eldevik et al. (2006) | 28 children (24 boys, four girls) with autism and mental retardation who were younger than 6 years old at the start of treatment | • Only measure on which groups differed significantly at intake was Vineland Socialization (in favor of the eclectic therapy group).
• Two years into treatment, the behavioral group demonstrated significantly greater gains than the eclectic group on intellectual functioning (*WPPSI-R, WISC-R, Stanford Binet, or Bayley Scales of Infant Development*), language comprehension and expressive language (*Reynell*), and *Vineland Communication*.
• Significant reduction in degree of mental retardation (MR) for 38% of the behavioral group versus 7% of the eclectic group.
• Significant difference in severe classification of MR at follow-up, with no child in the behavioral group but 40% of the children in the eclectic group receiving a severe MR classification.
• Statistically significant changes in overall pathology scores in favor of the behavioral group and on four of seven symptoms (affection, toy play, peer play, toilet training).
• Gains of behavioral group were more modest than those reported in other studies of intensive behavioral intervention. |

(Continued)

TABLE 5.1 (Continued)

Research design (SSED or group)	Study	Participants	Outcome
Controlled group comparison (behavioral treatment: group assignment made based on availability of supervisors)	Eikeseth et al. (2007)	25 children (19 boys, six girls) with autism, aged 4–7 years; deviation IQ of 50 or above on WPPSI-R or ratio IQ of 50 or more on the *Bayley Scales of Infant Development*	• Behavioral intervention group demonstrated significantly greater gains in adaptive behavior and IQ. • Behavioral group demonstrated significantly fewer social problems and aggressive behavior than the eclectic group at follow-up. • Significant differences in scores for *Vineland Composite, Socialization* between groups at follow-up. • 54% of children in the behavioral group performed in the average range in most or all measures at follow-up (IQ scores increased from a mean of 70 to a mean of 104); 17% of the eclectic group scored within one standard deviation of the mean on mean IQ and verbal IQ at follow-up. • Children with high intake IQ scored higher on outcome measures, but they did not make significantly greater gains in IQ, language, or adaptive scores.
Control group comparison (home-based EIBI in a community setting vs. autism-specific nursery services, group selected by parent)	Magiati et al. (2007)	44 children (27 boys, one girl) with ASD, ages 23–53 months	• Average hours of intervention per week were significantly higher for EIBI group (32.4 h) than the nursery group (25.6 h). • At 23–27-month follow-up, no group differences in cognitive, play, and language skills, or severity of autism. • Marginally statistically significant difference on *Vineland Daily Living Skills* standard score in favor of EIBI group. • No child was in a mainstream school without 1:1 support at follow-up. • Children who improved the most had intake IQs greater than 70 and all but one were verbal; none of the children who improved the least had intake IQs greater than 55 and all were non-verbal. • Initial IQ and receptive language raw scores were the strongest predictors of outcome after 2 years.

Control group comparison (based on parent selection of EIBI or "treatment as usual")	Remington et al. (2007)	44 children with autism, 30 to 42 months of age at intake	• Children in the comparison group were on average 3 months older than the children in the behavioral group at intake. • Behavioral intervention group received treatment for an average of 25.6 h per week over 2 years and demonstrated significantly higher scores on IQ, mental age, *Vineland Daily Living Skills*, and *Vineland Motor Skills* at 12-month follow-up, which were maintained at the 24-month follow-up. • At the 24-month follow-up, the behavioral intervention group demonstrated a significantly higher level of responding to joint attention than the comparison group, but there was no difference for initiating joint attention. • Behavioral intervention group demonstrated significantly higher performance on receptive and expressive language on the *Reynell* at 12 and 24 months. • More individual children in the behavioral intervention group than the comparison group demonstrated increases in IQ over time. • Children who responded the most to the behavioral intervention had higher IQ scores, higher mental age, and higher *Vineland Composite, Communication, and Social Skills* scores at baseline.
Comprehensive synthesis: descriptive analyses, effect size analyses, meta-analysis	Reichow and Wolery (2009)	373 children with autism, ASD, PDD, or PDD-NOS with a mean age less than 84 months (although most studies reported a mean age less than 42 months at onset of study)	• Descriptive analyses for school placement, psychopathology, and diagnostic reclassification suggested that EIBI is an effective intervention for many children with autism. • Effect size analysis suggests that post-intervention performance was generally higher than pre-intervention performance on multiple measures (IQ, adaptive behavior, expressive language, receptive language). • Between-group analyses of comparative studies suggest that children receiving EIBI made more gains than comparison groups (e.g., minimal behavioral intervention, eclectic intervention, treatment as usual). • Meta-analysis: EIBI is on average an effective intervention for increasing IQ scores among children with autism.

TABLE 5.2   Studies designed to improve social communication in individuals with ASD using joint attention (JA) training

Research design (SSED or group)	Study	Participants	Outcomes
RCT group comparison	Drew et al. (2002)	• 24 children under 2 years old with childhood autism, atypical autism, or PDD-NOS • Randomized to JA parent training group or local services only group	• Significantly more children in the parent training group went from non-verbal to having single-word or phrase speech (based on parent report in interview). • Marginally higher language comprehension in the parent training group at follow-up (but it did not reach significance).
SSED multiple baseline design, *intervention targeted at children with autism*	Whalen and Schreibman (2003)	• Five 4-year-old children with autism or PDD-NOS • Six typically developing children used for developmental norms of JA	• Intervention was effective for teaching correct responding to adult JA initiations (responding to showing and following a gaze and a point) for all children. • Teaching JA initiations (pointing and coordinated gaze shifting) was effective for four out of the five children. • Generalization to other contexts was shown for four out of the five children for initiation. • Positive changes in JA were noticeable to investigators and naïve observers.
RCT pre- and post-treatment group comparison	Aldred et al. (2004)	• 28 children (2;0 to 5;11 years old) with classic autism	• Significant reduction in autism symptoms as measured by the ADOS seen in the parent-training and routine care group compared with the routine care group alone. • All but two children in the treatment group showed significant increases in reciprocal social interaction, engagement, rapport, and social responses, and spontaneous initiation of social interaction. • Reduction in autism symptoms in the treatment group shown across all severity levels and all age groups, but a greater trend was seen in the younger subgroup. • Significant treatment effect mainly seen in the *reciprocal social interaction sub-domain* of the ADOS. • No significant treatment effect was found in the *communication sub-domain*; qualitatively, however, children in the treatment group were reported at post-treatment to use a variety of single words socially to seek attention, request and direct attention; the control group were more likely to use single words to label objects.

	Jones et al. (2006)	• Study 1: five children (2 to 3 years old); three with PDD-NOS, one with autism, one with ASD	• Children in the treatment group made significantly more progress in expressive language over the year as measured by the *MacArthur Communication Development Inventory* (MCDI) compared to the control group; no significant difference was found for comprehension.
			• A non-significant increase was seen for the treatment group compared to the control group on the *Vineland Communication* sub-domain.
			• There was no significant difference in levels of shared attention during the parent–child interaction.
			• The treatment group showed significantly better outcomes in parental positive synchronous communication and an increase in child communication acts during parent–child interaction.
• Study 1: SSED multiple probe design across behaviors (children taught JA)			• Study 1:All children mastered responding to and initiating JA during intervention implemented by teachers, although acquisition was at variable rates.
			• High levels of performance were seen for all children during generalization to novel stimuli and maintenance with original toys.
• Study 2: SSED clinical extension of skills learned with teacher (parents received JA instruction and taught to children)		• Study 2: two children from Study 1 (2;2 to 3;0 years old), one with autism and one ASD	• Study 2: Neither child demonstrated responding to or initiating JA with parent during baseline.
			• Both children mastered these skills with their parents for both toys and routines.
			• Generalization of both skills was seen to other toys, pictures, and routines for both children.

(Continued)

TABLE 5.2 (Continued)

Research design (SSED or group)	Study	Participants	Outcomes
• Study 3: investigation of collateral effects and social validity of intervention		• Study 3: four of the five children from Study 1	• Study 3: There was an increase in the number and variety of vocalizations seen for all four children during episodes of JA. • The two children from Study 2 were rated as appearing more interested in interacting and communicative with their mothers post-treatment; they were also rated as more similar to a typically-developing peer on social-communicative characteristics (interest, expressiveness, happiness, relationship) at post-treatment; one increased the amount of time he engaged in coordinated JA from pre- to post-treatment and one of the two generalized JA across setting and materials.
RCT group comparison	Kasari et al. (2006)	58 (46 boys and 12 girls) children with autism (3–4 year olds) in early intervention program	• JA group and play group showed significant improvement in initiating "shows" compared to control. • JA group showed greater improvement in responding to JA. • JA group made significant gains in giving compared to play group and more coordinated joint looks. • JA group engaged in more child-initiated JA than the control group.
SSED multiple baseline reversal across 3 participants, *treatment targeted at children with autism*	Martins and Harris (2006)	Three boys with autism, (3;10 to 4;8 years old)	• Responding to JA was defined as a 90-degree head turn for 2 s toward an object following an attention-getting phrase and head turn by the adult. • Following intervention, responding to JA skills increased for all children and were maintained without the presence of additional reinforcement. • Longer acquisition times were seen for all children when responding to "look," head turn, and eye gaze from adult. • Generalization to other settings and other individuals was observed for all three children. • There were minimal to no increases in initiating JA for any child following intervention. • Two of the children increased their requests for items from the adult following intervention.

SSED multiple baseline across participants, *intervention targeted at children with autism*	Whalen et al. (2006)	Four preschoolers (mean age 4;2) with autism	• There was an increase in social initiations and positive affect toward the experimenter at post-treatment but a decrease in positive affect at follow-up. • All four children showed increases in spontaneous speech at post-treatment; somewhat maintained at follow-up (remained above baseline).
RCT group comparison, *intervention targeted at children with autism*	Gulsrud et al. (2007)	35 children (28 males, seven females) with autism (33–54 months)	• Following intervention, significantly more children in the JA group acknowledged the novel probe (eye gaze or non-verbal gesture toward the probe and verbalization about the probe) compared to the symbolic play (SP) group. • Of those who acknowledged the probe in each group, significantly more children in the JA group engaged in coordinated joint looks between a person and the probe compared to the SP group; this engagement lasted significantly longer than that seen for the children in the SP group. • The JA group significantly increased their coordinated joint looks across the intervention, but the SP group did not. • There were no significant differences between the JA and the SP group on verbalizations and non-verbal gestures following intervention.
SSED multiple baseline design across participant pairs	Rocha et al. (2007)	• Three children with autism (26, 27, 42 months); two mothers and one father	• Children responded to parents' JA bids at baseline, during treatment, post-treatment, and follow-up. • Parents reported satisfaction with the treatment and initiated more JA bids during training than baseline. • Children responded to a greater number of JA bids during later phases of treatment and post-treatment than at baseline. • There was a generalized improvement in JA responding and initiation • All children showed greatest levels of coordinated JA during the last phase
Chronological age comparison group not receiving treatment (used to inform levels of JA)			
SSED multiple baseline design	Schertz and Odom (2007)	Three toddlers (22, 24, 33 months) with autism	• Two of the subjects showed steady improvement in all phases (focusing on faces, turn taking, responding to JA, initiating JA). • All three showed improvements over baseline. • Generalization was seen across home and community contexts. • Skills maintained five weeks post-treatment. • Parents indicated long-term child competence as result of intervention.

(Continued)

TABLE 5.2 (Continued)

Research design (SSED or group)	Study	Participants	Outcomes
RCT group comparison, randomized allocation to JA group, or control group	Kasari et al. (2008) (follow-up to Kasari et al. 2006)	• 58 children (3–4 years of age) with autism • Randomized allocation to JA group, symbolic play (SP) group, or control group • 56 children at 6 months post-treatment and 53 children at 12 months post-treatment	• JA and SP groups showed significantly greater growth in expressive language over time compared to control group. • There was no significant effect of treatment on receptive language growth over time. • Pre-intervention average of JA initiations, responding to JA, and duration of child-initiated JA episodes all significantly predicted expressive language growth. • Children with higher expressive language (more than five words and higher than 20 months on *Reynell*) at pre-treatment experienced more expressive language growth. • Children with low expressive language at pre-treatment showed significantly greater expressive language growth in the JA group compared to the SP and control groups. • There was a significantly greater rate of change in JA and SP skills over time for both experimental groups.

have been shown to be capable of providing effective intervention targeting language and communication (Moes and Frea 2002) and synchronous play, which lead to an increase in their children's language and communication (Siller and Sigman 2002).

In order to optimize parents' ability to interact in a facilitative way with their children with ASD, Sussman (1999) developed *More Than Words* (MTW). This program grows out of the tradition of "child-centered" or "responsive" interventions, building on the rationale that language is normally learned in the context of playful, affectively-positive interactions (Bloom 1993) in which adults follow the child's lead to maximize the child's attention, then say or do something for which the child shows an interest. This program trains parents to use specific interactive techniques to maximize their child's ability to pay attention, to find enjoyment in two-way communication, to imitate and understand what others say and do, to interact and have fun doing it, and to practice what has been learned. Parents also learn that their child's success depends on their ability to create activities that have a structure, are predictable and allow for repetition. Generally, the goals emphasized in the MTW program include increasing interaction and vocabulary. Specific objectives aimed at children at particular stages of communication are also provided. These stages are referred to in MTW as the "own agenda" (preintentional) stage, the "requester" (prelinguistic) stage, the "early communicator" (first words) user stage, and the "partner" (word combination) stage. Overall, parents are trained to teach new reasons for communicating and to facilitate a connection between what is being said and what is happening (Sussman 1999). Parents participating in the MTW program learn specific strategies to support their children's communication (e.g., observing, waiting and listening to their child; including their child's interests in play, imitating their

action, interpreting their intention and intruding on their activities; saying less, going slow, emphasizing or stressing critical information and showing their child what to focus on or how to do things). Two studies have examined the effectiveness of this intervention for families and children with ASD. McConachie et al. (2005) used the MTW program to facilitate parental understanding of ASD and the social communication of their children. As a result of participation in the program, parents increased their use of facilitative strategies and children with ASD increased their vocabulary size. A second study by Girolametto et al. (2007) found similar results for three families of children between 2.8 and 3.2 years of age, with parents increasing their use of responsive strategies and children increasing their vocabulary. Table 5.3 displays the details of these studies. Currently, randomized controlled trials investigating the effectiveness of the MTW program are underway at three different institutions.

Milieu communication training (MCT). This intervention has a strong empirical evidence base. It was developed to facilitate early communication and language of young children with developmental disabilities (Gilbert 2008) including those with ASD. MCT is derived from the behaviorist tradition, drawing on the strengths of behavioral programming including the use of task analysis, predictable structure and attention to antecedent and consequent events (Gilbert 2008; Yoder and Stone 2006a, b; Yoder and Warren 2001). It was, however, designed to address some of the shortcomings that characterize behavioral interventions, that is, the tendency for passive, prompt-dependent communication, and difficulties in generalization. MCT applies behaviorist principles in a naturalistic context and engineers the environment so that objects and activities that interest the child require adult assistance. Adults then follow the child's attentional

TABLE 5.3   Studies designed to improve communication in individuals with ASD using *More Than Words*

Research design (SSED or group)	Study	Participants	Outcome
Delayed control group study (groups based on availability of class, not random assign-ment)	McConachie et al. (2005)	51 preschool-aged children (24–48 months) with language delay and suspected autism; 57% diagnosed with autism, others with PDD-NOS or developmental language disorder (DLD); 49 mothers and two fathers	• Participants with autism in the intervention group had a significantly larger expressive vocabulary following intervention com-pared to those with autism in the control group. • The participants with PDD-NOS or DLD in the intervention group had the same result as the control group. • There was a significant difference between the autism intervention group and the control group in parents' use of facilitative strategies, with more strategies used among the parents of children in the autism inter-vention group. • There was no significant difference for children's social communication score, child behavior problems, parental stress, or adaptation.
Multiple case study	Girolametto et al. (2007)	Three families of children (2.8–3.2 years old) with ASD	• Parents showed increased use of responsive interaction strategies. • All children demonstrated increases in vocabulary size post-intervention, measured by the *MacArthur Communication Develop-ment Inventory* (MCDI). • An increase in lexical diversity was observed. • The rate of communicative acts and the number of social interaction sequences increased post-treatment. • Two of the three children demonstrated increases in initiations.

lead to procure these objects and activities in which the child demonstrates sponta-neous interest. Ultimately, the goal is to shape communicative behavior to develop functional language. MCT can be imple-mented at either the prelinguistic level, by means of prelinguistic milieu teaching (PMT) for children who do not yet use spoken language, or the enhanced milieu teaching (EMT) level, for children begin-ning to use their first words.

Several strategies are used in MCT to support the intentional communication in the prelinguistic phase for children with language delays, including those children with ASD. These strategies require arrang-ing the natural environment to promote communication, such as placing objects of interest in sight but out of reach and encouraging spontaneous communica-tion by using time delay or expectant wait-ing – refraining from verbal prompting and giving a child sufficient time to formulate a response. In addition, the communication partner might withhold objects or materials of interest or only give portions of needed materials or an inadequate supply to facilitate a spontaneous requesting and commenting. The communication partner might also sabotage or change a routine or violate expectations in a routine as well as protest actions or create unexpected situations to elicit a response. In the use of both PMT and EMT, the interventionist models the desired behavior, reinforces responses naturally and imitates words or actions in a contingent manner. Research suggests that parents can be taught to use MCT to facilitate their children's spontaneous communication and increase utterance length, as well as the number and diversity of words spoken (Hancock and Kaiser 2002; Kaiser et al. 2000; Hemmeter and Kaiser 1994), and that children generalize this learning to the home setting (Kaiser and Hester 1994). Further, children with ASD increase their spontaneous requests when using MCT (Olive et al. 2008). Research outcomes for PMT and EMT demonstrate similar increases in spontaneous requesting, turn-taking, and initiation of joint attention (Yoder and Stone 2006a, b). Table 5.4 presents the details of studies examining the outcomes of MCT for children with autism.

Picture Exchange Communication System (PECS). This intervention was developed for children with ASD and other social-communication deficits who exhibit limited or no functional communication (Frost and Bondy 1994). The goal is to teach functional communication (e.g., requesting) within a social context using intrinsic, non-social rewards (e.g., getting the item requested) (Prelock 2006). PECS was designed to circumvent problems associated with traditional language remediation including prerequisite attending and imitation skills, pointing, and initiation (Bondy and Frost 1994, 1998, 2001). PECS focuses on facilitating spontaneous communication while avoiding prompt dependency and extensive training is not required prior to the initiation of the system (Bondy and Frost 1998; Prelock 2006). PECS consists of six phases beginning with teaching the physically assisted exchange in Phase I, expanding spontaneity in Phase II, teaching picture discrimination in Phase III, building sentence structure in Phase IV, responding to questions in Phase V, and commenting in response to questions in Phase VI (Frost and Bondy 2002). Goals established for PECS are said to serve directive or regulatory (e.g., requesting, demanding, commanding) and social (e.g., commenting, describing, naming) communication functions (Prelock 2006), although the "social" functions are limited to scripted comments, such as "I see X."

Several studies have been implemented in the last 15 years to investigate the effectiveness of PECS as communication intervention for children with ASD. Table 5.5 provides a listing of those studies, summarizing the outcomes that have been achieved when implementing this intervention. Generally, PECS has been tested in small group and SSED studies. The research, conducted primarily without comparison to other intervention approaches, has examined the effectiveness of PECS for children with ASD between 18 months and 12 years of age. Outcomes of these uncontrolled studies suggest some facilitation of speech (Bondy and Frost 1994, 1998; Liddle 2001), vocabulary growth (Anderson et al. 2007; Magiati and Howlin 2003; Schwartz et al. 1998; Yoder and Stone 2006b), increased mean length of utterance (Charlop-Christy et al. 2002; Ganz and Simpson 2004), use of untrained communicative functions (Schwartz et al. 1998), maintenance of speech communication gains (Charlop-Christy et al. 2002; Yokoyama et al. 2006), gains in joint attention, eye contact and toy play with a reduction of problem behaviors (Charlop-Christy et al. 2002), increased spontaneous

TABLE 5.4   Studies designed to improve communication in individuals with ASD using milieu communication training

Research design (SSED or group)	Study	Participants	Outcome
SSED multiple probe design across families	Hemmeter and Kaiser (1994) (parent-implemented EMT)	Three boys (one with PDD), one girl (ages 25–49 months)	• Parents learned to use enhanced milieu teaching (EMT) strategies in the clinic and generalized them to home. • The child with PDD experienced increases in spontaneous utterances, total targets, and spontaneous targets following intervention in the clinic and at home. • The child with PDD increased in SICD-E and SICD-R scores from pre- to post-treatment; utterance length increased from one to three and the number of words increased from eight to 54.
SSED multiple baseline design across children	Kaiser and Hester (1994) (EMT)	Six children (51–86 months) with language delay; two children had autistic-like symptoms	• All six children showed increases in language in the treatment setting following introduction of EMT; the length of time to demonstrate performance varied among the children. • The results generalized to use of targets at home with parents; results of generalization to peers and teachers in classroom were more variable.
Randomized group experiment (PMT vs. responsive small group)	Yoder and Warren (1998) (PMT)	58 children (17–36 months) with developmental disabilities (two diagnosed with PDD-NOS) and their primary caregivers	• No main effect of treatment type on intentional communication was found. • During experimenter–child interaction, the PMT group had significantly more intentional communication than the RSG group for children with highly responsive mothers; the same effect was found for the mother–child interaction.
SSED design across children (EMT); data taken from a previous longitudinal study (Kaiser et al. 1998) Random assignment to the parent-implemented EMT group in the previous study	Kaiser et al. (2000) (EMT)	Six boys (32–54 months); three with autism, one with Asperger's, two with PDD	• All children showed increases in their total use of targets, both prompted and unprompted, and the number of target classes used during the intervention phase of parent-implemented EMT; all six continued to use their targets in the follow-up phase.utterances.utterances were the highest at follow-up. • There were modest changes in spontaneous use of • All six children displayed changes in MLU and word diversity at follow-up (only three children showed changes in either during intervention). • Generalization of the use of targets to home setting was seen for five of six children; all children used their targets more at home at the end of follow-up compared to the end of intervention. • There were general increases on developmental language measures throughout intervention and follow-up but results were variable.

Design	Study	Participants	Findings
Randomized group experiment (PMT vs. modified responsive small group)	Yoder and Warren (2001)	58 children (17–32 months) with developmental delays (two children diagnosed with PDD-NOS) and their primary caregivers	• Children whose mothers scored relatively high on pre-treatment responsivity and amount of formal education benefited the most from PMT; children whose mothers scored relatively low on these variables pre-treatment benefited the most from modified RSG. • Interaction between mothers' amount of formal education and the treatment group predicted all four language outcomes (lexical density, Reynell receptive- and expressive-age equivalency, comprehension of semantic relations). • Interaction between mothers' responsivity and the treatment group predicted lexical density and comprehension of semantic relations. • Effects grew over time (the last follow-up measure was 12 months post-treatment).
SSED multiple baseline design across children (EMT); data taken from a previous longitudinal study (Kaiser et al. 1998)	Hancock and Kaiser (2002) (EMT)	Four children (35–54 months); two children with autism, two with PDD; randomly assigned to trainer-implemented EMT condition in the previous study	• Following introduction of trainer-implemented EMT, all children showed an increase in the use of targets (a variety of two-word combinations and two- to three-word requests based on the child), both prompted and unprompted. • Three of the four children showed clear changes in spontaneous use of targets following introduction of intervention. • All children increased the total number of utterances from baseline to intervention and maintained these levels of target use during follow-up. • Three children showed increases in MLU during intervention and all four showed increases in word diversity. • Three children demonstrated generalization to the home setting, with the most generalization occurring shortly after follow-up, with less generalization at the 6-month follow-up. • A general increase on developmental language measures were observed during intervention, but results were variable.

(Continued)

TABLE 5.4 (Continued)

Research design (SSED or group)	Study	Participants	Outcome
RCT (Responsive education and prelinguistic milieu teaching)	Yoder and Warren (2002) (PMT)	39 toddlers (median age 22 months; SD 4 months) with DD (one child with autism) and their primary caregivers	• There were no main effects of RPMT on children's language. • RPMT accelerated growth in comments if children began treatment with low-frequency comments and it accelerated growth in lexical density if children began treatment with low-frequency canonical vocal communication (the opposite effect – deceleration – was seen for both if children began treatment with high-frequency comments and canonical vocal communication). • RPMT accelerated growth in requests if children did not have Down Syndrome (it appeared to decelerate growth in requests if children did have Down Syndrome).
RCT group comparison	Yoder and Stone (2006a) (PMT)	36 nonverbal children (18–60 months) with autistic disorder (33) or PDD-NOS (3)	• Both Responsive Education and Prelinguistic Milieu Teaching (RPMT) and PECS had positive effects on communication skills (turn taking, requesting, initiation of joint attention). • The RPMT group learned to take turns and initiate joint attention with an adult better than the PECS group. • The PECS group learned how to make requests more often than RPMT group.
RCT group comparison (Responsive education and prelinguistic milieu teaching (RPMT) and Picture Exchange Communication System (PECS))	Yoder and Stone (2006b) (PMT)	36 nonverbal children (18–60 months) with autistic disorder or PDD-NOS	• RPMT increased object exchange turns more than PECS. • PECS increased requests more than RPMT. • Children who used more initiating joint attention acts at pre-treatment benefited more from RPMT than PECS; children who used at most one initiating joint attention act at pre-treatment benefited more from PECS than RPMT.
SSED multiple probe across participants	Olive et al. (2007) (EMT)	Three children (45–66 months), two with autism, one with PDD-NOS	• All children increased VOCA use during intervention. • All children increased their total spontaneous requests during intervention (combination of independent VOCA use, gestures, verbal communication); only one child began vocalizing during the study.

TABLE 5.5 Studies designed to improve communication in individuals with ASD using the picture exchange communication system (PECS)

Research design (SSED or group)	Study	Participants	Outcome
Group longitudinal study	Bondy and Frost (1994)	85 children (under 5 years old) with autism and no functional speech or alternative communication systems when entering PECS treatment	• Of the 66 using PECS for more than 1 year, 39 (59%) acquired speech as their sole communication system. • 25 (29%) used a combination of speech and pictures or a complex printed word system after 5 years. • 41 (48%) used solely speech 5 years after training began. • 76% came to use speech as their sole communication system or augmented by a picture-based system. • Direct correlation found between development of speech and reduction in *Autism Behavior Checklist* (ABC) scores (those solely using speech had the greatest reduction in their ABC scores).
Case study	Bondy and Frost (1998)	Male (2;8 years old) with autism	• Child rapidly acquired pictures but did not say his first word until 11 months following training, at which point he was using over 50 pictures. • Over the next 6 months, the child continued to expand PECS use and speech production. • 18 months following the introduction of PECS, the child was using only speech to communicate.
Descriptive study	Schwartz et al. (1998)	• 31 preschool children (3–6 years); 16 diagnosed with autism or PDD-NOS; 15 diagnosed with Down syndrome, Angelman's syndrome, or other developmental disabilities • 18 children followed for a year (11 with autism)	• Vocabulary growth steadily increased for children identified as those who talked at the first observation; those who demonstrated fewer than five words at the first observation showed small gains in vocabulary growth. • Children who received training in one communicative function on PECS showed increased use of untrained communicative functions (e.g., commenting, requesting).
Descriptive study	Liddle (2001)	21 children with ASD or severe learning difficulties with little or no functional language	• Nine of the children increased attempts at spoken language. • Seven children were reported to be using single words.

(Continued)

Table 5.5 (Continued)

Research design (SSED or group)	Study	Participants	Outcome
SSED Multiple baseline design across participants	Charlop-Christy et al. (2002)	Three boys (3;8 Chinese-American, 5;9 Korean-American, and 12-year-old Ethiopian-American) with autism and limited to no spontaneous speech	• Gains in spontaneous speech in academic and free-play settings seen for all participants at post-training; gains maintained at 1 year follow-up for one participant (12 years old). • Gains in MLU observed for two children in academic setting at post-training and all three children in a free-play setting; further gains observed at one year follow-up for one child (12 years old). • All children made gains in joint attention, eye contact, or toy play at post-training, as well as in number of requests and initiations per session. • Reduction of problem behavior (tantrums, out of seat, disruptions, grabs) observed in all three children.
SSED multiple baseline design across settings	Kravitz et al. (2002)	Six-year-old girl with autism who used one- or two-word utterances when prompted, but speech was difficult to understand and limited initiations	• Significantly more initiations and verbalizations during training compared to baseline. • Increases seen in spontaneous language (i.e., requests and comments) including use of verbalizations and icons across settings in which PECS was implemented. • Increase observed in intelligible verbalizations in two of three settings.
Preliminary study to assess feasibility of controlled trial – no experimental control	Magiati and Howlin (2003)	34 children (29 boys, five girls), ages 5–12 years with autism or ASD and one with co-morbid hyperactivity	• Average PECS level rose from just below one before training to 4.6 by follow-up. • Increase in PECS vocabulary from less than one to between 20 and 50. • Average frequency with which children used PECS increased significantly. • Children showed increase in overall level of communication based on CSBS, from giving, pointing, using pictures to using single words or echoed words to communicate. • Increase in vocabulary size following training.

Design	Authors	Participants	Results
SSED design within subjects (changing criterion design – no baseline)	Ganz and Simpson (2004)	Three children (3;9 Caucasian, DD and SLI; 5;8 Asian, autism; 7;2 African-American, DD with autistic characteristics and SLI), 0–10 spoken words in functional contexts and no prior experience with PECS	• Average number of words per trial increased for all three participants, particularly in Phase III for two children and Phase IV for all three. • Utterance length increased for all participants by the end of Phase IV.
SSED alternating treatments design followed by best treatment phase	Tincani (2004)	• African American male (5;10) with autism & MR • Asian American female (6;8) with PDD-NOS • Both imitated some words but did not use speech to without prompts	• More vocalizations seen for both participants in sign language training compared to PECS training. • Procedural modification to PECS system increased vocalization to level similar to that in sign language training for one child. • Higher number of requests for preferred items seen in the PECS training phase.
• Study 1: SSED multiple baseline design across participants • Study 2: SSED multiple baseline	Tincani et al. (2006)	• Study 1: two boys (ages 10;2 and 11;9), with autism without functional speech or use of an AAC system • Study 2: 9;2 year-old boy with autism with some prior training in PECS, but lacked skills to functionally communicate with pictures	• Study 1: independent manding increased for both participants once PECS training began and similar levels were maintained during generalization; one participant made it to Phase IV in training, the other participant took longer to meet the criterion, so only reached Phase II. • No speech seen for one participant; the other participant made vocal approximations – these decreased from baseline throughout Phases I–III of PECS training, with a sharp increase in Phase IV and maintained at similar levels during generalization (reinforcement was provided at a 3–5-s delay in Phase IV compared to previous phases). • Study 2: No difference in rate of independent mands between the two conditions (Phase IV instruction with no reinforcement for speech vs. Phase IV instruction with a 3–5-s delay until delivery of the requested item, or until a word or vocal approximation was made). • Differentially higher percentage of vocal approximations noted in phases in which the reinforcement for speech was employed (3–5-s delay condition).

(Continued)

TABLE 5.5   (Continued)

Research design (SSED or group)	Study	Participants	Outcome
RCT group comparison	Yoder and Stone (2006a)	36 nonverbal children (18–60 months) with autistic disorder (33) or PDD-NOS (3)	• Both RPMT and PECS had positive effects on communication skills (turn taking, requesting, initiation of joint attention). • The RPMT group learned to take turns and initiate joint attention with an adult better than the PECS group. • The PECS group learned how to make requests more often than RPMT group.
RCT group comparison	Yoder and Stone (2006b)	36 nonverbal children (18–60 months) with autistic disorder or PDD-NOS (3)	• There was growth in both non-imitative, spoken communication acts and the number of words spoken for both PECS and RPMT. • Greater increases in both variables were seen for the PECS group. • The rate of growth in the number of different non-imitative words was faster in the PECS group compared to the RPMT group for children who began at a higher level of object exploration; a faster growth rate was seen in RPMT group than the PECS group for children who began at a lower level of object exploration
SSED multiple baseline design across participants and changing criterion design within participants	Yokoyama et al. (2006)	Three Japanese boys (aged 5, 5;11 and 7;11) with autism, none with functional vocalizations	• All three boys demonstrated acquisition of PECS in Phases I–IV and generalization of use at a distance (from desired object), with a different communicative partner, or after a time delay. • Maintenance of PECS over time was seen at six- or 8-month follow-up for both trained and untrained contexts. • Improvement in intelligibility of vocalizations was observed during PECS training compared to free play. • Intelligible vocalizations during PECS training occurred most frequently when time delay was used. • Verbal behavior acquired during PECS training was under the functional use of the command (all three boys had a high rate of correct responses when offered an item they did not request).

Design	Authors	Participants	Results
SSED A-B-C-D design A: Baseline, observations only B: Baseline, assessment of readiness for intervention C: Compliance training D: PECS training up to Phase IV	Anderson et al. (2007)	Six-year-old boy with severe autism; no functional language, but some echolalic speech	• No mands were observed in the first three phases of the study, but were observed on 12 of 17 days during the PECS training phase. • No verbal initiations (other than mands) were observed during baselines 1 or 2: seven times on the first day of compliance training and once on each of the last 2 days; during PECS training there was an increase in the number of days on which child made initiations and in the rate of initiations each day. • One new word was spoken on baseline 1; 16 new words were spoken on the first day of compliance training (from a single phrase of echolalic speech from TV); once PECS training began, new words were observed on 15 of 17 days, expanding observed spoken vocabulary to 89 words.
Within-subjects measure and between-subjects control group comparison (group membership based on distance from researchers)	Carr and Felce (2007a)	Children with a diagnosis of autism (3–7 years) and no previous PECS teaching beyond Phase I (24 participants in the PECS group, 17 in the control group)	• There was a significant increase in frequency of child-to-adult initiations for the intervention group following PECS training to Phase III; no significant change for the control group between Time 1 and Time 2. • There was a significant increase in child-to-adult linguistic communicative initiations from Time 1 to Time 2 for the PECS group, not for the control group; at Time 2, the frequency of these initiations was significantly greater in the PECS group. • Adult response to child initiations increased significantly from Time 1 to Time 2 for the PECS group, not for control group; frequency of this behavior was significantly greater in the PECS group at Time 2 compared to the control. • There was a significant increase in adult-to-child initiations with opportunity for child response in the control group from Time 1 to Time 2, but not a significant difference in frequency between the groups at Time 2. • Child responses to adult initiations increased significantly from Time 1 to Time 2 in the PECS group, not the control group, and between-group differences were significant at Time 2 (a higher percentage of responding was seen in the PECS group). • There was a significant decrease in adult initiations with no opportunity for the child to respond in the PECS group from Time 1 to Time 2; frequency was significantly lower in the PECS group at Time 2 compared to control.

(Continued)

TABLE 5.5 (Continued)

Research design (SSED or group)	Study	Participants	Outcome
Within-subjects in treatment group and between-subjects control group comparison	Carr and Felce (2007b) *(follow-up to Carr and Felce 2007a)	Children (3–7 years) with autism and no previous PECS teaching beyond Phase I (24 participants in the PECS group, 17 in the control group)	• Results are based on five children in each group who used single words in at least one of the three observations. • Only one of the five children in the control group made slight increases in the total number of words uttered; total word production decreased at Time 2 for all other control group children. • In the PECS group, two children did not produce any words at Time 0 and Time 1 but began producing words following treatment; one child showed a similar increase in words spoken between Times 1 and 2 as between Times 0 and 1; two children showed a decrease in words produced between Times 0 and 1 but then demonstrated an increase following PECS intervention.
RCT group comparison (treatment, delayed treatment, no treatment)	Howlin et al. (2007)	85 children with autism or ASD on the ADOS-G, ages 4–11 years with little or no functional language	• Immediately post-treatment, those children receiving PECS training demonstrated a higher rate of initiations than those who had not and a higher rate of PECS use within the classroom. • At the 10-month follow-up, the immediate treatment group demonstrated a significant reduction in ADOS-G reciprocal social interaction severity scores (there was no effect on the communication severity scores). • There was no significant effect of treatment on the raw scores of standardized language tests (EOWPVT, BPVS).
SSED multiple baseline design across participants	Ganz et al. (2008)	Two boys (aged 4;5 and 3;1) with autism; one girl (age 5;1) with a seizure disorder, significant global delays and autism	• Two of the participants mastered PECS through Phase IV (the third child needed significant modifications and never mastered PECS according to protocol). • PECS resulted in a functional communication system for the two participants who mastered it. • PECS training did not significantly increase expressive speech.

language and use of verbalizations across settings (Kravitz, Kamps et al. 2002), and increased initiations (Carr and Felce 2007a; Howlin, Gordon et al. 2007) for children with ASD using PECS. This intervention appears to be an appropriate strategy for helping preintentional and prelinguistic children at preschool and elementary ages achieve their first steps in communication. More research is needed to demonstrate its effectiveness for older children, the degree to which the completion of all phases enhance outcomes over completion of initial phases only, and the relative efficacy and efficiency of PECS as opposed to more straightforward speech-focused interventions. In addition, more research is needed to learn which children will derive the most benefit from PECS and which will have greater success using other intervention methods. A few studies have made direct comparisons between PECS and other intervention methods. The work of Yoder and Stone (2006a, b), for example, found that PECS was more effective than MCT in eliciting requests from children with little ability to initiate joint attention before treatment, whereas more turn-taking and initiation was seen in children who received MCT when they began intervention with some joint attention behavior. Thus, for PECS, as for all interventions, more needs to be learned to find the most effective match between the child and the selected intervention method.

EARLY LANGUAGE LEVEL

Early Language in Typical Development

Typical children say their first word, on average, at 12–15 months of age. At this age, children also show clear evidence of understanding some words or even simple phrases, responding appropriately to specific words outside the context of routine games (Huttenlocher 1974; Tomasello 1992). During the 12-to 18-month period, there is a gradual increase in both receptive and expressive vocabulary. The words children learn in this period are names for objects and people, usually those on which the child acts (e.g., "daddy," "mommy," "cookie," "ball") and words to describe relationships among objects (e.g., "all gone," "more") (Fenson et al. 1993, 2007). Children also learn social words to be used in rituals such as greetings ("hi," "bye-bye"). First words are generally used to express the same basic functions – regulating others' behavior, attaining social interaction, and establishing joint attention – that were expressed earlier with gestures and vocalizations.

By the age of 18 months, expressive vocabulary size typically reaches an average of about 50–100 words (Fenson et al. 2007; Nelson 1973). This period may be punctuated by many requests from children for adults to label things in the world around them ("Whazzat?") and words are learned very quickly, often after only a single exposure without explicit instruction. This stage marks an important turning point as children are no longer learning via association; instead, they understand the referential nature of words (Nazzi and Bertoncini 2003) and are able to use words to get new information about the world (Halliday 1975). By 16–19 months, infants are able to use nonverbal cues, such as an adult's eye gaze, to make distinctions between an object that an adult is naming and another object that happens to be present (Baldwin 1991), suggesting that they can understand the intentions of others within language contexts. Similar findings for learning words to describe actions have been reported for 2 year-olds (Tomasello 1992; Tomasello and Kruger 1992).

Between 18 and 24 months, typical children begin combining words to form two-word "telegraphic" sentences (Brown 1973) encoding a small set of meanings. Children talk about objects by naming them, and by discussing their locations or attributes, who owns them, and who is doing things to them. They also talk about other people, their actions, their locations, their own actions on objects, and so forth. Objects, people, actions, and their interrelationships preoccupy the young typically developing child. Thus, early language development, from gestures to single words to beginning sentences, reflects both how young children think about the world (e.g., recognition of the coming and going of things and people) and what is important to them (e.g., things that they can act on or interesting events, such as going outside or wiping up a spill).

The period of 18–24 months is also a time of important developments in conversational ability. Children now begin to understand the "conversational obligation" to reply to speech with speech (Chapman 2000). They reliably ask and answer routine questions ("Where's the doggy?" "What's this?" "What's the cow say?") and can genuinely take their own part in a back-and-forth exchange. Individual differences exist among typically developing children, but language development follows a generally consistent pattern, with forms being acquired in order to interact more elaborately with others.

Early Language Development in ASD

Parents' most pressing concerns in the second year of life for children with ASD are typically around speech. Acquisition of first words is usually delayed. Paul et al. (2007b), for example, reported that 36% of children with ASD over the age of two still had no expressive language. Parents may also become concerned at this time because their child learned a few words but never progressed or lost the early words acquired. About 20% of children who end up on the autism spectrum are reported to experience a regression in skills, usually loss of the ability to say words, during their second year (Hoshino et al. 1987; Kobayashi 1993; Kobayashi and Murata 1998; Kurita 1985; Rogers and DiLalla 1990; Tuchman and Rapin 1997). Even when children begin acquiring words, expressive vocabulary size tends to lag about 6 months behind nonverbal mental age for toddlers on the ASD spectrum with both average and delayed nonverbal cognitive development (Paul et al. 2007b).

Children with ASD are also delayed in making the transition to multiword speech. Paul et al. (2007b) reported that even children who had begun using single words and who had, on average, over 100 words in their expressive vocabulary, were not routinely combining words by 28 months of age, even though typically developing children with this expressive vocabulary size do use multiword utterances (Fenson et al. 2007). Children who were not speaking at age two but had acquired some speech by age four were just beginning to combine words in their utterances at the latter age. Moreover, throughout the second and third years of life, children with ASD continue to show deficits in the use of gaze, imitation, joint attention, conventional gestures, attention to speech and faces, and in sharing interests and feelings (Chawarska and Volkmar 2005; Mundy and Burnette 2005; Wetherby et al. 2004).

In addition to showing slow growth in the acquisition of words and word combinations, children with ASD also show some unusual behaviors when they begin speaking. Pronoun reversals may be heard, in which the child says, for example, "You want cookie," when he means he does (Fay 1979). In addition, when children with ASD begin to speak, they may produce *echolalia*, imitations of the speech of others. Both immediate echolalia, repeating just what a speaker says upon hearing it, and delayed echolalia, reproducing learned scripts from television shows or jingles, may be heard. Although typically developing children do some echoing in the early stages of language acquisition (Bloom 1993; Tager-Flusberg and Calkins 1990; Yule and Rutter 1987), it is short-lived and represents a small part of their output. For children with ASD, however, echolalia may serve as the bulk of their speech production and persist long beyond early childhood. Although some instances of echolalia may serve a communicative function (McEvoy et al. 1988; Prizant and Rydell 1984), others appear self-directed and without communicative intent (Tager-Flusberg et al. 2005). However, research does suggest that, as language skills increase, echolalia decreases in children with ASD (McEvoy et al. 1988; Tager-Flusberg and Calkins 1990), just as it does in typical development.

In developing language interventions for children with ASD, then, it is important not only to teach new words and sentence forms, but to provide opportunities and extended practice in using those words and forms to share attention, interests, and feelings with others, and to attend to others' faces, voices, and speech in interactive contexts.

Treatments to Enhance Early Language

As we have seen, once children with ASD begin to use words or other conventional forms to express their intent, challenges remain in the development of communicative competence. Several communication approaches have been designed to improve the maturity with which children with ASD use language forms and to enable more effective communication use. Three intervention strategies with an evidence base for supporting the production of first words and word combinations, using verbal, signed and voice output modes of communication have been selected for review: verbal behavior,

functional communication training, and augmentative alternative communication.

Verbal behavior. This is a traditional Skinnerian approach to intervention that emphasizes verbal imitation through reinforcement. This intervention approach provides a sequenced curriculum for teaching language to children emerging as early communicators through more advanced language forms (Paul and Sutherland 2005). Verbal behavior incorporates a highly structured behavioral approach using techniques such as errorless learning, prompting, fading and DTI in both intensive teaching sessions and in more naturalistic contexts (Sundberg et al. 1995). Language goals include Skinnerian categories of verbal behavior, such as echoes (practice imitating verbal behavior), mands (requests), tacts (labels), reception by feature, function and class (responding to commonly used words), and intraverbals (conversational responses) (Paul and Sutherland 2005). A modest amount of literature exists to support the use of the verbal-behavior approach for acquisition of verbal operants although there is no outcome research to directly support its long-term application to children with autism (Carr and Firth 2005). The lack of generalization to natural settings and unprompted environments as well as the poor imitation ability of many children with ASD create some notable challenges for interventionists implementing this approach to communication. Table 5.6 presents a series of recent studies that provide evidence supporting the verbal-behavior approach to increase verbal production in children with ASD. Some studies have examined the use of verbal behavior to increase vocalizations and sound productions with varying results; in one study, production increased during treatment and returned to baseline after treatment (Miguel et al. 2002). In another, no increases in target vocalizations were observed (Normand and Knoll 2006). In a third, increased vocalizations in response

TABLE 5.6 Studies designed to improve communication in individuals with ASD using a verbal-behavior approach

Research design (SSED or group)	Study	Participants	Outcome
SSED simultaneous treatment design with probes before and after treatment in each phase	Partington et al. (1994)	Six-year-old girl with autism	• *Phase 1 (objects):* When the verbal stimulus was changed from "What is that?" to saying the child's name and pointing to an object in a box, she acquired the tacts in both correction procedures (imitative: experimenter producing the sign; and intraverbal: experimenter saying "Say X"); acquisition was slightly faster in the imitative condition. • When the verbal stimulus "What is that?" was reintroduced in the final phase, performance decreased and child produced her stereotypic response – verbal stimulus blocked the establishment of nonverbal stimulus control. • *Phase 2 (pictures):* Criterion was met faster with the verbal presentation "What is that?" versus saying the child's name and pointing to the picture. • Fewer prompts were required for the "What's that?" condition and, overall, for Phase 2 compared to Phase 1. • When a delay procedure was introduced, the child quickly acquired tacts for pictures and objects, although acquisition was faster for objects; in the final sessions of this phase all tacts occurred solely under the control of the nonverbal stimuli.
Descriptive case study	Drash et al. (1999)	Three nonverbal boys (ages 2;6 to 3;6) with autism	• Mand repertoire (90% responses to prompts) was acquired by all children by Session 6; children received preferred reinforcers for appropriate vocalizations only in response to a preferred toy or food item just out of the child's reach. • Echoic repertoire of 70% accuracy (on four or more sounds and nine or more words) was acquired by Session 7 for all children. • Two children began to tact toys and picture cards by Session 10. • The percentage of no response or inappropriate behavior significantly decreased as the percentage of reinforced mand and echoic responses increased for two children (this behavior remained low for the third child throughout training sessions).

Study	Design	Participants	Findings
Sundberg et al. (2000)	SSED multi-element design with a between-subjects replication	Two boys (4 and 5 years old) with autism	• Participants acquired sign tacts in the intraverbal prompt condition ("Say [name of object]") to criterion; these responses stabilized throughout treatment and were maintained. • Participants did not acquire tacts in the standard prompt procedure ("What is that?"). • When objects trained in the intraverbal condition were presented in the standard condition, responses deteriorated; when object trained in the standard procedure were presented with the intraverbal prompt, tacting immediately improved. • Both participants acquired pure tacts and eventually were able to respond to the traditional prompt ("What is that?").
Finkel and Williams (2001)	SSED multiple baseline design across stimuli (three sets of questions)	Six-year-old boy with autism who had few intraverbal skills and did not answer direct questions	• Full-sentence answers were not given for three sets of questions during baselines for the echoic prompt fading procedure or textual prompt fading procedure. • Following introduction of the echoic prompt fading procedure, improvements in correct partial responses were seen for all three sets of questions; behavior was maintained and increased slightly during post-fading and follow-up for two sets of questions, while third set saw a decrease. • Following implementation of the textual prompt fading procedure, immediate increases in the number of questions answered correctly using full-sentence responses and partial responses were seen for all three sets of questions; these levels were maintained throughout post-fading and follow-up.
Miguel et al. (2002)	SSED multiple baseline design across vocal behaviors with a reversal to baseline	Three boys (3–5 years old) with autism	• Increase in production of target sounds following a stimulus–stimulus pairing procedure seen for both target sounds for one child, one of two sounds for another child, and neither sound for third child. • Increased rates of production returned to baseline levels following termination of the intervention.

(Continued)

TABLE 5.6 (Continued)

Research design (SSED or group)	Study	Participants	Outcome
SSED multiple baseline and multi-element design with a between-subject replication	Sundberg et al. (2002)	• Study 1: two boys with autism (5 and 6 years old) who were not using the "where?" mand • Study 2: two boys with autism (6 and 8 years old, one from Study 1, but a year later) who were using the "where?" mand but not the "who?" mand	Study 1: • Following intervention both participants acquired the "where?" mand to criterion (100% over two sessions), one child in five sessions the other in eight sessions. • Children acquired the mand faster for more desirable than less desirable items. • One participant generalized manding to two desirable untrained objects, but not to two less desirable untrained objects; the other participant did not generalize to any untrained objects. • Eventually both participants were able to mand for undesirable objects. Study 2: • Participants acquired the "who?" mand following three and five training sessions. • One participant demonstrated a chain of three mands (where, who, and requesting the object) in the experimental context. • Neither participant showed a differential amount of manding between desired and undesired objects.
SSED with two multiple baseline designs, across three participants with a 3-month follow-up and a multiple baseline design across two participants	Ross and Greer (2003)	Five children (ages 5;5 to 7;8) with autism, who did not spontaneously vocalize nor imitate vocal speech	• Mand training during baseline was unsuccessful at eliciting mands from any of the five participants. • When children participated in rapid imitation of modeled motor behaviors during treatment prior to vocal imitation, generalized vocal imitation was observed for all five participants. • Vocal imitation of words and subsequent mands were taught using a fading procedure (an opportunity to respond without imitation of motor behavior was immediately followed by an opportunity to respond with no vocal model). • Immediate follow-up and 3-month probes demonstrated that four of the five children continued to mand.

SSED multiple baseline design across three sets of 10 tacts (behaviors)	Barbera and Kubina (2005)	Seven-year-old boy with moderate autism and mild intellectual disability	• Participant did not make any correct tacts for any of the three sets during baseline. • Following a receptive to echoic to tact procedure with picture cards of objects appropriate for his age, the participant learned 30 tacts over 60 teaching sessions (the three sets were staggered; criterion for a set was 100% for three consecutive days). • Child consistently increased number of tacts correctly produced after the 5-min teaching sessions were introduced.
Descriptive case study	Hartman and Klatt (2005)	Two boys (age 2;6) diagnosed with autism; could echo a few words but did not mand to obtain tangible objects	• One child learned to mand faster for toys that he did not have access to for 23 h before the session versus those that he got to play with for 5 min pre-session following a stimulus-pairing procedure. • The same child acquired mands in only slightly fewer sessions for highly preferred toys versus those preferred at medium or low levels. • The other child's acquisition of mands was determined more by preference level than the 23-h deprivation vs. five min. pre-session exposure, but data was not robust. • One child did not learn to mand at all in the less effective establishing operations condition; the other child still acquired mands, but at a much slower rate than his more motivating establishing operations.
SSED multiple baseline design across two target phonemes	Normand and Knoll (2006)	Three-year-old boy with autism	• No increase in target vocalizations ("ah" and "ee") was seen in the stimulus-pairing condition either immediately post-session or at a 60-min follow-up. • Three inexplicable observations of high-vocalization follow-up sessions were observed, one in baseline and two during intervention.

(Continued)

TABLE 5.6 (Continued)

Research design (SSED or group)	Study	Participants	Outcome
SSED multiple baseline design across participants	Yi et al. (2006)	Three children (two boys, one girl), 8 to 11 years old and diagnosed with autism	• All three participants engaged in challenging behavior 100% of the time when an undesired item was presented in baseline (no child-produced mands). • Manding increased and challenging behaviors decreased during mand training with time delay and physical prompting, although levels were variable. • During the mixed presentation (block presentation of three non-preferred items) and random rotation (randomized presentation of three items) phase manding reached 100% and challenging behaviors 0% for two of the three participants; challenging behavior remained at or below 20% for the third child. • Generalization to non-preferred untrained items was seen for all three participants.
SSED multiple probe design across three semantic categories	Goldsmith et al. (2007)	Three boys (4 to 7 years old) with autism	• All three children acquired the targeted intraverbal repertoires with varying trials to criterion. • Faster acquisition was observed with subsequently trained categories compared to the first. • Generalization to a fourth untrained category and maintenance effects were limited.
SSED multiple baseline across responses	Kelley et al. (2007)	Three boys with developmental disabilities; the participant of interest is a boy (aged 10;10) with autism	*Results for the participant with autism:* • Low levels of tacting and manding observed in baseline. • Tact training produced tacting on 100% of trials for all three responses in the first set; "tune" and "chocolate" generalized during mand generalization assessment but he never acquired manding for "book." • Tacting and manding acquired following training for all three words in the second set; mand training only generalized to tacting for one of three words; tacting for the other two words acquired immediately following initiation of tact training. • Mand training did not generalize to tacting for the last two words.

SSED multiple baseline design across behaviors	Sweeney-Kerwin et al. (2007)	Two boys (3 and 7 years old) with autism	• Both participants demonstrated baseline levels of motivating operation (MO) controlled mands of zero mands per session. • Following introduction of a rolling time-delay procedure, both participants began using MO controlled mands within the first session or after one experimental session. • Fading of stimulus item reflected a transfer of the stimulus control of the participants' manding repertoire from the control of a discriminative stimulus and an MO to an MO and a listener.
SSED multiple probe design across sounds (stimuli) and participants	Ward et al. (2007)	Two girls with autism (3;4 and 3;5 years)	• Occurrences of target vocalizations increased immediately from baseline when they were paired with desirable stimuli. • Development of correct echoic production of the first sound trained was much slower than the second sound for one child (presumably because of the history of learning from the first sound).

to desirable stimuli were seen (Ward et al. 2007). Generally positive results have been reported for the increased use of tacts in response to pictures or objects (Barbera and Kubina 2005; Partington et al. 1994) as well as increased use of mands and echoics with decreases in inappropriate behaviors (Drash et al. 1999; Yi et al. 2006), especially when mand training was focused on acquiring desired items (Hartman and Klatt 2005; Ross and Greer 2003; Sundberg, Loeb et al. 2002). Sundberg et al. (2000) also reported an increase in signed tacts that were maintained following intervention with children successfully responding to "What's that?" Research investigating verbal behavior has also probed the use of partial and full sentences that were maintained in response to questions (Finkel and Williams 2001) contrasted with increased use of intraverbals but limited maintenance (Goldsmith et al. 2007).

Functional communication training. The deficits children with ASD experience in their speech and language often contribute to their challenging behavior and can become a primary mode for communicating wants and needs. Functional communication training (FCT) is a systematic intervention in which a child's challenging behavior is replaced by more socially appropriate behavior, presuming the challenging behavior is an attempt to communicate a particular intent. Frequently the replacement behavior includes vocalizations, manual signs and gestures or graphic symbols. FCT is often used in combination with other interventions such as speech-generating devices (SGDs) as described in Tables 5.7 and 5.8 (Durand 1999; Olive et al. 2008). A recent review indicated that FCT leads to a decrease in challenging behaviors with a corresponding increase in communication in children with ASD (Mancil, Conroy et al. 2006). As presented in Table 5.7, FCT results in significant changes in aberrant behavior following functional analysis and the replacement of

challenging behavior with more appropriate communication responses including mands (Brown et al. 2000; ÓNeill and Sweetland-Baker 2001) and increased spontaneous and more appropriate verbal communication (Mancil et al. 2006; Ross 2002). These results are typically maintained (Casey and Merical 2006) and generalize to untrained activities (Olive et al. 2008; Wacker et al. 2005). It should be noted that, unlike verbal behavior and the programs at the prelinguistic level that aim to expand the range of communicative intents expressed by children with ASD, FCT focuses only on the expression of regulatory intentions and does not include aims to expand the functions of the child's communicative behaviors. Its use, in addition, is confined to those students who evidence maladaptive forms of communication.

Augmentative alternative communication – voice output devices and sign. Several systematic research reviews have been done in the last 10 years examining the evidence for the use of augmentative alternative communication (AAC) to support the communication needs of children with autism spectrum disorders who have limited speech production. These reviews have focused on the use of signs, as well as on aided and unaided systems including voice output communication aids (VOCAs) or devices. The results have been mixed for facilitating speech production in children with ASD with earlier reviews indicating little improvement (Schlosser and Blischak 2001) and more recent reviews reporting modest gains (Millar et al. 2006; Schlosser and Wendt 2008). The research has also reported variable results for ease of learning and using manual signs versus aided AAC approaches, although children with autism who demonstrate adequate fine motor and verbal imitation abilities are seen as good candidates for using total communication approaches that target speech development (Mirenda 2003). The literature also suggests that aided communication techniques have

TABLE 5.7 Studies designed to improve communication in individuals with ASD using functional communication training

Research design (SSED or group)	Study	Participants	Outcome
SSED multiple baseline across participants	Durand (1999)	Five children (aged 3;6 to 15); two with autism (aged 9;6 and 11;6)	• All children demonstrated unprompted communication in the classroom following functional communication training with vocal output communication devices, after not using the devices at all before FCT. • None of the participants used their devices in the community before FCT, but all used it to some extent without prompting outside the classroom following FCT. • All five children demonstrated reductions in problem behavior inside and outside the classroom following FCT in the classroom.
SSED multiple baseline across behaviors	Braithwaite and Richdale (2000)	Seven-year-old boy with autism and intellectual disability	• Reductions in target behaviors occurred in both access to preferred objects and escape conditions. • Corresponding increase in target phrase (requesting) was also observed.
SSED alternating treatments	Brown et al. (2000)	Four children (5–13 years old) with multiple disabilities; one child (7 years old) with autism and severe intellectual disability and possible seizure disorder; one child (5 years old) with PDD and moderate intellectual disability	• FCT used different mands across conditions: establishing operation (EO) that was relevant to the function of the aberrant behavior; one condition in which EO was absent, and play condition. • Mands used in the EO-present condition served the same function as aberrant behavior and a corresponding decrease in frequency of aberrant behavior was observed across all contexts. • Mands used in the EO-absent context served a different function than the ones identified in the functional analysis. • Increases in relevant mands were observed in the EO-present condition for three of the children. • Low levels of manding were observed in the play context.
Case study	Durand and Merges (2001)	11 ½-year-old boy with autism and severe mental retardation	• Following a month of FCT on a communication device, the participant's self-injurious behavior was reduced dramatically in the classroom and he appropriately used the device to ask for help.
SSED multiple probe across three communicative functions	Keen et al. (2001)	Four children with autism (3;7 to 7;7 years old)	• Intervention was associated with a reduction in prelinguistic behaviors and an increase in replacement behaviors for all four children.

(Continued)

TABLE 5.7 (Continued)

Research design (SSED or group)	Study	Participants	Outcome
SSED multiple baseline across participants	Óneill and Sweetland-Baker (2001)	Two boys (6 and 15 years old) with autism	• Decreases in disruptive behavior and increases in unprompted requesting to take a break were seen in the initially trained tasks compared to baseline. • Results were generalized to some untrained tasks; once FCT and escape extinction was introduced in these tasks, levels of disruptive behavior were near zero for both participants.
SSED reversal design (A–B–A)	Ross (2002)	Two girls, one boy with autism (9;0 to 14;10 years old)	• Functional analysis indicated that attention was maintaining faulty responses (delayed echolalia, perseverative responses, unusually lengthy or brief responses). • Faulty responses decreased immediately following introduction of FCT. • Correct responses and conversational exchanges increased and were maintained during reversal to baseline and subsequent probe sessions.
SSED alternating treatments	Solis et al. (2003)	Twelve-year-old boy with autism and developmental delays	• Functional analysis indicated that problem behaviors were maintained by escape. • FCT reduced rate of aberrant behaviors.
Descriptive case study	Fisher et al. (2005)	Two girls (13 and 14 years old) with autism	• Behavior was maintained by escape from demand for participant 1 and by attention and escape from certain tasks for participant 2. • Participant 1 consistently chose positive reinforcement in both restricted choice (when she could only choose one) and unrestricted choice (when she could choose one or the other or both) conditions, therefore positive reinforcement lessened her motivation to escape demands. • Participant 2 only decreased destructive behavior when punishment was introduced; she did not consistently prefer one type of reinforcement over the other.
SSED A–B–C	Martin et al. (2005)	Ten year-old nonverbal boy with autism	• FCT was successful at teaching the child to reject items by touching an icon instead of pushing them away. • Intervention had little effect on other problem behaviors that were used for rejecting.
SSED adapted concurrent multiple baseline across settings	Schindler and Horner (2005)	Three children with autism (4–5 years old)	• FCT was successful at reducing problem behaviors in the three participants in the primary training setting; did not initially generalize to secondary settings. • When low-effort intervention was introduced in these settings following FCT in the primary setting, problem behaviors were reduced and competing behaviors (functional communication skills) increased; the low-effort intervention was not effective at reducing problem behaviors in the secondary settings before FCT was introduced in the primary setting.

Design	Citation	Participants	Results
Five-phase lon-gitudinal design (5-year period) with embedded SSED multiple probe	Wacker et al. (2005)	23 children (aged 1;4 to 6;6) with developmental delays and problem behaviors; five with PDD, one with autism	• Total problem behavior in the sample was reduced by 83% on average following functional analysis and FCT carried out by parent. • Generalization of these results was seen across persons, settings, and tasks.
SSED multiple baseline across classrooms	Casey and Merical (2006)	11-year-old male with autism	• Self-injurious behavior was low during the first phase of treatment but the child only used the target verbal response once. • When gestural response was introduced into the classroom, self-injurious behavior decreased to zero in the classroom in which treatment was taking place for 3 days. • When treatment was introduced in a second classroom there was an increase in self-injurious behavior and communication in both classrooms in which intervention was taking place; by the end of each class period, he exclusively used communication. • Intervention was introduced into a third classroom and self-injurious behavior remained low in all three classrooms associated with FCT. • There were no changes in self-injurious behavior in any classrooms where intervention was not taking place. • Follow-up at 5, 12, and 24 months revealed no occurrences of self-injurious behavior.
SSED multiple baseline across mands	Mancil et al. (2006)	Four-year-old boy with PDD	• Tantrums decreased to zero during mand training. • Spontaneous verbalizations increased from 38 to 50 words. • Communication (measured by the number of spontaneous verbalizations and latency to respond during training) increased and aberrant behavior decreased in the home setting following FCT in the home; child also began using two- and three-word combinations. • Generalization from experimenter to mother and across tangible objects (which were maintaining the tantrums) occurred.
SSED mul-tiple probe across activities	Olive et al. (2008)	Four year-old girl with ASD	• There was an immediate decline in challenging behavior following implementation of FCT with a VOCA. • Requesting increased in activities in which FCT and VOCA intervention was implemented, and this behavior generalized to untrained activities. • An increase in correct pronoun use was observed following intervention.

TABLE 5.8 Studies designed to improve communication in individuals with ASD using augmentative and alternative communication approaches

Research design (SSED or group)	Study	Participants	Outcome
SSED interactional experimental design, both additive (A–B–BC–B–BC) and reductive (A–BC–B–BC–B)	Parsons and La Sorte (1993)	Six children (five males, one female) with autism (4;8 to 6;8 years old)	• Computer-assisted communication intervention alone did not increase spontaneous verbalizations over baseline. • Frequency of spontaneous utterances increased for all participants when synthesized speech was added; when synthesized speech was removed, a marked decrease in spontaneous utterances occurred. • Results were seen in both the additive and reductive designs (three participants in each); number of spontaneous utterances increased from baseline to computer with synthesized speech condition, and decreased to baseline levels when synthesized speech was removed.
SSED multiple probe design across time and across two participants in two classroom routines (snack and play), and two participants in one routine (snack)	Schepis et al. (1998)	Four children (3–5 years old) with autism	• All participants increased their communicative interactions during Voice Output Communication Aid (VOCA) and naturalistic teaching intervention compared to baseline in a snack and play routine. • There was no decrease in non-VOCA communicative behaviors (gestures, nonword vocalizations, words) during intervention; behaviors increased slightly in VOCA conditions, except for word vocalizations; only one child demonstrated increased word vocalizations. • No child-to-child interactions were observed in baseline or intervention for three of the children and seven occurrences were observed for the fourth child in the VOCA snack condition. • Interactions observed in the intervention condition were rated as appropriate for all children by classroom staff and unfamiliar observers. • Communicative intents expressed through VOCA use included requesting, responding to questions, and social commenting.
SSED multiple baseline design across participants	Durand (1999)	Five children, two with autism (9½ and 11½ years old)	• All children demonstrated unprompted communication in the classroom following functional communication training with vocal output communication devices. • All five children demonstrated reductions in problem behavior in and outside the classroom following FCT using voice output devices. • None of the participants used their devices in the community before FCT, but all used it to some extent without prompting outside the classroom following FCT.

Design	Author	Participants	Results
Case study	Brady (2000)	Five-year-old female with autism	• Following VOCA instruction to request objects or actions, the participant learned six symbols in requesting routines. • After learning to select the graphic symbols for six target objects with the VOCA, comprehension for the object names increased to 100%.
Case study: pictures in the classroom setting	Cafiero (2001)	Thirteen-year-old African American male with autism (non-verbal)	• Student increased his functional vocabulary from four to 29 pictures following implementation of natural aided language with interactive language boards by staff. • Following intervention, the student initiated with picture symbols; motor imitation was observed prior to intervention. • Student began combining pictures following intervention.
SSED multiple baseline across two groups of children and three activities	DiCarlo et al. (2001)	12 children (15 to 36 months old) with developmental disabilities (Down syndrome, autism, cerebral palsy)	• Increases in the use of manual signs by toddlers with and without disabilities were observed during the signing condition (teacher added the use of manual signs to her verbalizations and labeling with a VOCA to highlight key words during an art activity in the classroom) versus the control condition (verbalizations and VOCA use by the teacher). • No decreases in verbalizations observed for either group of toddlers in the signing condition compared to the control condition. • VOCA use among toddlers was infrequent throughout study.
SSED multiple probe across participants	Johnston et al. (2003)	Three males, ages 4;3, 5;3, and 5;1years with autism or PDD	• All three children were taught to use symbolic communication (a graphic symbol – Mayer Johnson picture for "Can I play?" – or verbal language) to gain entrance to play activities and increased their percentage of correct use of symbolic communication (e.g., graphic symbol or graphic symbol and verbalization) to gain entrance into play activities following intervention. • Results were maintained and generalized to untrained activities.
SSED multiple baseline across participants	Sigafoos et al. (2003)	Three males, ages 3, 4, and 13 years old; two with severe autism, one with Leber's Congenital Amaurosis and demonstrating autistic-like behaviors	• No participants purposefully activated a speech-generating device (SGD) programmed to produce "I want more" during baseline. • All three children acquired ten unprompted requests with the SGD that were maintained post-acquisition phases, both when speech output was turned ON and when it was turned OFF; access to the desired objects facilitated maintenance of SGD use. • One participant increased the number of vocalizations from baseline to post-acquisition phases; the other two participants maintained similar levels of vocalizations throughout the study; thus, SGD use did not inhibit vocalizations.

(Continued)

TABLE 5.8 (Continued)

Research design (SSED or group)	Study	Participants	Outcome
SSED multiple baseline across participants	Sigafoos et al. (2004)	16-year-old male with PDD-NOS; 20-year-old female with autism, intellectual disability, and severe bilateral hearing loss	• Neither participant used a VOCA to initiate a request or repair a breakdown during baseline. • During intervention, both participants independently used the VOCA within 10 s of an ignored initial response to repair the communication breakdown 80–100% of the time. • Both participants also began using the VOCAs alone and in combination with behavioral indications to initiate requests. • One participant went back to the use of behavioral indications (e.g., pointing, gesturing, moving toward object) to make initial requests by the end of the study but consistently used the VOCA to correct communication repairs. • The other participant relied exclusively on her VOCA to make initial requests by the end of intervention and consistently used it to repair breakdowns.
SSED alternating treatments followed by best-treatment phase (most effective training modality)	Tincani (2004)	5;10 African American male with diagnoses of autism and mental retardation 6;8 Asian American female diagnosed with autism	• More vocalizations seen for both participants in sign language training compared to PECS I training. • Procedural modification to PECS system increased girl's vocalization to a level similar to that in sign language training. • A higher number of requests for preferred items (using the augmentative system) was seen in the PECS training phase.
SSED alternating treatments	Preis (2006)	Five children (three girls, two boys) between 5 and 7 years old diagnosed with autism	• There was no significant difference in command acquisition between the two conditions (commands presented with or without picture symbols). • Generalization of acquired commands to a novel examiner was greater (with border-line significance) when examiner presented child with a picture symbol versus a verbal directive alone. • Participants retained a significantly greater number of commands in the treatment phase that used pictures to support commands.

Design	Author	Participants	Findings
SSED alternating treatments	Son et al. (2006)	Two children with autism and one child with PDD, ages 3;8, 5;5	• Acquisition rates (measured by correct requesting) for VOCA and picture exchange were similar. • Two children showed consistent preference for picture exchange and the third showed preference for VOCA. • Level of proficiency with their respective AAC systems following intervention was consistent with that during intervention (maintenance).
SSED multiple probe across participants	Olive et al. (2007)	Two children with autism, one child with PDD-NOS, 45–66 months	• All children increased VOCA use during intervention targeting VOCA use through enhanced milieu teaching. • All children increased their total spontaneous requests during intervention (combination of independent VOCA use, gestures, verbal communication); only one child began vocalizing during the study.
SSED adapted alternating treatments across participants	Schlosser et al. (2007)	Five children, ages 8–10 years, with autism (four boys, one girl)	• Two children requested more accurately in the treatment condition in which a speech-generating device with speech output was provided. • One child requested more effectively in the treatment condition in which a speech-generating device without speech output was provided (the speech output was turned off and the child told it was broken, but used the same method of requesting as the speech output condition, by pushing the keys). • The remaining two children demonstrated similar levels of accurate requesting in the speech vs. no-speech conditions. • Only one child demonstrated limited increase in elicited vocalizations.
Mixed methods case study analysis of four participants in one or two activities	Thunberg et al. (2007)	Two boys with autism and two boys with PDD-NOS, ages 4;11 to 7;6	• Introduction of a speech-generating device resulted in an increase in communication effectiveness (measured by partner response to participants) in three different home activities (mealtime, story reading, sharing experiences of the preschool day). • The greatest increase in communicative effectiveness was seen in sharing experiences of the preschool day; smallest increase in mealtime.
SSED multiple probe across activities	Olive et al. (2008)	Four year-old girl with ASD	• There was an immediate decline in challenging behavior following implementation of FCT with a VOCA. • Requesting increased in activities in which FCT and VOCA intervention was implemented, and this behavior generalized to untrained activities. • An increase in correct pronoun use was observed following intervention.

(Continued)

TABLE 5.8 (Continued)

Research design (SSED or group)	Study	Participants	Outcome
Systematic review: SSED and RCT	Schlosser and Wendt (2008)	• Nine SSEDs with 27 participants (23 males, four females), 37 to 144 months (mean 81 months), with autism • Two RCTs, 98 participants with autism, mean age of 60 months and 33 months in the two studies	• No study reported a decline in speech production following AAC intervention (PECS, VOCAs, manual signs). • Most studies reported modest gains in speech production following intervention.

an advantage of making fewer memory and cognitive demands on learners and foster ease of use with communication partners. Specifically, VOCAs and computers with communication software have been used to support the communication of students in school settings (Mirenda 2003) although more research is needed regarding the use of VOCAs in community and home settings. Table 5.8 provides a summary of intervention studies completed in the last 15 years that used symbolic communication in the form of pictures, graphic symbols and signs or voice output devices to facilitate object comprehension, requesting, communication repairs and spontaneous communication in children with ASD between 15 months and 13 years of age. As indicated in the reported outcomes, studies using computer assistance demonstrate improvement in comprehension, increases in requesting, unprompted spontaneous verbalizations and effective communicative interactions (Durand 1999; Olive et al. 2008; Parsons and LaSorte 1993; Schepis et al. 1998; Sigafoos et al. 2003, 2004; Thunberg et al. 2007) without decreases in other gesture and verbal communication. The use of speech-generating devices, in particular, appears to have the most consistent evidence for positive communication support that leads to spontaneous initiations and requests, and repair of communication breakdowns that are maintained post-treatment (Olive et al. 2007; Sigafoos et al. 2003; Thunberg et al. 2007).

THE ACQUISITION OF LANGUAGE

Basic Language Acquisition in Typical Development

The preschool period (from 2 to 5 years old) is the time during which the child's language evolves from simple telegraphic utterances to fully grammatical forms. In addition to rapidly acquiring new vocabulary, the child also goes through a process of approximating more and more closely the grammar of the language spoken in the home. There is evidence of the child's active role as a hypothesis-generator in the frequent occurrence of overgeneralized forms, such as "goed," "comed," and "mouses" (Cazden 1968). These errors are taken as evidence that the child is indeed acquiring a rule-governed system, rather than learning these inflections by imitation or on a word-by-word basis.

As the child's grammar becomes more complex, sentence length increases (Brown 1973; Loban 1976; Miller and Chapman 1981) and children begin to use a variety of sentence forms including statements, negation, and questions. As structures in simple sentences approach the adult model, complex sentences using embedded clauses ("Whoever wins can go first") and conjoined clauses ("Then it broke and we didn't have it any more") emerge (Miller 1981). The abilities to encode ideas grammatically ("Daddy's shoe" vs. "Daddy shoe") and to relate ideas within one utterance ("I'll go get it if you give me a bite of your candy") free the child's language from dependence on nonlinguistic contexts for interpretation. Whereas an adult has to use knowledge of the child and the situation to interpret "Daddy shoe" (The shoe that belongs to Daddy? Daddy put on the shoe?), the morphologically marked "Daddy's shoe" is unambiguous and interpretable by anyone.

In addition to changing their use of grammatical form, children between three and 5 years of age also change the ideas that they express in their sentences. Earlier utterances generally describe actions and objects that are immediately present. During later preschool years, sentence content expands to allow for reference to events that are remote in time and space. Children begin to use their language in more diverse ways (Dore 1978) to include imaginative, nonliteral, interpretive, and logical functions.

At this time, a variety of more advanced conversational and other discourse skills emerge and become refined. Children increase their ability to maintain and add new information to the conversational topic; to clarify and request clarification of misunderstood utterances; to make their requests or comments using polite or indirect forms; and to choose the appropriate speech style on the basis of the speaker's role and the listener's status (Bates 1976). Children also begin to engage in different types of discourse, including story-telling, recounting events, and personal narratives, all of which follow cultural conventions for these diverse genres of linguistic reporting.

Although children have acquired most of the sentence structure of their language by age five, syntactic development continues into the school years as children learn devices for elaborating their utterances, expressing co-reference relations using pronouns (e.g., "When Mom wakes up, she'll help me dress"), and for condensing more information into each sentence by increasing the proportion of dependent clauses (Loban 1976). Children also gradually learn to use and to comprehend the more complex, optional sentence types in their language, such as passives ("The boy was hit by the car"; Lempert 1978). They learn to use syntactic cues not only to decode semantic relations within sentences but also to identify the connections between sentence elements and those given previously in the discourse (Paul 1985). Semantic and conversational abilities also continue to develop during the school years. Vocabulary size is still increasing and new words are learned from reading as well as from conversation. School-aged children gradually acquire the ability to communicate with precision, to take the listener's viewpoint into account in formulating an utterance, and to tell more complex well-structured narratives (Peterson and McCabe 1983).

Basic Language Acquisition in Children with ASD

Although they begin to speak late and show slow growth in language during the preschool period, most children with ASD do develop some functional use of spoken language. Unlike children with typical acquisition, they may go through an extended period of echolalic speech and echolalia may persist even when spontaneous use emerges. There are few longitudinal studies of language acquisition among verbal children with autism to describe in detail the course of their language acquisition. However, the research that does exist suggests that during the preschool years, progress within each domain of language (e.g., vocabulary, syntax) follows pathways similar to those seen in typically developing children (Tager-Flusberg et al. 1990). Tager-Flusberg (1995) has identified the basic pattern of language development in children with ASD, characterizing it as showing a dissociation between form and function. That is, when children with ASD begin to talk, they show development generally consistent with overall mental age in the areas of syntax (sentence structure), morphology (word structure), and phonology (pronunciation), with prominent deficits in the areas of pragmatics (appropriate use of language) and prosody (the musical aspects of language, including intonation, rhythm, and emphasis that convey meaning above and beyond words and sentences). There may be certain classes of words that are under-represented in the vocabularies of children with autism, including mental states (think, know, remember, pretend) and social–emotional terms (Hobson and Lee 1989; Tager-Flusberg 1992) but, for most speakers with ASD, vocabulary size is a relative strength. Tager-Flusberg and Joseph (2003) found that there is a subset of speakers with ASD who show patterns of language development that are similar to those seen in developmental language disorders, with persistent deficits relative to mental age expectations in syntax and morphology, but in most cases speakers with ASD will show relatively preserved language form (syntax, morphology, phonology) with significant problems in language function (pragmatics and prosody), or the ability to use language to accomplish social goals. Thus, interventions for speakers with ASD must aim not only to expand vocabulary and sentence structure but also to focus intensely on developing social uses of language and conversational skills.

Treatments to Advance Language Development

Because of the centrality of language development in general, and social language use in particular, in the successful adaptation of children with ASD, a variety of programs have been developed and marketed that purport to address these areas of disability. One example from an ABA framework is *Teach Me Language* (Freeman and Dake 1997), a comprehensive curriculum with guidelines and intervention activities that support the development of grammar, syntax, and narrative skills. The program also addresses social language, general knowledge, advanced language and academic concepts. Methods employed include table-based activities, modeling of correct responses, repetition of language drills, visual and auditory instructions, and cuing strategies. Although a popular curriculum, no evidence has yet been published to support the use of *Teach Me Language*.

Another popular intervention for verbal children with high-functioning autism and Asperger syndrome is ILAUGH (Winner 2000, 2002). This is a "social thinking" approach designed to help individuals with ASD understand the relationship between social interaction and problem solving. The program focuses on (Winner 2002, 2004, 2005, 2007): (1) *Initiating language (I)* to

seek assistance or information; (2) *Listening with Eyes and Brain (L)* to encourage integration of visual and auditory information in order to decide whether messages should be interpreted literally; (3) *Abstract and Inferential Language/Communication (A)* which focuses on gleaning meaning from both verbal and nonverbal cues and context; (4) *Understanding Perspective (U)* which works on taking another's point of view; (5) *Gestalt Processing/Getting the Big Picture (G)* in order to help children see the "forest" of meaning and not just the "trees" of literal detail; and, (6) *Humor and Human Relatedness (H)* to foster a sense of humor and minimize anxiety (Winner 2002, 2004, 2005, 2007). In contrast to the behavioral framework and focus on language structure used in *Teach Me Language*, the *ILAUGH* approach attempts to teach pragmatic principles through meta-linguistic and meta-cognitive strategies. Like *Teach Me Language*, however, the *ILAUGH* approach has yet to establish any empirical evidence to demonstrate its efficacy.

Other intervention strategies that facilitate more advanced language use and have a research base to support their implementation for children with ASD are available to practitioners. Three of these with the most extensive empirical data (script fading, Social Stories, and video modeling) are described here. These programs are also noteworthy for their accessibility to practitioners and the broad range of communicative skills that they address.

Scripting and fading. Children engaged in early routines (e.g., getting ready for bed) develop an understanding of predictable sequences of events and the language (what is said or talked about) used at particular points in the event (Nelson 1973; Prelock 2006). Over time, they internalize a mental script, or *schema*, that represents the actions, actors, words, and props involved in familiar routines. Children often learn scripts not only through observation but through explicit adult guidance

(Goodman, Duchan, and Sonnenmeier 1994); using scripts facilitates the ability to communicate (Nelson 1973).

Intervention for developing script knowledge and use involves providing perceptual supports (e.g., relevant objects, written text, picture sequences, and audio recordings) to represent relevant aspects of an event and practice in reenacting scripts with decreasing levels of external support. Sonnenmeier (1994) recommends setting up the environment with the appropriate props and then introducing the theme of the script as a play topic (e.g., a doctor's office). The adult assigns each participant a role in the event structure (e.g., patient) and the child with ASD practices that role by relying on pictured or written cues and props. Other roles (e.g., doctor or nurse) may be assigned, initially to the adult and later to typically developing peers. Over time, roles are switched so the target child gains experiences with multiple roles within the event structure, and the script is reenacted numerous times with decreasing support from the adult and increasing involvement with typical peers. Krantz and McClannahan (1998) showed that fading scripts, by gradually removing increasingly larger chunks of the external support, that is, literally cutting off portions of a written script, was effective in leading to unscripted interactions and generalization to new topics among children with ASD and peers. Table 5.9 highlights a range of studies that utilize this technique and the outcomes reported. Scripting and fading has been used successfully to increase initiations and bids for joint attention (Krantz and McClannahan 1993; MacDuff et al. 2007), to increase scripted statements about trained and untrained stimuli (Sarokoff et al. 2001), to increase and maintain scripted, elaborated and unscripted interactions across participants and settings (Charlop-Christy and Kelso 2003; Krantz and McClannahan 1998; Stevenson et al. 2000), and to

generalize conversational interactions to community settings (Brown et al. 2008) in children with ASD between three and 13 years old. McClannahan and Krantz (2005) have provided a detailed guide to the use of these evidence-based techniques, including procedures for addressing communication from the prelinguistic level up through procedures that are appropriate for fluent readers. These activities apply scripting and fading to basic interactions through words and VOCAs, more complex conversations, peer interactions, and problem solving.

Social Stories. Social Stories incorporate directions and explicitly stated guidelines aimed at providing children with ASD a way of understanding the daily interactions and routines they find confusing or troublesome. As such, they are a form of scripting that employs repeated practice, rather than fading, to help the child internalize the sequence. Social Stories are usually composed of several short sentences that use printed words or words paired with pictures. Typically they take the form of a *descriptive* sentence that provides information about the setting, people, or activities; a *directive* sentence that informs children what they need to do in a given setting; a *perspective* sentence that describes the feelings, beliefs, or reactions of others; and a *control* sentence that identifies strategies the child might use to recall the information in a Social Story (Gray 1995; Gray and Garand 1993; Prelock 2006). During intervention, a Social Story targeting specific behaviors is developed in collaboration with the child, then read to the child prior to an activity or event targeted in the story. Data are collected to determine effectiveness and strategies are used to ensure that the targeted behavior is maintained and generalized (Prelock 2006).

Unlike the scripting and fading procedure of McClannahan and Krantz (2005), which is aimed at teaching appropriate ways to talk in particular social situations,

TABLE 5.9 Studies designed to improve communication in individuals with ASD using scripting and fading

Research design (SSED or group)	Study	Participants	Outcome
SSED multiple baseline across participants	Krantz and McClannahan (1993)	Four children with autism	• Children rarely initiated to peers during baseline. • Peer initiations increased when the script addressed peer initiations related to recently completed, current, and future activities. • Unscripted initiations increased as the script was faded. • During the fading phase, only minimal written prompts were available and initiations generalized across setting, time, teacher, and activity. • Once the script was faded, participants' initiations were similar to a normative sample of three children without autism. • Peer initiations were maintained by three of the four children at a 2-month follow-up.
SSED multiple baseline across participants	Krantz and McClannahan (1998)	Three boys (4–5 years old) with autism	• None of the boys talked to a familiar teacher during baseline. • Text cues "Look" and "Watch me" were paired with images in activity schedules children already used and were gradually faded. • One child required an adaptation to his script procedure (i.e., attaching textual cues to his wrist band before he approached a teacher). • Elaborations and scripted conversations increased over the teaching period. • Unscripted interactions increased during script teaching, maintenance and new activities. • All scripted and unscripted interactions and elaborations increased and were maintained across a new adult.
SSED multiple probe across participants	Stevenson et al. (2000)	Four boys (10–15 years old) with autism	• Three of the participants did not engage in any interaction during two 10-min baseline sessions; three instances of interaction were recorded across two baselines for the fourth participant. • Scripted interactions increased slightly with teaching and were maintained at these low levels following fading of the scripts. • Unscripted interactions remained high across maintenance sessions following fading of audio-taped scripts.
SSED multiple baseline across three sets of stimuli	Sarokoff et al. (2001)	Two boys (8 and 9 years old) with autism	• Both children demonstrated increases in scripted and unscripted statements about the stimuli following introduction of scripts with embedded text. • Statements were maintained when the scripts were faded. • Scripted statements generalized to novel stimuli and novel peers and were maintained in the absence of adults.

(Continued)

TABLE 5.9 (Continued)

Research design (SSED or group)	Study	Participants	Outcome
SSED multiple baseline across participants	Charlop-Christy and Kelso (2003)	Three boys (8;6 to 11;7 years old) with autism	• The amount of appropriate conversation increased during cue-card and written-script conversation intervention for all three boys. • Maintenance was observed for all three participants following withdrawal of cue cards. • Generalization occurred to novel topics and across settings and conversation partners.
SSED multiple probe across participants	MacDuff et al. (2007)	Three boys (3–5 years old) with autism	• All three boys were pre-taught verbal imitation of single syllable words (different from the one used in intervention, i.e., "see") and pointing. • No participant initiated bids for joint attention during baseline. • All three participants met the criterion for saying the script ("see") without prompts during teaching (children were taught to point to activate a button-activated recorder next to an object that produced the message "see"). • When the script was faded in two steps (removing the message "see" from the recorder and then removing the recorder), unscripted bids for joint attention increased. • Unscripted bids remained stable during maintenance, when no prompts or rewards were given. • Bids for joint attention generalized to untrained materials and environments. • Pointing increased during teaching (required to activate the recorders) but was inconsistent across participants during maintenance and did not consistently generalize across materials and settings; decreases in behavior were seen for two children.
SSED multiple baseline across settings	Brown et al. (2008)	Three boys (7–13 years old) with autism	• Participants were pre-taught the stimulus materials used in the study and pre-taught to read all words that were used in the scripts. • Intervention began with response-contingent modeling and scripts were attached to stimulus items in mock stores set up in the classroom, faded from last word to first. • Scripted interactions with the conversation partner immediately increased with the introduction of the scripts; as scripts were faded, unscripted interactions systematically increased during simulated shopping trips. • Generalization of conversational interactions to untrained stimuli was observed after the introduction of the script-fading procedure. • No child demonstrated interactions in the community settings during baseline, but all demonstrated increases in interactions in community stores following treatment.

Social Stories primarily target managing behavior and anxiety, and often focus on internal states and behaviors ("If I get angry, I can count to ten;" "I can stand in line and wait my turn") rather than language production. Table 5.10 highlights recent studies that were designed to assess the effectiveness of Social Stories for facilitating communication skills. Social Stories have been used to increase appropriate greetings (Swaggart et al. 1995) and compliments (Dodd et al. 2008), increase verbal interactions (Crozier and Tincani 2007) and decrease inappropriate social interactions (Norris and Dattilo 1999). In addition, they have been used to increase initiation of comments and requests with variable generalization and maintenance across social behaviors (Delano and Snell 2006; Scattone et al. 2006; Thiemann and Goldstein 2001). Further, Social Stories have been used to decrease echolalia and excessive voice volume (Brownell 2002), to decrease tantrums and ineffective communication (Lorimer et al. 2002), to increase appropriate use of words (Adams et al. 2004) and labeling and explaining of emotions (Bernad-Ripoll 2007), and to increase conversational abilities (Sansosti and Powell-Smith 2006, 2008). Maintenance of skills taught using this method is inconsistent. More research is needed to demonstrate generalized effects across communication behaviors and social contexts.

Video modeling. This intervention requires a child to watch the behavior of another and use what was observed on the video in their own interactions. Generally video models are produced by individual clinicians, using either peers or children with ASD themselves as "actors." There are also some commercially produced materials designed for use in video-modeling activities (e.g., "My School Day" by Silver Lining Multimedia). Video modeling helps focus the attention of the child with ASD on the relevant behaviors in the video so

that, with practice and rehearsal, the child retains and displays the targeted language and behavior that was modeled (Prelock 2006). Video modeling also fosters a child's ability to take what is learned in a video-modeling session and helps generalize that information to aspects of daily life (Shipley-Benamou et al. 2002). Charlop-Christy et al. (2000) showed that video modeling resulted in faster acquisition of skills than did modeling from live demonstrations and was effective in promoting generalization.

When designing a video model, it is important to incorporate motivating themes in the conversational language being modeled as well as desirable objects of play or activities of interest. Depending on the video's emphasis, the camera might be strategically placed to present a facial expression or show an actor's hands carrying out a particular task or activity (Charlop-Christy and Kelso 1997). The video can be paused to point out specific information that the child is expected to consider followed by a debriefing to review what was seen and heard, identify any new language heard as well as note the prosody and emotional expression of the models (Charlop and Milstein 1989). Research suggests that in addition to watching the video, generalization and maintenance are increased when children watch the video interaction, then rehearse it verbally before re-enacting the scenario (Paul 2003).

There are several considerations when developing a video and using video modeling as an intervention strategy to support the learning of a child with ASD. First, the team needs to select and define the target behavior which should be operationally defined so that is it measurable, observable, and specific to the child with ASD (Charlop-Christy 2004). Second, a task analysis is completed in which the steps for the video model are itemized. This should be guided by an observation of whatever target script has been identified in children who are

TABLE 5.10 Studies designed to improve communication in individuals with ASD using Social Stories

Research design (SSED or group)	Study	Participants	Outcome
SSED A–B design	Swaggart et al. (1995)	• Child 1: 11-year-old female with autism; some expressive language skills, but difficult to understand; greeting behaviors and aggression targeted for intervention	*Child 1*: At baseline, 7% of greetings were judged to be appropriate, 82% involved touch, 9% were judged to be aggressive and there were no instances of ignores; Following treatment, 74% of greetings were judged to be appropriate, touches decreased to 26%, and no aggression was observed.
		• Child 2: 7-year-old male with PDD; some expressive language but difficult to understand	*Child 2*: During 10 baseline sessions, aggression was not shown in 70%, parallel play was shown in 80%, but the child did not share in any session and screamed in all sessions; Following treatment, aggression was not shown on 94% of days, parallel play was exhibited on 94% of days, the child independently shared on 22% of days and screamed on 56% of days.
		• Child 3: 7-year-old male with autism; used mostly echolalia	*Child 3*: At baseline, there was no aggression in 80% of sessions, parallel play in 80%, grabbing in 100%, and no instances of sharing; Following treatment, there was no aggression and engagement in parallel play on 94% of the days; independently shared on 35% and grabbed toys on 35%.
SSED A–B	Norris and Dattilo (1999)	Eight-year-old African American female with mild to moderate autism	• Number of inappropriate social interaction behaviors at lunchtime began to decrease 5 days after the Social Story intervention was introduced. • 48% reduction in inappropriate social interactions between the first data point in baseline and the last data point taken. • When inappropriate interactions decreased, absence of social interactions increased. • No change observed in the number of appropriate interaction behaviors throughout the study.
SSED multiple baseline across social communication skills and across triads	Thiemann and Goldstein (2001)	• Five children with social impairments (aged 6;6 to 12;2); four with autism, one with language impairment • Ten age-matched peers without disabilities	• Improved and more consistent rates of targeted social behaviors (initiating comments and requests, securing attention, contingent responses) seen in the children with social impairments following treatment compared to baseline. • Generalization across targeted behaviors seen for some behaviors in all participants • General lack of maintenance seen across social behaviors.

	Study	Participants	Findings
SSED multiple baseline across presentation methods (music or reading)	Brownell (2002)	Four boys (6–9 years old) with autism	• Child 1: Significant decrease in TV/movie echolalia in both treatment conditions compared to baseline, but no significant difference between the two interventions. • Child 2: Significant increase in following directions in both treatment conditions compared to baseline, but no significant difference between the two interventions. • Child 3: Significantly decreased loud voice behavior in both treatment conditions compared to baseline measures; target behavior significantly lower in music condition compared to reading. • Child 4: Significant reduction in loud voice occurrences in both treatment conditions compared to baselines; no significant difference between treatment conditions.
SSED multiple baseline	Lorimer et al. (2002)	Five-year-old boy with mild to moderate autism	• Target behavior: ineffective communication prior to tantrums (through "talking with adults" and "waiting" Social Stories). • Initial baseline: tantrums on 5 out of 7 days; initial treatment: tantrums on one out of 7 days. • Second baseline: tantrums on two out of 3 days; second intervention: tantrums on one out of 7 days. • Precursor behaviors several times a day during baseline, began to decrease with introduction of stories, dramatic increase during second baseline, downward trend when stories reintroduced.
SSED withdrawal design (A–B–A–B)	Adams et al. (2004)	Seven-year-old male with Asperger syndrome	• Frequency of crying, screaming, falling, and hitting all decreased during homework time. • Qualitative parent report: decreased frustration during homework, child able to find appropriate words and understood he could ask for help; parents learned to communicate better with son.
SSED multiple probe across participants	Delano and Snell (2006)	• Three boys (6–9 years old, one African American, two Caucasian) with autism who used functional verbal communication and demonstrated impairments in social functioning • Six age-matched nondisabled peers	• All children increased duration of time spent socially engaged with both the training peer and novel peer. • All children showed gains in use of targeted social behaviors (esp. contingent responding and initiating comments) with training peer and novel peer. • Two children demonstrated generalization to their classroom setting.

(Continued)

TABLE 5.10 (Continued)

Research design (SSED or group)	Study	Participants	Outcome
SSED multiple baseline across participants	Sansosti and Powell-Smith (2006)	Three boys (9;9 to 11;6 years old) diagnosed with Asperger syndrome	• Target behavior: social engagement (characterized as sportsmanship, maintaining conversation, joining in). • Intervention was effective for increasing social engagement skills for two of the participants. • There was no demonstration of maintenance.
SSED multiple baseline across participants	Scattone et al. (2006)	Three boys (8–13 years old) with ASD; all had intelligible speech and spoke in complete sentences	• Two students showed an increase in appropriate social interactions (verbal, physical or gestural initiation or response to a peer; a comment or question related to the activity or conversation; continued engagement in activity with a peer; response to a peer's comment or question; physical gesture to indicate approval or disappointment).
SSED A–B design	Bernad-Ripoll (2007)	One boy (9;8 years old) with Asperger syndrome	• Labeling and explaining emotions and determining action responses increased following intervention and maintained during generalization phases.
SSED A–B–A–B for two participants SSED A–B–A–B–C–B–C for one participant	Crozier and Tincani (2007)	Three boys (aged 3;9 to 5;1) with ASD	• One participant showed an increase in unprompted verbal interactions.
SSED multiple baseline across behaviors and participants	Dodd et al. (2008)	Two boys (9;10 and 12;7 years old) with PDD-NOS	• Target behaviors: giving directions to others and giving compliments. • *Child 1*: Stable trend of excessive directions during baseline, dropped immediately following introduction of Social Story and continued to decrease when story was withdrawn; no compliments given during baseline, increasing trend once Social Story introduced. • *Child 2*: Only exhibited one compliment during eight baseline sessions; this quickly increased to seven once the Social Story was introduced but a decreasing trend was seen throughout the treatment phase.

| SSED multiple baseline across participants | Sansosti and Powell-Smith (2008) | Three boys (6;6 to 10;6 years old) with autism or Asperger syndrome | • Target behaviors: joining in and maintaining conversations.
• Immediately following introduction of video modeled Social Stories treatment, target behaviors increased; decline was then seen for two participants, until teacher prompting and child confederates were introduced, when skills were regained and maintained; the third participant did not require modifications and demonstrated steady increases.
• Some degree of maintenance was seen two weeks following intervention.
• Some generalization across settings and across time was seen for only one participant. |

typically developing (Prelock 2006). Input to guide the development of the video models should also be gathered from parents, teachers, and the child. When preparing the video, actors should speak slowly and clearly, and exaggerate target behaviors as appropriate while facing the camera. In addition, there should be minimal distractors in the video to ensure the child's focus when watching the video will be on the relevant cues. Finally, the target behavior should be demonstrated about 75–80% of the time before determining acquisition and at least two observations of the video should occur before the child's acquisition of learning is assessed (Charlop-Christy 2004).

Several explanations have been given for the value of this method of intervention for children with ASD including their rote memory strengths, which makes remembering target language behaviors a reasonable expectation, and the tendency for delayed echolalia in verbal children with ASD when they hear the language targets on the video. In addition, watching a video is often a motivating activity for the child with ASD (Charlop-Christy and Daneshvar 2003; Charlop-Christy et al. 2000). Further, visual and auditory distractions are minimal with video modeling (Charlop-Christy and Kelso 1997) in that the video focuses on the relevant and critical information and capitalizes on the visual strengths reported for individuals with ASD.

Video modeling appears to be an appropriate intervention across a range of developmental levels; Charlop-Christy (2004) describes using this strategy with children as young as 4 years of age through older adults. It is a strategy reported to generalize across settings and can be used to support the conversational skills of individuals with ASD (Charlop and Walsh 1986). Table 5.11 presents studies using video modeling that have focused on supporting the communication skills of individuals with ASD from 3 to 15 years of age. Video modeling has been used to increase appropriate responses to questions (Buggey et al. 1999; Sherer et al. 2001), to increase play comments and social language in both scripted and unscripted play schemes (D'Ateno et al. 2003; Maione and Mirenda 2006; Taylor et al. 1999), to increase spontaneous requests (Wert and Neisworth 2003), and to teach complimenting others, though not initiating interaction (Apple et al. 2005). In addition, studies that have shown generalization and maintenance include those aimed at increasing social initiation and time engaged with others and decreasing latency to social initiations (Buggey 2005; Nikopoulos and Keenan 2003, 2004a, 2004b, 2007), joining in and maintaining conversation (Sansosti and Powell-Smith 2008), generalizing conversational speech across topics (Charlop and Milstein 1989; Charlop-Christy et al. 2000), increasing perspective taking (Charlop-Christy and Daneshvar 2003; LeBlanc Coates et al. 2003), and increasing time spent looking at people while decreasing looking at objects. The latter study also demonstrated concomitant improvement in scores for the *Vineland Adaptive Behavior Scale* and the *MacArthur Communication Development Inventory* (Baharav and Darling 2008). In sum, video modeling is practice with a relatively strong evidence base for supporting the development of several language and social communication skills in individuals with ASD that has promise for generalized learning and skill maintenance.

TABLE 5.11 Studies designed to improve communication in individuals with ASD using video modeling

Research design (SSED or group)	Study	Participants	Outcome
SSED multiple baseline across children and within subjects across conversations; multiple probe design across conversations for each child	Charlop and Milstein (1989)	Three boys (6;10 to 7;10 years old) with autism; all children considered high functioning, answering basic questions in three- or four-word phrases	• All participants acquired conversational speech during video-modeling intervention and generalization observed across topics of conversation, conversation partners, settings, stimuli; generalization not seen for any child to the abstract conversation. • Maintenance effects seen for all children during follow-up probes 1, 2, 3, 6, and 15 months following acquisition. • Increase in number of unmodeled, new responses provided during conversations with the therapist after implementation of video modeling. • Increase in the number of appropriate questions asked after introduction of video modeling. • Significant positive difference in social validation measure following intervention.
SSED multiple baseline across participants	Buggey et al. (1999)	Three children (7–12 years old) with autism	• All three children showed increases in appropriate responses to questions during play activities. • Following withdrawal from treatment, two children showed slight decreases in responding behavior. • Two children's parents expressed that they observed increases in appropriate responses to questions before knowing what behavior was being targeted in intervention.
SSED multiple baseline probe across three play activities (two experiments)	Taylor et al. (1999)	Experiment 1: 6-year-old boy with autism Experiment 2: 9-year-old boy with autism	• Experiment 1: Child met criterion for producing scripted comments in three play contexts after not demonstrating any during baseline (sibling produced the scripted comments in probe contexts); child did not demonstrate any unscripted comments. • Experiment 2: Child increased number of play comments (scripted and unscripted) in three play contexts following a forward-chaining procedure during training (sibling did not produce scripted comments in probe contexts).
SSED multiple baseline across subjects, within subject across modeling condition, and within modeling condition across tasks	Charlop-Christy et al. (2000)	Five children (7–11 years old) with autism and enrolled in an after-school behavior therapy program for children with autism	• Overall video modeling led to faster acquisition of skills compared to in vivo modeling. • Generalization across persons, settings or stimuli occurred for behaviors following video modeling but not after in vivo modeling. • Behaviors included expressive labeling of emotions, independent play, spontaneous greetings, oral comprehension, cooperative play, conversational speech, daily living skills, and social play.

(Continued)

TABLE 5.11 (Continued)

Research design (SSED or group)	Study	Participants	Outcome
SSED multiple baseline and alternating treatments	Sherer et al. (2001)	Five boys (3;11 to 11;2 years old), four diagnosed with autism and one diagnosed with PDD-NOS	• Two children reached the criterion for responding accurately to personal questions in the self-video condition. • Three children reached the criterion in the other-video condition (two children did not reach the criterion in either condition after several months of treatment). • Using another as model was just as effective as using self; not a strong preference for one versus the other among the children.
SSED multiple baseline across participants and within subject across tasks	Charlop-Christy and Daneshvar (2003)	Three boys (6–9 years old) with autistic disorder	• All participants failed the pretest perspective-taking task. • Two of the three passed the posttest and consistently met criterion on primary tasks in maintenance and showed generalization; the third participant demonstrated inconsistent generalization during maintenance. • One participant required only one viewing of the video to pass the first two tasks, two viewings to pass the third, and then the child met criterion on the remaining tasks.
SSED multiple baseline across play sequences	D'Ateno, Mangiapanello, and Taylor (2003)	Girl (3;8 year old) with autism who rarely verbalized during play activities	• Scripted verbal responses increased in all play sequences following video modeling. • Novel verbal responses remained low throughout both baseline and intervention sessions; experimental control was not achieved for novel verbal responses.
SSED multiple baseline across tasks and participants	LeBlanc et al. (2003)	Three boys (7–13 years old) with autism	• All children failed perspective-taking tasks in baseline, but mastered them and passed novel variants of the task even when they required novel vocal or motor responses. • Two children passed the Sally and Anne task (untrained) following intervention on two different tasks after all children failed it at baseline.
SSED multiple treatment for six children and an A-B design for one child	Nikopoulos and Keenan (2003)	Six boys with autism and one girl with Asperger syndrome (9–15 years old)	• Social initiation effectiveness was seen for four of the seven children. • Social initiation responding of these four children was generalized across settings, peers, and toys and results were maintained at 1- and 2-month follow-ups.
SSED multiple baseline across participants	Wert and Neisworth (2003)	Four children (3–6 years old) with autism and limited or nonexistent spontaneous requests	• There was a marked increase in spontaneous requests made by children in their preschool settings during intervention. • Three children continued to show an increased number of spontaneous requests during maintenance phase (the fourth child did not remain in the study long enough for maintenance data to be taken).

Design	Study	Participants	Findings
SSED multiple probe across matrices and testing	Dauphin et al. (2004)	Boy (3;1 years old) with ASD and ADHD	• Child imitated 25% of modeled language during training, but imitated nearly all "say" components of computer schedule by Session 6. • During testing, child perfectly imitated all "say" components of the three trained activities. • Upon first viewing of each test computer schedule, child completed three of six activities with 100% accuracy and performed 88% of the novel "say" components correctly.
SSED multiple baseline across participants	Nikopoulos and Keenan (2004a)	Three boys (7 and 9 years old) with autism	• Decrease in latency to social initiation and increase in duration of reciprocal play observed for all participants. • Result maintained at 1- and 3-month follow-ups.
SSED multiple baseline across participants	Nikopoulos and Keenan (2004b)	Two boys and one girl (7;5–10.5 years old) with autism	• All participants demonstrated decreased latency to social initiation and increased time engaged in reciprocal play following video modeling when only one object was present. • Results generalized to four different toys in the absence of video modeling and any experimenter prompts or consequences.
SSED multiple baseline across participants	Apple et al. (2005)	• Experiment 1: two boys(5;0 and 5;1 years old) with Asperger syndrome and autism, respectively • Experiment 2: two boys with Asperger syndrome and one girl with autism (all aged between 4;1 and 5;9)	• Experiment 1: Participants acquired compliment-giving responses during video-modeling phase, but neither acquired compliment-giving initiations. • Following a video and reinforcement phase, both children began to make initiations, but only compliment-giving responses were maintained when the reinforcement and video were withdrawn in the final phase. • Experiment 2: Increase seen in compliment-giving responses upon introduction of video for all children. • All met criteria for compliment-giving initiations on the first day of the self-management teaching phase. • Rapid generalization of compliment-giving responses across settings observed. • Self-management system in Experiment 2 led to greater performance in compliment-giving initiations (compared to Experiment 1). • Children observed to give compliments in the absence of self-management devices. • Small increase in teacher ratings of social skills for three of the four children following treatment (across the two experiments).

(Continued)

TABLE 5.11 (Continued)

Research design (SSED or group)	Study	Participants	Outcome
SSED multiple baseline across participants and behaviors	Buggey (2005)	• Study 1: two boys (11;3 and 9;11 years old) with autism and Asperger syndrome • Study 3: 1 boy (5;5 years old) with PDD	• Study 1 (social initiations): substantial gains in frequency of social initiations following intervention, and maintained through maintenance phase. • Study 3 (pushing and language production): small increase in rate of responding to questions; no unprompted utterances noted after one week of observation. The method was modified and a new video made; a larger increase was then seen in the rate of responding to questions and also an increase in the number of unprompted verbalizations.
SSED multiple baseline across activities	Maione and Mirenda (2006)	One boy (5;7 years old) with autism	• Three video vignettes with adult models for each set of toys (three) were made to demonstrate talking and playing in the context of those toys; different scripts used in each vignette. • Both a video feedback condition and a prompting condition were added for one play condition because the participant was not showing increases in verbalizations, and he perseverated on the toy. • Increases in total social language verbalizations, scripted and unscripted language, and initiations and responses all increased following video modeling; in one play condition, behaviors did not increase reliably until video feedback and prompting was added. • A greater number of unscripted verbalizations were observed compared to scripted verbalizations.
Experiment 1: SSED multiple baseline across participants	Nikopoulos and Keenan (2007)	• Experiment 1: three boys (6.5–7 years old) with autism	• Experiment 1: Latency to social initiation and to imitative responses decreased in all children following introduction of video modeling targeting social initiation; these results generalized across peers, and were maintained at 1-month follow-up for one participant and at 1- and 2-month follow-ups for two participants. • Time spent in reciprocal play initially increased for all participants following video modeling but was generally variable across the course of the study.
Experiment 2: SSED A-B		• Experiment 2: 1 girl (7.5 years old) with autism	• Experiment 2: Latency to social initiation and to imitative responses decreased following video modeling, generalized to peers, and was maintained at 1- and 2-month follow-ups. • Time spent in reciprocal play increased following video modeling and was maintained at 1- and 2-month follow-ups.

Design	Study	Participants	Outcomes
SSED A-B	Baharav and Darling (2008)	One boy (5;8 years old) with autism	• No change in ADOS and MacArthur outcomes between two baseline phases (four weeks apart), but changes seen following video modeling (parent's face speaking or singing to child while performing familiar activities) listened to via an FM system. The total algorithm score on ADOS post-treatment was at cutoff for communication and well below cut-off for reciprocal social interaction and total score. On the MacArthur test, the number of words produced doubled and the number of words understood improved from the 40th percentile to the 85th percentile. • Significant decrease in time spent looking at objects and significant increase in time spent looking at people following treatment. • Scores on Vineland II for communication and socialization increased from pre-treatment to three weeks post-withdrawal; increase reflected change from the 60th to the 80th percentile.
SSED multiple baseline across participants	Sansosti and Powell-Smith (2008)	Three boys (6;6 to 10;6 years old) with autism or Asperger syndrome	• Target behaviors: social communication in the form of joining in and maintaining conversations. • Immediately following introduction of video modeled Social Stories treatment, target behaviors increased; decline seen for two participants, until teacher prompting and child confederates were introduced, when skills were regained and maintained; the third participant did not require modifications and demonstrated steady increases. • Some degree of maintenance seen two weeks following intervention. • Some generalization across setting, across time was seen for only one client.

CONCLUSION

The interventions reviewed here demonstrate that a range of methods show promise for improving the social communication skills of children with autism spectrum conditions. Methods that employ highly structured and didactic interactions, such as DTI, and operant approaches, such as verbal behavior, have demonstrated efficacy for eliciting early communication, first words, and more elaborated language structures. More naturalistic methods that have evolved out of the ABA tradition, such as MCT, PECS, video modeling, and scripting and fading have also demonstrated success at both the earlier and more advanced communication levels. Approaches aimed at following the child's lead and increasing the contingency of input, such as MTW, have also shown some promise but have a less well-established track record.

Training in AAC and FCT appear useful in increasing adaptive and decreasing maladaptive communicative acts in the early stages of communication, but have yet to demonstrate the ability to lead to any elaborated forms of communication in this population. Replacing oral–aural communication with more temporally stable, visual communication modalities has not led to dramatic increases in communicative competence in children with ASD, as was hoped when sign and other AAC approaches were first introduced to this population (Fay and Schuler 1980; Grove and Dockrell 2000; Yoder and Layton 1988). One of the most robust prognostic findings in the ASD literature is the connection between the acquisition of spoken language by the beginning of the school years and improved long-term outcome (Gillberg and Steffenburg 1987; Howlin 2005; Howlin et al. 2004; Paul and Cohen 1984; Venter et al. 1992). Both the increasing proportion of children with ASD who have acquired some spoken language in recent years (Rogers 2006;

Tager-Flusberg et al. 2005) – most likely as a result of earlier identification and intervention (Dawson and Osterling 1997; Koegel and Koegel 1988; Rogers 2006; Rogers and Vismara 2008) – and recent emphasis from parental and governmental agencies on working toward increasing this proportion still further (Tager-Flusberg et al. 2009) highlight the need for research that directly contrasts both the efficacy and efficiency of methods for engendering early language development. Such research will be most useful when it makes use of randomized controlled trials to perform direct contrasts among AAC methods such as PECS and VOCA training, more direct speech approaches such as DTI, and naturalistic methods such as MCT and MTW.

For children who acquire a basic platform in spoken language, interventions will be needed to foster both the more abstract, mature language skills that will support academic development, as well as the rich, varied and nuanced forms that will enable participation in developmentally appropriate interactions with others. Social Stories, video modeling, and scripting and fading all take an essentially script-based approach to expanding the ability to use language to accomplish social goals once children with ASD acquire basic language structure. The main differences among these approaches concern the form scripts take, whether based in dynamic visual samples (video modeling), static pictured or written text (scripting and fading), or written text that adheres to a specific format (Social Stories). The problem with all script-based approaches is that they inevitably teach a narrow range of social behaviors appropriate for a small number of social situations. Even when they demonstrate generalization and maintenance, these approaches do not fundamentally change the capacity of the child with ASD to engage fluidly and competently in the rapidly shifting, dynamic world of normal social interaction. White et al. (2007) discuss the need for research on interventions for children with ASD that move closer to enabling these more broadly-applicable social interaction skills, but at this point in the development of our field, we are able to effect changes on only small slices of behavior.

Thus, the picture of the state of the art in ameliorating social communication skills in children with ASD reveals a landscape with some encouraging vistas, but with many areas that remain to be filled in. We know of some techniques that appear effective for increasing simple communication behaviors, that can help bridge the gap between wants and needs and their expression until more elaborated forms emerge, and that can provide basic skills in some constrained aspects of conversation. Although we are a long way from fully overcoming the significant disabilities in social communication that constitute a core symptom of ASD in children at all levels of functioning, this review suggests that beginning steps have been made toward attaining this distant but essential goal.

ACKNOWLEDGEMENTS

- Maternal and Child Health Bureau Grant 6T73 MC 00039
- National Institute of Child Health and Development P01-HD03008
- National Institute of Deafness and Communication Disorders R01 DC07129
- NIDCD MidCareer Development Award K24 HD045576
- NIMH Autism Center of Excellence Grant P50 MH81756
- National Alliance for Autism Research and the Autism Speaks Foundation

REFERENCES

Acredolo, L. P., & Goodwyn, S. (1988). Symbolic gesturing in normal infants. *Child Development, 59*(2), 450–466.

Adams, L., Gouvousis, A., VanLue, M., & Waldron, C. (2004). Social Story intervention: Improving communication skills in a child with autism spectrum disorders. *Focus on Autism and Other Developmental Disabilities, 19*(2), 87–94.

Aldred, C., Green, J., & Adams, C. (2004). A new social communication intervention for children with autism: Pilot randomized controlled treatment study suggesting effectiveness. *Journal of Child Psychology and Psychiatry, 45*(8), 1420–1430.

Anderson, S. R., Avery, D. L., DiPietro, E. K., Edwards, G. L., & Christian, W. P. (1987). Intensive home-based early intervention with autistic children. *Education and Treatment of Children, 10*, 352–366.

Anderson, A., Moore, D., & Bourne, T. (2007). Functional communication and other concomitant behavior change following PECS training: A case study. *Behaviour Change, 24*(3), 173–181.

Apple, A. L., Billingsley, F., & Schwartz, I. S. (2005). Effects of video modeling alone and with self-management on compliment-giving behaviors of children with high-functioning ASD. *Journal of Positive Behavior Interventions, 7*(3), 33–46.

Baharav, E., & Darling, R. (2008). Case report: Using an auditory trainer with caregiver Video modeling to enhance communication and socialization behaviors in autism. *Journal of Autism and Developmental Disorders, 38*, 771–775.

Baldwin, D. A. (1991). Infants' contribution to the achievement of joint reference. *Child Development, 62*, 875–890.

Barbera, M., & Kubina, R. (2005). Using transfer procedures to teach tacts to a child with autism. *The Analysis of Verbal Behavior, 21*, 155–161.

Bates, E. (1976). *Language and context: The acquisition of pragmatics.* New York: Academic.

Bernad-Ripoll, S. (2007). Using a self-as-model video combined with Social Stories™ to help a child with Asperger syndrome understand emotions. *Focus on Autism and Other Developmental Disabilities, 22*(2), 100–106.

Bibby, P., Eikeseth, S., Martin, N., Mudford, O., & Reeves, D. (2001). Progress and outcomes for children with autism receiving parent-managed intensive interventions. *Research in Developmental Disabilities, 22*, 425–447.

Birnbrauer, J. S., & Leach, D. J. (1993). The Murdoch early intervention program after 2 years. *Behaviour Change, 10*, 63–74.

Bloom, L. (1993). *The transition from infancy to language: Acquiring the power of expression.* New York: Cambridge University Press.

Bondy, A. S., & Frost, L. A. (1994). The picture exchange communication system. *Focus on Autistic Behavior, 9*(3), 1–19.

Bondy, A. S., & Frost, L. A. (1998). The picture exchange communication system. *Seminars in Speech and Language, 19*(4), 373–388.

Bondy, A. S., & Frost, L. A. (2001). The picture exchange communication system. *Behavior Modification, 25*(5), 725–744.

Boyd, R., & Corley, M. (2001). Outcome survey of early intensive behavioral intervention for young children with autism in a community setting. *Autism, 5*, 430–441.

Brady, N. (2000). Improved comprehension of object names following voice output communication aid use: Two case studies. *Augmentative and Alternative Communication, 16*, 197–204.

Braithwaite, K., & Richdale, A. (2000). Functional communication training to replace challenging behaviors across two behavioral outcomes. *Behavioral Interventions, 15*, 21–36.

Brown, R. (1973). *A first language: The early stages.* Cambridge, MA: Harvard University Press.

Brown, K., Wacker, D., Derby, K., Peck, S., Richman, D., Sasso, G., et al. (2000). Evaluating the effects of functional communication training in the presence and absence of establishing operations. *Journal of Applied Behavior Analysis, 33*, 53–71.

Brown, J., Krantz, P., McClannahan, L., & Poulson, C. (2008). Using script fading to promote natural environment stimulus control of verbal interactions among youths with autism. *Research in Autism Spectrum Disorders, 2*, 480–497.

Brownell, M. (2002). Musically-adapted Social Stories to modify behaviors in students with autism: Four case studies. *Journal of Music Therapy, 39*(2), 117–144.

Buggey, T. (2005). Video self-modeling applications with students with autism spectrum disorder in a small private school setting. *Focus on Autism and Other Developmental Disabilities, 20*(1), 52–63.

Buggey, T., Toombs, K., Gardener, P., & Cervetti, M. (1999). Training responding behaviors in students with autism: Using videotaped self-modeling. *Journal of Positive Behavior Interventions, 1*(4), 205–214.

Cafiero, J. (2001). The effect of an augmentative communication intervention on the communication, behavior, and academic program of an adolescent with autism. *Focus on Autism and Other Developmental Disabilities, 16*(3), 179–189.

Carpenter, M., & Tomasello, M. (2000). Joint attention, cultural learning, and language acquisition. In A. M. Wetherby & B. M. Prizant (Eds.), *Autism spectrum disorders* (pp. 31–54). Baltimore: Brookes.

Carpenter, M., Nagell, K., & Tomasello, M. (1998). Social cognition, joint attention, and communicative competence from 9 to 15 months of age. *Monographs of the Society for Research in Child Development, 63*(4), 176.

Carr, D., & Felce, J. (2007a). The effects of PECS teaching to Phase III on the communicative interactions between children with autism and their teachers. *Journal of Autism and Developmental Disorders, 37*(4), 724–737.

Carr, D., & Felce, J. (2007b). Brief report: Increase in production of spoken words in some children with autism after PECS teaching to phase III. *Journal of Autism and Developmental Disorders, 37*(4), 780–787.

Carr, J., & Firth, A. (2005). The verbal behavior approach to early and intensive behavioral intervention for autism: A call for additional empirical support. *Journal of Early and Intensive Behavior Intervention, 2*(1), 18–27.

Casey, S., & Merical, C. (2006). The use of functional communication training without additional treatment procedures in an inclusive school setting. *Behavioral Disorders, 32*(1), 46–54.

Cazden, C. B. (1968). The acquisition of noun and verb inflections. *Child Development, 39*(2), 433–448.

Chapman, R. (2000). Children's language learning: An interactionist perspective. *Journal of Child Psychology and Psychiatry, 41*, 33–54.

Charlop, M. H., & Milstein, J. P. (1989). Teaching autistic children conversational speech using video modeling. *Journal of Applied Behavioral Analysis, 22*, 275–285.

Charlop, M. H., & Walsh, M. E. (1986). Increasing autistic children's spontaneous verbalizations of affection: An assessment of time delay and peer modeling procedures. *Journal of Applied Behavior Analysis, 19*, 307–314.

Charlop-Christy, M. H. (2004, June). *Using video modeling to teach perspective taking to children with autism.* Presentation at the annual Vermont Summer Autism Institute, Burlington, VT.

Charlop-Christy, M. H., & Daneshvar, S. (2003). Using video modeling to teach perspective taking to children with autism. *Journal of Positive Behavior Interventions, 5*(1), 12.

Charlop-Christy, M. H., & Kelso, S. E. (1997). *How to treat the child with autism.* Claremont, CA: Claremont Autism Center.

Charlop-Christy, M. H., & Kelso, S. E. (2003). Teaching children with autism conversational speech using a cue card/written script program. *Education and Treatment of Children, 26*(2), 108–127.

Charlop-Christy, M. H., Le, L., & Freeman, K. A. (2000). A comparison of video modeling with in vivo modeling for teaching children with autism. *Journal of Autism and Developmental Disorders, 30*(6), 537–552.

Charlop-Christy, M. H., Carpenter, M., Le, L., LeBlanc, L. A., & Kellet, K. (2002). Using the picture exchange communication system (PECS) with children with autism: Assessment of PECS acquisition, speech, social-communicative behavior, and problem behavior. *Journal of Applied Behavior Analysis, 35*(3), 213–231.

Charman, T. (2003). Why is joint attention a pivotal skill in autism? *Philosophical Transactions of the Royal Society of London. Series B: Biological Sciences, 358*(1430), 315–324.

Charman, T., Howlin, P., Aldred, C., Baird, G., Degli Espinosa, F., & Diggle, T. (2003). Research into early intervention for children with autism and related disorders: Methodological and design issues. Report on a workshop funded by the Welcome Trust, Institute of Child Health, London, UK, November 2001. *Autism, 7*(2), 217–225.

Chawarska, K., & Volkmar, F. (2005). Autism in infancy and early childhood. In F. R. Volkmar, R. Paul, A. Klin, & D. J. Cohen (Eds.), *Handbook of autism and pervasive developmental disorders* (3rd ed., pp. 223–246). Hoboken, NJ: Wiley.

Cohen, H., Amerine-Dickens, M., & Smith, T. (2006). Early intensive behavioral treatment: Replication of the UCLA model in a community setting. *Developmental and Behavioral Pediatrics, 27*, S145–S155.

Crozier, S., & Tincani, M. (2007). Effects of Social Stories on prosocial behavior of preschool children with autism spectrum disorders. *Journal of Autism and Developmental Disorders, 37*(9), 1803–1814.

D'Ateno, P., Mangiapanello, K., & Taylor, B. (2003). Using video modeling to teach complex play sequences to a preschooler with autism. *Journal of Positive Behavior Interventions, 5*, 5–11.

Dauphin, M., Kinney, E., & Stromer, R. (2004). Using video-enhanced schedules and matrix training to teach sociodramatic play to a child with autism. *Journal Positive Behavior Interventions, 6*, 238–250.

Dawson, G., & Osterling, J. (1997). Early intervention in autism: Effectiveness of common elements of current approaches. In M. J. Guralnick (Ed.), *The effectiveness of early intervention: Second generation research* (pp. 302–326). Baltimore: Brooks.

Dawson, G., Meltzoff, A., Osterling, J., & Rinaldi, J. (1998). Neuropsychological correlates of early symptoms of autism. *Child Development, 69*(5), 1276–1285.

Dawson, G., Toth, K., Abbott, R., Osterling, J., Munson, J., Estes, A., et al. (2004). Early social attention impairments in autism: Social orienting, joint attention, and attention to distress. *Developmental Psychology, 40*(2), 271–283.

Delaney, E. M., & Kaiser, A. P. (2001). The effects of teaching parents blended communication and behavior support strategies. *Behavioral Disorders, 26*, 93–116.

Delano, M., & Snell, M. E. (2006). The effects of Social Stories on the social engagement of children with autism. *Journal of Positive Behavior Interventions, 8*, 29–42.

DiCarlo, C., Stricklin, S., Banajee, M., & Reid, D. (2001). Effects of manual signing on communicative verbalizations by toddlers with and without disabilities in inclusive classrooms. *Journal of the Association for Persons with Severe Handicaps, 26*, 120–126.

Dodd, S., Hupp, S., Jewell, J., & Krohn, E. (2008). Using parent and siblings during a Social Story intervention for two children diagnosed with PDD-NOS. *Journal of Developmental and Physical Disabilities, 20*, 217–229.

Dore, J. (1978). Requestive systems in nursery school conversations: Analysis of talk in its social context. In R. Campbell & P. Smith (Eds.), *Recent advances in the psychology of language*. New York: Plenum.

Drash, P., High, R., & Tudor, R. (1999). Using mand training to establish an echoic repertoire in young children with autism. *The Analysis of Verbal Behavior, 16*, 29–44.

Drew, A., Baird, G., Baron-Cohen, S., Cox, A., Slonims, V., et al. (2002). A pilot randomized control trial of a parent training intervention for pre-school children with autism: Preliminary findings and methodological challenges. *European Child & Adolescent Psychiatry, 11*, 266–272.

Durand, V. (1999). Functional communication training using assistive devices: Recruiting natural communities of reinforcement. *Journal of Applied Behavior Analysis, 32*, 247–267.

Durand, V., & Merges, E. (2001). Functional communication training: A contemporary behavior analytic intervention for problem behaviors. *Focus on Autism and Other Developmental Disabilities, 16*(2), 110–119.

Eikeseth, E., Smith, T., Jahr, E., & Eldevik, S. (2002). Intensive behavioral treatment at school for 4-to 7-year-old children with autism. *Behavior Modification, 26*, 49–68.

Eikeseth, E., Smith, T., Jahr, E., & Eldevik, S. (2007). Outcome for children with autism who began intensive behavioral treatment for autism between ages 4 and 7: A comparison controlled study. *Behavior Modification, 31*, 264–278.

Eldevik, S., Eikeseth, E., Jahr, E., & Smith, T. (2006). Effects of low-intensity behavioral treatment for children with autism and mental retardation. *Journal of Autism and Developmental Disorders, 36*, 211–224.

Fay, W. (1979). Personal pronouns and the autistic child. *Journal of Autism and Developmental Disorders, 9*(3), 247–260.

Fay, W., & Schuler, A. (1980). *Emerging language in autistic children.* Baltimore: University Park Press.

Fenson, L., Dale, P., Reznick, J., Thal, D., Bates, E., Hartung, J. P., et al. (1993). *The MacArthur communicative development inventories: User's* guide and technical manual. San Diego: Singular Publishing Group.

Fenson, L., Dale, P., Reznick, J., Thal, D., Bates, E., Hartung, J. P., et al. (2007). *The MacArthur-Bates communicative development inventories*. Baltimore: Brookes.

Fernald, A. (1983). The perceptual and affective salience of mothers' speech to infants. In L. Feagans (Ed.), *The origins and growth of communication* (pp. 5–29). New Brunswick, NJ: Alex.

Finkel, A., & Williams, R. (2001). A comparison of textual and echoic prompts on the acquisition of intraverbal behavior in a six-year-old boy with autism. *The Analysis of Verbal Behavior, 18*, 61–70.

Fisher, W., Adelinis, J., Volkert, V., Keeney, K., Neidert, P., & Hovanetz, A. (2005). Assessing preferences for positive and negative reinforcement during treatment of destructive behavior with functional communication training. *Research in Developmental Disabilities, 26*, 153–168.

Freeman, S., & Dake, L. (1997). *Teach me language: A manual for children with autism, asperger's syndrome and related developmental disorders*. Langley, BC: SKF Books.

Frost, L. A., & Bondy, A. (1994). *The picture exchange communication system training manual*. Cherry Hill, NJ: Pyramid Educational Consultants.

Frost, L. A., & Bondy, A. S. (2002). *The picture exchange communication system training manual* (2nd ed.). Newark, DE: Pyramid Educational Products.

Ganz, J. B., & Simpson, R. L. (2004). Effects on communicative requesting and speech development of the Picture Exchange Communication System in children with characteristics of autism. *Journal of Autism and Developmental Disorders, 34*(4), 395–409.

Ganz, J. B., Simpson, R. L., & Corbin-Newsome, J. (2008). The impact of the Picture Exchange Communication System on requesting and speech development in preschoolers with autism spectrum disorders and similar characteristics. *Research in Autism Spectrum Disorders, 2*, 157–169.

Gilbert, K. (2008). Milieu communication training for late talkers. *Perspectives on Language Learning and Education, 15*, 112–118.

Gillberg, C., & Steffenburg, S. (1987). Outcome and prognostic factors in infantile autism and similar conditions: A population-based study of 46 cases followed through puberty. *Journal of Autism and Developmental Disorders, 17*(2), 273–287.

Girolametto, L., Sussman, F., & Weitzman, E. (2007). Using case study methods to investigate the effects of interactive intervention for children with autism spectrum disorders. *Journal of Communication Disorders, 40*(6), 470–792.

Goldsmith, T., LeBlanc, L., & Sautter, R. (2007). Teaching intraverbal behavior to children with autism. *Research in Autism Spectrum Disorders, 1*, 1–13.

Goodman, G., Duchan, J., & Sonnenmeier, R. (1994). Children's development of scriptal knowledge. In J. Duchan, L. Hewitt, & R. M. Sonnenmeier (Eds.), *Pragmatics: From theory to practice* (pp. 120–133). Englewood Cliffs, NJ: Prentice-Hall.

Gray, C. A. (1995). *Social stories and comic strip conversations: Unique methods to improve social understanding*. Jenison, MI: Carol Gray.

Gray, C. A., & Garand, J. D. (1993). Social Stories: Improving responses of students with autism with accurate social information. *Focus on Autistic Behavior, 8*(1), 1–10.

Grove, N., & Dockrell, J. (2000). Multisign combinations by children with intellectual impairments: An analysis of language skills. *Journal of Speech, Language, and Hearing Research, 43*(2), 309.

Gulsrud, A. C., Kasari, C., Freeman, S., & Paparella, T. (2007). Children with autism's response to novel stimuli while participating in interventions targeting joint attention or symbolic play skills. *Autism, 11*, 535–546.

Halliday, M. (1975). *Learning how to mean: Explorations in the development of language*. New York: Arnold.

Hancock, T., & Kaiser, A. (2002). The effects of trainer-implemented enhanced milieu teaching on the social communication of children with autism. *Topics in Early Childhood Special Education, 22*(1), 39–54.

Hartman, E., & Klatt, K. (2005). The effects of deprivation, presession exposure, and preferences on teaching manding to children with autism. *The Analysis of Verbal Behavior, 21*, 135–144.

Hemmeter, M., & Kaiser, A. (1994). Enhanced milieu teaching: An analysis of parent-implemented language intervention. *Journal of Early Intervention, 18*(3), 269–289.

Hobson, R., & Lee, A. (1989). Emotion-related and abstract concepts in autistic people: Evidence from the British picture vocabulary scale. *Journal of Autism and Developmental Disorders, 19*(4), 601–623.

Hoshino, Y., Kaneko, M., Yashima, Y., Kumashiro, H., Volkmar, F. R., & Cohen, D. J. (1987). Clinical features of autistic children with setback course in their infancy. *The Japanese Journal of Psychiatry and Neurology, 41*, 237–245.

Howlin, P. (2005). Outcome in autism spectrum disorders. In F. R. Volkmar, R. Paul, A. Klin, & D. J. Cohen (Eds.), *Handbook of autism and pervasive developmental disorders* (3rd ed., pp. 201–222). Hoboken, NJ: Wiley.

Howlin, P., Goode, S., Hutton, J., & Rutter, M. (2004). Adult outcomes for children with autism. *Journal of Autism and Developmental Disorders, 34*, 212–229.

Howlin, P., Gordon, R., Pasco, G., Wade, A., & Charman, T. (2007). The effectiveness of picture exchange communication system (PECS) training for teachers of children with autism: A pragmatic, group randomized controlled trial. *Journal of Child Psychology and Psychiatry, 48*, 473–481.

Huttenlocher, J. (1974). *The origins of language comprehension.* Paper presented at the Theories in cognitive psychology: The Loyola Symposium, Chicago, IL.

Johnston, S., Nelson, C., Evans, J., & Palazolo, K. (2003). The use of visual supports in teaching young children with autism spectrum disorder to initiate interactions. *Augmentative and Alternative Communication, 19*, 86–103.

Jones, E., Carr, D., & Feeley, K. (2006). Multiple effects of joint attention intervention for children with autism. *Behavior Modification, 30*, 782–834.

Kaiser, A., & Hester, P. (1994). Generalized effects of enhanced milieu teaching. *Journal of Speech and Hearing Research, 37*, 1320–1340.

Kaiser, A., Hancock, T., & Nietfeld, J. (2000). The effects of parent-implemented enhanced milieu teaching on the social communication of children who have autism. *Early Education and Development, 11*(4), 423–446.

Kaiser, A. P., Hancock, T. B., & Hester, P.P. (1998). Parents as co-interventionists: Research on applications of naturalistic language teaching procedures. *Infants and Young Children, 11* 10(4), 1–11.

Kasari, C., Freeman, S., & Paparella, T. (2006). Joint attention and symbolic play in young children with autism: A randomized controlled intervention study. *Journal of Child Psychology and Psychiatry, 47*(6), 611–620.

Kasari, C., Paparella, T., Freeman, S., & Jahromi, L. (2008). Language outcome in autism: Randomized comparison of joint attention and play interventions. *Journal of Consulting and Clinical Psychology, 76*(1), 125–137.

Keen, D., Sigafoos, J., & Woodyatt, G. (2001). Replacing prelinguistic behaviors with functional communication. *Journal of Autism and Developmental Disorders, 31*(4), 385–398.

Kelley, M. E., Shillingsburg, M. A., Castro, M. J., Addison, L. R., & LaRue, R. H. (2007). Further evaluation of emerging speech in children with developmental disabilities: Training verbal behavior. *Journal of Applied Behavior Analysis, 40*, 431–445.

Kobayashi, R. (1993). Setback phenomena and the long-term prognoses for autistic children. *Japanese Journal of Child and Adolescent Psychiatry, 34*(3), 239–248.

Kobayashi, R., & Murata, T. (1998). Setback phenomenon in autism and long-term prognosis. *Acta Psychiatrica Scandinavica, 98*(4), 296–303.

Koegel, R. L., & Koegel, L. K. (1988). Generalized responsivity and pivotal behaviors. In R. H. Horner & G. Dunlap (Eds.), *Generalization and maintenance: Life-style changes in applied settings* (pp. 41–66). Baltimore: Brookes.

Koegel, R. L., & Koegel, L. K. (Eds.). (2006). *Pivotal response treatments for autism: Communication, social, and academic development.* Baltimore: Brookes.

Krantz, P. J., & McClannahan, L. E. (1993). Teaching children with autism to initiate to peers: Effects of a script-fading procedure. *Journal of Applied Behavior Analysis, 26*, 121–132.

Krantz, P. J., & McClannahan, L. E. (1998). Social interaction skills for children with autism: A script-fading procedure for beginning readers. *Journal of Applied Behavior Analysis, 31*(2), 191–202.

Kravitz, T. R., Kamps, D. M., Kemmerer, K., & Potucek, J. (2002). Brief report: Increasing communication skills for an elementary-aged student with autism using the picture exchange communication system. *Journal of Autism and Developmental Disorders, 32*(3), 225–230.

Kurita, H. (1985). Infantile autism with speech loss before the age of thirty months. *Journal of the American Academy of Child Psychiatry, 24*(2), 191–196.

LeBlanc, L. A., Coates, A. M., Daneshvar, S., Charlop-Christy, M. H., Morris, C., & Lancaster, B. M. (2003). Using video modeling and reinforcement to teach perspective-taking skills to children with autism. *Journal of Applied Behavior Analysis, 36*, 253–257.

Lempert, H. (1978). Extrasyntactic factors affecting passive sentence comprehension in young children. *Child Development, 49*, 694–699.

Liddle, K. (2001). Implementing the picture exchange communication system (PECS). *International Journal of Language & Communication Disorders, 36*, 391–395.

Loban, W. (1976). *Language development: Kindergarten through grade twelve.* Urbana, IL: National Council of Teachers of English.

Lorimer, P., Simpson, R. L., Smith Myles, B., & Ganz, J. B. (2002). The use of Social Stories as a preventative behavioral intervention in a home setting with a child with autism. *Journal of Positive Behavior Interventions, 4*(1), 53–60.

Lovaas, O. I. (1987). Behavioral treatment and normal educational and intellectual functioning in young autistic children. *Journal of Consulting and Clinical Psychology, 55*(1), 3–9.

MacDuff, J., Ledo, R., McClannahan, L., & Krantz, P. (2007). Using scripts and script-fading procedures to promote bids for joint attention by young children with autism. *Research in Autism Spectrum Disorders, 1*, 281–290.

Magiati, I., & Howlin, P. (2003). A pilot evaluation study of the Picture Exchange Communication System for children with autistic spectrum disorders. *Autism, 7*, 297–320.

Magiati, I., Charman, T., & Howlin, P. (2007). A two-year prospective follow-up study of community-based early intensive behavioural intervention and specialist nursery provision for children with autism spectrum disorders. *Journal of Child Psychology and Psychiatry, 48*, 803–812.

Mahoney, G., & Perales, F. (2003). Using relationship-focused intervention to enhance the social-emotional functioning of your children with autism spectrum disorders. *Topics in Early Childhood Special Education, 23*, 77–89.

Maione, L., & Mirenda, P. (2006). Effects of video modeling and video feedback on peer-directed social language skills of a child with autism. *Journal of Positive Behavior Interventions, 8*(2), 106–118.

Mancil, G., Conroy, M., Nakao, T., & Alter, P. (2006). Functional communication training in the natural environment: A pilot investigation with a young child with autism spectrum disorder. *Education and Treatment of Children, 29*(4), 615–633.

Martin, C., Drasgow, E., Halle, J. W., & Brucker, J. M. (2005). Teaching a child with autism and severe language delays to reject: Direct and indirect effects of functional communication training. *Educational Psychology, 25*, 287–304.

Martins, M., & Harris, S. (2006). Teaching children with autism to respond to joint attention initiations. *Child and Family Behavior Therapy, 28*(1), 51–68.

McClannahan, L., & Krantz, P. (2005). *Teaching conversation to children with autism: Scripts and script fading*. Bethesda, MD: Woodbine House.

McConachie, H., Val Randle, V., Hammal, D., & LeCouteur, A. (2005). A controlled trial of a training course for parents of children with suspected autism spectrum disorders. *The Journal of Pediatrics, 147*, 335–340.

McDuffie, A., Yoder, P., & Stone, W. (2005). Prelinguistic predictors of vocabulary in young children with autism spectrum disorders. *Journal of Speech, Language, and Hearing Research, 48*, 1080–1097.

McEachin, J. J., Smith, T., & Lovaas, O. I. (1993). Long-term outcome for children with autism who received early intensive behavioral treatment. *American Journal of Mental Retardation, 97*(4), 359–372.

McEvoy, R. E., Loveland, K. A., & Landry, S. H. (1988). The functions of immediate echolalia in autistic children: A developmental perspective. *Journal of Autism and Developmental Disorders, 18*(4), 657–668.

Miguel, C., Carr, J., & Michael, J. (2002). The effects of a stimulus-stimulus pairing procedure on the vocal behavior of children diagnosed with autism. *The Analysis of Verbal Behavior, 18*, 3–13.

Millar, D., Light, J., & Schlosser, R. (2006). The impact of augmentative and alternative communication intervention on the speech production of individuals with developmental disabilities: A research review. *Journal of Speech, Language, and Hearing Research, 49*, 248–264.

Miller, J. (1981). *Assessing language production in children: Experimental procedures*. Baltimore: University Park Press.

Miller, J., & Chapman, R. (1981). The relation between age and mean length of utterance in morphemes. *Journal of Speech and Hearing Research, 24*, 154–162.

Mirenda, P. (2003). Toward functional augmentative and alternative communication for students with autism: Manual signs, graphic symbols, and voice output communication aids. *Language, Speech, and Hearing Services in Schools, 34*, 203–216.

Moes, D. R., & Frea, W. D. (2002). Contextualized behavioral support in early intervention for children with autism and their families. *Journal of Autism and Developmental Disorders, 32*, 519–533.

Mundy, P., & Burnette, C. (2005). Joint attention and neurodevelopmental models of autism. In F. R. Volkmar, R. Paul, A. Klin, & D. J. Cohen (Eds.), *Handbook of autism and pervasive developmental disorders* (3rd ed., pp. 650–681). Hoboken, NJ: Wiley.

Mundy, P., & Stella, J. (2000). Joint attention, social orienting, and nonverbal communication in autism. In A. M. Wetherby & B. M. Prizant (Eds.), *Autism spectrum disorders: A transactional developmental perspective, Communication and language intervention series, 9:55–77*. Baltimore: Brookes.

Mundy, P., Sigman, M., & Kasari, C. (1990). A longitudinal study of joint attention and language development in autistic children. *Journal of Autism and Developmental Disorders, 20*(1), 115–128.

National Research Council. (2001). *Educating young children with autism*. Washington, DC: National Academy Press.

Nazzi, T., & Bertoncini, J. (2003). Before and after the vocabulary spurt: Two modes of word acquisition? *Developmental Science, 6*(2), 136–142.

Nelson, K. (1973). Structure and strategy in learning to talk. *Monographs of the Society for Research in Child Development, 38*, 1–2.

Nikopoulos, C. K., & Keenan, M. (2003). Promoting social initiation in children with autism using video modeling. *Behavioral Interventions, 18*(2), 87–108.

Nikopoulos, C. K., & Keenan, M. (2004a). Effects of video modeling on social initiations by children with autism. *Journal of Applied Behavior Analysis, 37*, 93–96.

Nikopoulos, C. K., & Keenan, M. (2004b). Effects of video modeling and generalization of social initiation and reciprocal play by children with autism. *European Journal of Applied Behavior Analysis, 5*, 1–13.

Nikopoulos, C. K., & Keenan, M. (2007). Using video modeling to teach complex social sequences to children with autism. *Journal of Autism and Developmental Disorders, 37*, 678–693.

Normand, M., & Knoll, M. (2006). The effects of a stimulus-stimulus pairing procedure on the unprompted vocalizations of a young child diagnosed with autism. *The Analysis of Verbal Behavior, 22*, 81–85.

Norris, C., & Dattilo, J. (1999). Evaluating effects of a Social Story on a young girl with autism. *Focus on Autism and Other Developmental Disabilities, 14*, 180–186.

Olive, M., de la Cruz, B., Davis, T. N., Chan, J. M., Lang, R. B., et al. (2007). The effects of enhanced milieu teaching and a voice output communication aid on the requesting of three children with autism. *Journal of Autism and Developmental Disorders, 37*, 1505–1513.

Olive, M. L., Lang, R. B., & Davis, T. N. (2008). An analysis of the effects of functional communication and a voice output communication aid for a child with autism spectrum disorder. *Research in Autism Spectrum Disorders, 2*, 223–236.

ÓNeill, R., & Sweetland-Baker, M. (2001). Brief report: An assessment of stimulus generalization and contingency effects in functional communication training with two students with autism. *Journal of Autism and Developmental Disorders, 31*, 235–240.

Osterling, J., & Dawson, G. (1994). Early recognition of children with autism: A study of first birthday home videotapes. *Journal of Autism and Developmental Disorders, 24*(3), 247–257.

Parsons, C., & La Sorte, D. (1993). The effect of computers with synthesized speech and no speech on the spontaneous communication of children with autism. *Australian Journal of Human Communication Disorders, 21*, 12–31.

Partington, J., Sundberg, M., Newhouse, L., & Spengler-Schelley, M. (1994). Overcoming an autistic child's failure to acquire a tact repertoire. *Journal of Applied Behavior Analysis, 27*, 733–734.

Paul, R. (1985). The emergence of pragmatic comprehension: Children's understanding of sentence-structure cues to given/new information. *Journal of Child Language, 12*, 161–180.

Paul, R. (2003). Promoting social communication in high functioning individuals with autistic spectrum disorders. *Child and Adolescent Psychiatric Clinics of North America, 12*(1), 87–106. vi–vii.

Paul, R., & Cohen, D. (1984). Outcomes of severe disorders of language acquisition. *Journal of Autism and Developmental Disorders, 14*(4), 405–421.

Paul, R., & Sutherland, D. (2005). Enhancing early language in children with autism spectrum disorders. In F. R. Volkmar, R. Paul, A. Klin, & D. J. Cohen (Eds.), *Handbook of autism and pervasive developmental disorders* (3rd ed., pp. 946–976). Hoboken, NJ: Wiley.

Paul, R., Chawarska, K., Fowler, C., Cicchetti, D., & Volkmar, F. (2007a). Listen, my children and you shall hear: Auditory preferences in toddlers with ASD. *Journal of Speech, Language, and Hearing Research, 50*, 1350–1364.

Paul, R., Chawarska, K., Klin, A., & Volkmar, F. (2007b). Dissociations in the development of early communication in ASD. In R. Paul (Ed.), *Language disorders from a developmental perspective: Essays in honor of Robin Chapman*. Hillsdale, NJ: Erlbaum.

Paul, R., Chawarska, K., Klin, A., & Volkmar, F. (2008). Language outcomes in toddlers with ASD: A 2 year follow-up. *Autism Research, 1*, 97–107.

Peterson, C., & McCabe, A. (1983). *Developmental psycholinguistics: Three ways of looking at a child's narrative*. New York: Plenum.

Preis, J. (2006). The effect of picture communication symbols on the verbal comprehension of commands by young children with autism. *Focus on Autism and Other Developmental Disabilities, 21*(4), 194–210.

Prelock, P. A. (2006). *Autism spectrum disorders: Issues in assessment and intervention*. Austin, TX: Pro-Ed.

Prizant, B. M., & Rydell, P. J. (1984). Analysis of functions of delayed echolalia in autistic children. *Journal of Speech and Hearing Research, 27*(2), 183–192.

Reichow, B., & Wolery, M. (2009). Comprehensive synthesis of early intensive behavioral interventions for young children with autism based on the UCLA young autism project model. *Journal of Autism and Developmental Disorders, 39*, 23–41.

Reichow, B., Paul, R., Lewis, M., & Schoen, E. (2009, May) *Randomized study contrasting behavioral and naturalistic approaches to inducing speech in prelinguistic children with autism spectrum disorders: Preliminary analysis.* Paper presented at the international meeting for autism research, Chicago.

Remington, B., Hastings, R., Kovshoff, H., Degli Espinosa, F., Jahr, E., Brown, T., et al. (2007). Early intensive behavioral intervention: outcomes for children with autism and their parents after two years. *American Journal of Mental Retardation, 112,* 418–438.

Rocha, M. L., Schreibman, L., & Stahmer, A. C. (2007). Effectiveness of training parents to teach joint attention in children with autism. *Journal of Early Intervention, 29*(2), 154–172.

Rogers, S. (2006). Evidence-based intervention for language development in young children with autism. In T. Charman & W. Stone (Eds.), *Social and communication development in autism spectrum disorders: Early identification, diagnosis, and intervention* (pp. 143–179). New York: Guilford.

Rogers, S. J., & DiLalla, D. L. (1990). Age of symptom onset in young children with pervasive developmental disorders. *Journal of the American Academy of Child and Adolescent Psychiatry, 29*(6), 863–872.

Rogers, S. J., & Vismara, L. A. (2008). Evidence-based comprehensive treatments for early autism. *Journal of Clinical Child and Adolescent Psychology, 37,* 8–38.

Rogers, S., Hepburn, S., Stackhouse, T., & Wehner, E. (2003). Imitation performance in toddlers with autism and those with other developmental disorders. *Journal of Child Psychology and Psychiatry, 44*(5), 763–781.

Rogers, S., Cook, I., & Meryl, A. (2005). Imitation and play in autism. In F. R. Volkmar, R. Paul, A. Klin, & D. J. Cohen (Eds.), *Handbook of autism and pervasive developmental disorders* (3rd ed., pp. 382–405). Hoboken, NJ: Wiley.

Ross, D. (2002). Replacing faulty conversational exchanges for children with autism by establishing a functionally equivalent alternative response. *Education and Training in Mental Retardation and Developmental Disabilities, 37*(4), 343–362.

Ross, D. E., & Greer, R. (2003). Generalized imitation and the mand: Inducing first instances of speech in young children with autism. *Research in Developmental Disabilities, 24*(1), 58–74.

Sallows, G., & Graupner, T. (2005). Intensive behavioral treatment for children with autism: four-year outcome and predictors. *American Journal of Mental Retardation, 110,* 417–438.

Sansosti, F. J., & Powell-Smith, K. A. (2006). Using Social Stories to improve the social behavior of children with Asperger syndrome. *Journal of Positive Behavior Interventions, 8*(1), 43–57.

Sansosti, F. J., & Powell-Smith, K. A. (2008). Using computer-presented Social Stories and video models to increase the social communication skills of children with high-functioning autism spectrum disorders. *Journal of Positive Behavior Interventions, 10*(3), 162–178.

Sarokoff, R., Taylor, B., & Poulson, C. (2001). Teaching children with autism to engage in conversational exchanges: Script fading with embedded textual stimuli. *Journal of Applied Behavior Analysis, 34*(1), 81–84.

Scattone, D., Tingstrom, D. H., & Wilczynski, S. M. (2006). Increasing appropriate social interactions of children with autism spectrum disorders using Social Stories™. *Focus on Autism and Other Developmental Disabilities, 21*(4), 211–222.

Schepis, M., Reid, D., Behrmann, M., & Sutton, K. (1998). Increasing communicative interactions of young children with autism using a voice output communication aid and naturalistic teaching. *Journal of Applied Behavior Analysis, 31,* 561–578.

Schertz, H. H., & Odom, S. L. (2007). Promoting joint attention in toddlers with autism: A parent-mediated developmental model. *Journal of Autism and Developmental Disorders, 37*(8), 1562–1575.

Schindler, H., & Horner, R. (2005). Generalized reduction of problem behavior of young children with autism: Building trans-situational interventions. *American Journal of Mental Retardation, 110*(1), 36–47.

Schlosser, R., & Blischak, D. (2001). Is there a role for speech output in interventions for persons with autism? A review. *Focus on Autism and Other Developmental Disabilities, 16*(3), 170–178.

Schlosser, R., & Wendt, O. (2008). Effects of augmentative and alternative communication intervention on speech production in children with autism: A systematic review. *American Journal of Speech-Language Pathology, 17,* 212–230.

Schlosser, R., Sigafoos, J., Luiselli, J., Angermeier, K., Harasymowyz, U., et al. (2007). Effects of synthetic speech output on requesting and natural speech production in children with autism: A preliminary study. *Research in Autism Spectrum Disorders, 1,* 139–163.

Schwartz, I. S., Garfinkle, A. N., & Bauer, J. (1998). The picture exchange communication system: Communicative outcomes for young children with disabilities. *Topics in Early Childhood Special Education, 18*(3), 144–159.

Sheinkopf, S., & Siegel, B. (1998). Home-based behavioral treatment of young children with autism. *Journal of Autism and Developmental Disorders, 28*, 15–23.

Sheinkopf, J., Mundy, P., Oller, D. K., & Steffens, M. (2000). Vocal atypicalities of preverbal autistic children. *Journal of Autism and Developmental Disorders, 30*, 345–354.

Sherer, M., Pierce, K. L., Paredes, S., et al. (2001). Enhancing conversation skills in children with autism via video technology: Which is better, "self" or "other" as a model? *Behavior Modification, 25*(1), 140–158.

Shipley-Benamou, R., Lutzker, J. R., & Taubman, M. (2002). Teaching daily living skills to children with autism through instructional video modeling. *Journal of Positive Behavior Interventions, 4*(3), 166–177.

Sigafoos, J., Didden, R., & ÓReilly, M. (2003). Effects of speech output on maintenance of requesting and frequency of vocalizations in three children with developmental disabilities. *Augmentative and Alternative Communication, 19*, 37–47.

Sigafoos, J., Drasgow, E., Halle, J., ÓReilly, M., Seeely-York, S., et al. (2004). Teaching VOCA use as a communicative repair strategy. *Journal of Autism and Developmental Disorders, 34*, 411–422.

Sigman, M., & Ruskin, E. (1999). Continuity and change in the social competence of children with autism, Down syndrome, and developmental delays. *Monographs of the Society for Research in Child Development, 64*(1), 1–14.

Siller, M., & Sigman, M. (2002). The behaviors of parents of children with autism predict the subsequent development of their children's communication. *Journal of Autism and Developmental Disorders, 32*(2), 77–89.

Smith, T., Eikeseth, S., Klevstrand, M., & Lovaas, O. I. (1997). Intensive behavioral treatment for preschoolers with severe mental retardation and pervasive developmental disorder. *American Journal of Mental Retardation, 102*, 238–249.

Smith, T., Buch, J., & Gamby, T. (2000a). Parent-directed, early intensive intervention for children with pervasive developmental disorder. *Research in Developmental Disabilities, 21*, 297–309.

Smith, T., Groen, A. D., & Wynn, J. W. (2000b). Randomized trial of intensive early intervention for children with pervasive developmental disorder. *American Journal of Mental Retardation, 105*(4), 269–285.

Smith, V., Mirenda, P., & Zaidman-Zait, A. (2007). Predictors of expressive vocabulary growth in children with autism. *Journal of Speech, Language, and Hearing Research, 50*, 149–160.

Solis, T., Derby, K. M., & McLaughlin, T. F. (2003). The effects of precision teaching techniques and functional communication training on problem behavior for a 12-year old male with autism. *International Journal of Special Education, 18*(1), 49–54.

Son, S., Sigafoos, J., ÓReilly, M., & Lancioni, G. E. (2006). Comparing two types of augmentative and alternative communication systems for children with autism. *Pediatric Rehabilitation, 9*, 389–395.

Sonnenmeier, R. M. (1994). Script-based language intervention: Learning to participate in life events. In J. Duchan, L. Hewitt, & R. M. Sonnenmeier (Eds.), *Pragmatics: From theory to practice* (pp. 134–148). Englewood Cliffs, NJ: Prentice-Hall.

Stevenson, C., Krantz, P., & McClannahan, L. (2000). Social interaction skills for children with autism: A script-fading procedure for nonreaders. *Behavioral Interventions, 15*, 1–20.

Stokes, K. S. (1977). Planning for the future of a severely handicapped autistic child. *Journal of Autism and Childhood Schizophrenia, 7*(3), 288–302.

Stone, W. L., Ousley, O. Y., Yoder, P. J., Hogan, K. L., & Hepburn, S. L. (1997). Nonverbal communication in two- and three-year-old children with autism. *Journal of Autism and Developmental Disorders, 27*(6), 677–696.

Sundberg, M., Michael, J., Partington, J., & Sundberg, C. (1995). The role of automatic reinforcement in early language acquisition. *The Analysis of Verbal Behavior, 13*, 21–37.

Sundberg, M., Endicott, K., & Eigenheer, P. (2000). Using intraverbal prompts to establish tacts for children with autism. *The Analysis of Verbal Behavior, 17*, 89–104.

Sundberg, M., Loeb, M., Hale, L., & Eigenheer, P. (2002). Contriving establishing operations to teach mands for information. *The Analysis of Verbal Behavior, 18*, 15–29.

Sussman, F. (1999). *More than words: Helping parents promote communication and social skills in children with autism spectrum disorders.* Toronto, Canada: A Hanen Centre Publication.

Swaggart, B., Gagnon, E., Jones Bock, S., Earles, T., Quinn, C., Smith Myles, B., et al. (1995). Using Social Stories to teach social and behavioral skills to children with autism. *Focus on Autistic Behavior, 10*, 1–16.

Sweeney-Kerwin, E., Carbone, V., ÓBrien, L., Zecchin, G., & Janecky, M. N. (2007). Transferring control of the mand to the motivating operation in children with autism. *The Analysis of Verbal Behavior, 23*, 89–102.

Tager-Flusberg, H. (1992). Autistic children's talk about psychological states: Deficits in the early acquisition of a theory of mind. *Child Development, 63,* 161–172.

Tager-Flusberg, H. (1995). Dissociation in form and function in the acquisition of language by autistic children. In H. Tager-Flusberg (Ed.), *Constraints on language acquisition: Studies of atypical children* (pp. 175–194). Hillsdale, NJ: Erlbaum.

Tager-Flusberg, H., & Calkins, S. (1990). Does imitation facilitate the acquisition of grammar? Evidence from a study of autistic, Down's syndrome and normal children. *Journal of Child Language, 17*(3), 591–606.

Tager-Flusberg, H., & Joseph, R. M. (2003). Identifying neurocognitive phenotypes in autism. *Philosophical Transactions of the Royal Society of London, B, 358,* 303–314.

Tager-Flusberg, H., Calkins, S., Nolin, T., Baumberger, T., Anderson, M., & Chadwick-Dias, A. (1990). A longitudinal study of language acquisition in autistic and Down syndrome children. *Journal of Autism and Developmental Disorders, 20*(1), 1–21.

Tager-Flusberg, H., Paul, R., & Lord, C. (2005). Language and communication in autism. In F. R. Volkmar, R. Paul, A. Klin, & D. J. Cohen (Eds.), *Handbook of autism and pervasive developmental disorders* (3rd ed., pp. 335–364). Hoboken, NJ: Wiley.

Tager-Flusberg, H., Rogers, S., Cooper, J., Landa, R., Lord, C., Paul, R., et al. (2009). Defining spoken language benchmarks and selecting measures of expressive language development for young children with autism spectrum disorders. *American Journal of Speech-Language Pathology, 52,* 643–652.

Taylor, B. A., Levin, L., & Jasper, S. (1999). Increasing play-related statements in children with autism toward their siblings: Effects of video modeling. *Journal of Developmental and Physical Disabilities, 11,* 253–264.

Thal, D. J. (1991). Language and cognition in normal and late-talking toddlers. *Topics in Language Disorders, 11*(4), 33–42.

Thiemann, S., & Goldstein, H. (2001). Social Stories, written text cues, and video feedback: Effects on social communication of children with autism. *Journal of Applied Behavior Analysis, 34,* 425–446.

Thunberg, G., Ahlsen, E., & Sandberg, A. (2007). Children with autistic spectrum disorders and speech-generating devices: Communication in different activities at home. *Clinical Linguistics & Phonetics, 21*(6), 457–479.

Tincani, M. (2004). Comparing the picture exchange communication system and sign language training for children with autism. *Focus on Autism and Other Developmental Disabilities, 19*(3), 152–163.

Tincani, M., Crozier, S., & Alazetta, L. (2006). The picture exchange communication system: Effects on manding and speech development for school-aged children with autism. *Education and Training in Developmental Disabilities, 41*(2), 177–184.

Tomasello, M. (1992). The social bases of language acquisition. *Social Development, 1*(1), 67–87.

Tomasello, M., & Kruger, A. C. (1992). Joint attention on actions: Acquiring verbs in ostensive and non-ostensive contexts. *Journal of Child Language, 19*(2), 311–333.

Tsiouri, I., & Greer, R. (2003). Inducing vocal verbal behavior in children with severe language delays through rapid motor imitation responding. *Journal of Behavioral Education, 12*(3), 185–206.

Tuchman, R. F., & Rapin, I. (1997). Regression in pervasive developmental disorders: Seizures and epileptiform electroencephalogram correlates. *Pediatrics, 99,* 560–566.

Venter, A., Lord, C., & Schopler, E. (1992). A follow-up study of high-functioning autistic children. *Journal of Child Psychology and Psychiatry, 33*(3), 489–507.

Volkmar, F. R., Carter, A., Grossman, J., & Klin, A. (1997). Social development in autism. In D. J. Cohen & F. R. Volkmar (Eds.), *Handbook of autism and pervasive developmental disorders* (2nd ed., pp. 173–194). New York: Wiley.

Wacker, D., Berg, W., Harding, J., Barretto, A., Rankin, B., & Ganzer, J. (2005). Treatment effectiveness, stimulus generalization, and acceptability to parents of functional communication training. *Educational Psychology, 25,* 233–256.

Ward, S. P., Osnes, P., & Partington, J. (2007). The effects of a delay of noncontingent reinforcement during a pairing procedure in the development of stimulus control of automatically reinforced vocalizations. *The Analysis of Verbal Behavior, 23,* 103–111.

Warren, S., & Yoder, P. (1998). Facilitating the transition to intentional communication. In A. Wetherby, S. Warren, & J. Riechle (Eds.), *Transitions in prelinguistic communication* (Vol. 7, pp. 365–385). Baltimore: Brookes.

Weiss, M. (1999). Differential rates of skill acquisition and outcomes of early intensive behavioral intervention for autism. *Behavioral Interventions, 14,* 3–22.

Wert, B. Y., & Neisworth, J. T. (2003). Effects of video self-modeling on spontaneous requesting in children with autism. *Journal of Positive Behavior Interventions, 5,* 30–34.

Wetherby, A. M. (1986). Ontogeny of communicative functions in autism. *Journal of Autism and Developmental Disorders, 16,* 295–319.

Wetherby, A. M., & Prizant, B. M. (1992). Profiling young children's communicative competence. In S. F. Warren & J. Reichle (Eds.), *Communication and language intervention series* (Causes and effects in communication and language intervention, Vol. 1, pp. 217–253). Baltimore: Brookes.

Wetherby, A. M., Prizant, B. M., & Hutchinson, T. A. (1998). Communicative, social/affective, and symbolic profiles of young children with autism and pervasive developmental disorders. *American Journal of Speech-Language Pathology, 7,* 79–91.

Wetherby, A. M., Prizant, B. M., & Schuler, A. L. (2000). Understanding the nature of communication and language impairments. In A. M. Wetherby & B. M. Prizant (Eds.), *Autism spectrum disorders: A transactional developmental perspective* (pp. 109–141). Baltimore: Brooks.

Wetherby, A. M., Woods, J., Allen, L., Cleary, J., Dickinson, H., & Lord, C. (2004). Early indicators of autism spectrum disorders in the second year of life. *Journal of Autism and Developmental Disorders, 34*(5), 473–493.

Whalen, C., & Shreibman, L. (2003). Joint attention training for children with autism using behavior modification procedures. *Journal of Child Psychology and Psychiatry, 44,* 456–468.

Whalen, C., Schreibman, L., & Ingersoll, B. (2006). The collateral effects of joint attention training on social initiations, positive affect, imitation, and spontaneous speech for young children with autism. *Journal of Autism and Developmental Disorders, 36*(5), 655–664.

White, S., Koenig, K., & Scahill, L. (2007). Social skills development in children with autism spectrum disorders: A review of intervention research. *Journal of Autism and Developmental Disorders, 37*(10), 1858–1868.

Winner, M. (2000). *Inside out: What makes the person with social cognitive deficits tick?* San Jose, CA: Think Social Publishing.

Winner, M. (2002). Assessment of social skills for students with Asperger syndrome and high-functioning autism. *Assessment for Effective Intervention, 27,* 73–80.

Winner, M. (2004). Perspective taking across the school and adult years for persons with social cognitive deficits: A proposal for a perspective taking spectrum and related critical curriculum and support to facilitate adult success. *The Educational Therapist, 25*(1), 6–12.

Winner, M. (2005). *Think social! A social thinking curriculum for school age students.* San Jose, CA: Think Social Publishing.

Winner, M. (2007). *Thinking about you thinking about me* (2nd ed.). San Jose, CA: Think Social Publishing.

Yi, J., Christian, L., Vittimberga, G., & Lowenkron, B. (2006). Generalized negatively reinforced manding in children with autism. *The Analysis of Verbal Behavior, 22,* 21–33.

Yoder, P. J. (2006). Predicting lexical density growth rate in young children with autism spectrum disorders. *American Journal of Speech-Language Pathology, 15*(4), 378.

Yoder, P., & Layton, T. L. (1988). Speech following sign language training in autistic children with minimal verbal language. *Journal of Autism and Developmental Disorders, 18*(2), 217–229.

Yoder, P. J., & McDuffie, A. S. (2006). Treatment of responding to and initiating joint attention. In T. Charman & W. Stone (Eds.), *Social and communication development in autism spectrum disorders: Early identification, diagnosis, and intervention* (pp. 117–142). New York: Guilford.

Yoder, P., & Stone, W. (2006a). A randomized comparison of the effect of two prelinguistic communication interventions on the acquisition of spoken communication in preschoolers with ASD. *Journal of Speech, Language, and Hearing Research, 49,* 698–711.

Yoder, P., & Stone, W. (2006b). Randomized comparison of two communication interventions for preschoolers with autism spectrum disorders. *Journal of Consulting and Clinical Psychology, 74*(3), 426–435.

Yoder, P., & Warren, S. (1998). Maternal responsivity predicts the prelinguistic communication intervention that facilitates generalized intentional communication. *Journal of Speech, Language, and Hearing Research, 41,* 1207–1219.

Yoder, P., & Warren, S. (2001). Relative treatment effects of two prelinguistic communication interventions on language development in toddlers with developmental delays vary by maternal characteristics. *Journal of Speech, Language, and Hearing Research, 44,* 224–237.

Yoder, P., & Warren, S. (2002). Effects of prelinguistic milieu teaching and parent responsivity education on dyads involving children with intellectual disabilities. *Journal of Speech, Language, and Hearing Research, 45,* 1158–1174.

Yokoyama, K., Naoi, N., & Yamamoto, J. (2006). Teaching verbal behavior using the picture exchange communication system (PECS) with children with autism spectrum disorders. *Japanese Journal of Special Education, 43*(6), 485–503.

Yule, W., & Rutter, M. (1987). *Language development and disorders.* London: MacKeith.

CHAPTER 6

Treatments to Increase Social Awareness and Social Skills

Suzannah J. Ferraioli and Sandra L. Harris

ABBREVIATIONS

ADHD	Attention deficit hyperactivity disorder
ADI-R	Autism Diagnostic Interview – revised
ADOS	Autism Diagnostic Observation Schedule
ASDs	Autism spectrum disorders
CARS	Childhood Autism Rating Scale
CBT	Cognitive behavioral therapy
CGI	Clinical global improvement
DSM-IV-TR	Diagnostic and Statistical Manual of Mental Disorders 4th edition
MBD	Multiple baseline design
NIMH	National Institutes of Mental Health
OCD	Obsessive–compulsive disorder
ODD	Oppositional defiant disorder
PCIT	Parent–child interaction therapy
PDD-NOS	Pervasive developmental disorder not otherwise specified
RCT	Randomized control trial
RUPP	Research Units on Pediatric Psychopharmacology
SRS	Social Responsiveness Scale
SSED	Single subject experimental design
SST	Social skills training

INTRODUCTION

There is an extensive literature on methods for increasing the social awareness and social skills of people with autism spectrum disorders (ASDs) of every diagnostic category and every age. This work varies in research quality from the mediocre to the exemplary, although the exemplary are outnumbered by the less rigorous. One reason for the focus on treating social behaviors is that

B. Reichow et al. (eds.), *Evidence-Based Practices and Treatments for Children with Autism*,
DOI 10.1007/978-1-4419-6975-0_6, © Springer Science+Business Media, LLC 2011

qualitative impairments in social interaction are intrinsic to ASDs (APA 2000). To support people on the autism spectrum in learning sufficient social behavior to move with reasonable comfort within the wider "neurotypical" society, a great deal of work needs to be done by them and by us to help them master sufficient knowledge and skills to handle social encounters. Our teaching methods should be efficient and effective.

Our goal in the present chapter is to review research about several social domains including joint attention, imitation, in vivo and video modeling, peer training, social skills groups for children and adolescents, and Social Stories. That is not an inclusive list of research in social skills and cognition, but a sample of some of the empirically best and weakest. Although we included many articles under each heading some articles may have escaped our notice and we apologize for any serious omission.

Along with descriptions of various single subject experimental designs (SSED) and group designs used to investigate the domains we reviewed, we have rated the articles using the evaluative method of Reichow et al. (2008). A rating of "weak" in their system does not mean that the intervention is ineffective, but that the methods used do not allow one to conclude that the intervention meets the standards of evidence-based practice. Preliminary, innovative research in science is often weak when initial hypotheses are explored. It is not until well-controlled studies are done which verify the hypotheses that the method reaches the stage where one can be satisfied that it should be considered established evidence-based practice. To move our understanding of evidence-based practices for social skills and knowledge into wide use we need to go well beyond uncontrolled case studies to the randomized control trials (RCT) and rigorous SSED that are the gold standard of research.

In each of the sections, there is a brief description of the technique under study, commentaries on the studies we read, and a table summarizing the ratings. We conclude the chapter with a summary of our findings and recommendations for future work.

JOINT ATTENTION

It is not surprising that children with ASDs miss opportunities to learn from modeling of social behaviors such as joint attention (JA) that are critical for appropriate social development. JA is a social-communicative behavior (see Chapter 5) that is generally defined as a child's ability to use gestures and eye contact to coordinate attention with another person to share the experience of an interesting object or event. Because JA is considered a pivotal skill and is universally impaired in children with autism, many researchers have developed interventions targeting JA skills. This section reviews the variety of behavioral interventions specifically targeting JA; a summary of findings can be found in Table 6.1.

Whalen and Schreibman (2003) created an intervention to progressively target individual elements of JA (e.g., giving, showing, eye contact, and following gaze) in five children with autism and included separate procedures to teach responding to and initiating JA. Acquisition criteria were developed from observations of typically developing preschoolers, a major strength of this study. All five participants increased in their responding to JA (e.g., following a point, following a gaze shift), and four demonstrated increased initiations (e.g., protodeclarative pointing). These results were maintained at a 3-month follow-up and generalized across settings. The findings from the 2003 study are impressive but limited in social significance. The intervention was done in a laboratory setting and treatment was provided by trained interventionists.

TABLE 6.1   Summaries and ratings for studies on joint attention

Study	Design	Outcome	Rating
Kasari et al. (2006)	RCT: JA versus play interventions	Improvements in social skills for both groups; JA-specific gains for the JA intervention	Strong
Martins and Harris (2006)	MBD with reversal of JA response training	Increase in JA responding; minimal increase in initiating	Strong
Rocha et al. (2007)	MBD of parent-mediated JA training	Increases in JA responding and initiating	Strong
Whalen and Schreibman (2003)	MBD of JA training	Increases in JA responding; increases in initiations for four out of five participants	Strong
Whalen et al. (2006)	MBD of JA training	Improvements in affects, imitation, and spontaneous speech	Strong
Zercher et al. (2001)	MBD of integrated play group	Increases in JA, play, and language	Adequate

To enhance the social and external validity of the training, Rocha et al. (2007) did a follow-up to determine if parents of children with autism could implement the same intervention. Three parent–child pairs successfully completed the intervention and all children increased their rates of initiating and responding to JA. The benefits also generalized to unfamiliar adults on a structured assessment of JA.

In 2006, Whalen, Schreibman, and Ingersoll published data on collateral social behaviors tracked during the 2003 study. In addition to improvements in JA, children from the 2003 study demonstrated ancillary gains in social initiations, positive affect, imitation, and spontaneous speech. These results supported the conceptualization of JA as a pivotal behavior and evidenced generalization across social skills.

In the studies discussed thus far, the use of participants who were already demonstrating some emerging JA skills limited the external validity of the intervention procedures. From these results, it is unclear whether the training procedures are useful for the acquisition of JA or just the improvement of existing skills. Martins and Harris (2006) attempted to fill this

gap in the literature. Three children with autism with marked JA deficits increased their responding to social bids following an adult-mediated behavioral intervention. In this case, the response did not automatically generalize to initiations, suggesting that initiating skills may need to be explicitly targeted in the acquisition phase.

In typically developing children, JA emerges as a preverbal behavior. Considering the link between JA and language development, some of the effects of JA training on children with autism may be masked by an intervention's use of verbal cues or instruction or by varying verbal abilities among participants. Hwang and Hughes (2000) used social interactive training with three preverbal children with autism to parse out the effects of language on JA outcomes. All participants demonstrated increases in eye contact, JA and imitation responses, which were maintained at follow-up probes. Although this study was effective in isolating the effects of a JA intervention from verbal ability, the use of multiple targeted behaviors may have confounded the results. The authors did not control for the effects of teaching the imitation response versus the JA response; it is therefore possible that imitation training alone could have accounted for gains in JA. Indeed, such findings were obtained by Ingersoll and Schreibman (2006).

Only one RCT has been published on the use of JA training. Kasari et al. (2006) randomly assigned 65 children with autism to a JA treatment group, a symbolic play treatment group, or a control group (treatment as usual). Both treatment groups performed better than the controls on measures of coordinated joint gaze and did not differ from each other. The JA group demonstrated responding to JA, giving, and showing that was superior to both the control and the symbolic play groups. As expected, the play group did significantly better on measures of play. These results provide some information on the specificity of the treatments. In general, the outcomes of these participants matched the target of treatment, but there was some overlap (e.g., gains in joint gaze for the play group). The lack of improvement in the control group supports the efficacy of JA training as a whole. One significant limitation to this study is the small number of participants. Although the group differences were statistically significant, the results have limited power and small effect sizes. Regardless, considering the dearth of controlled group studies in the area of social skills, this is an encouraging base for replication with larger samples.

IMITATION

Although not considered a core deficit, imitation skills are almost ubiquitously impaired in children with ASDs. Typically developing children rely heavily on observational learning from adults and peers to acquire overt social skills (e.g., sharing, initiating conversation or play) and more subtle or complex social behavior (e.g., JA, reciprocity, descriptive gestures); therefore, the failure of children with ASDs to flexibly imitate may contribute significantly to overall deficits in socialization. Imitation has also been strongly linked to language and cognitive ability; it may represent a non-specific mechanism for the atypical development of a variety of skills (Ingersoll and Schreibman 2006). This section describes results from two types of widely used teaching procedure: in vivo modeling and video modeling. A summary of findings can be found in Table 6.2.

In vivo Modeling

In observational learning, children must attend to multiple cues, including model behavior, context, and consequences of the behavior (Garfinkle and Schwartz 2002). The use of modeling procedures to teach social skills raises some significant challenges for skills acquisition and generalization. For example, social behavior is less rote and less easily operationalized than other skills, such as object discrimination and self-care routines. In vivo modeling provides a good method for addressing this obstacle because it can occur in the actual social situation and because the modeled response can vary from trial to trial.

The generalization challenge has also been addressed in the in vivo modeling literature by using models who are likely to engage in developmentally appropriate behavior in the natural environment. Peers have been shown to be effective models and training peers can lead to increases in both the frequency of social initiation and the quality of social interactions (Kamps et al. 2002; McGrath et al. 2003). Peer-trained social skills are found to be more robust and facilitate more generalization than adult-centered training (Kamps et al. 2002). The studies discussed below use peers as models unless otherwise specified.

Garfinkle and Schwartz (2002) looked at the effects of a peer imitation intervention

TABLE 6.2   Summaries and ratings for studies on imitation

Study	Design	Outcome	Rating
Bellini et al. (2007)	MBD of video self-modeling	Increases in social interactions for two participants	Adequate
Charlop-Christy and Daneshvar (2003)	MBD of video modeling to teach perspective taking	Increases in correct responding to perspective-taking tasks	Adequate
Garfinkle and Schwartz (2002)	MBD of peer imitation training	Improvements in social interactions and initiations	Adequate
Gena et al. (2005)	MBD with reversal to compare in vivo and video modeling	Increases in appropriate affective responding for both treatments	Strong
Ingersoll et al. (2007)	MBD of reciprocal imitation training	Increases in imitation and spontaneous use of descriptive gestures	Strong
Ingersoll and Schreibman (2006)	MBD of reciprocal imitation training	Improvements in joint attention, pretend play, and language	Strong
Jahr et al. (2000)	Nonconcurrent MBD of in vivo modeling to engage in play	Increases in initiating and responding to cooperative play	Strong
Kroeger et al. (2007)	Group comparison of video modeling versus play group	Overall improvements in prosocial skills; larger gains reported in the treatment group	Adequate
Maione and Mirenda (2006)	MBD of video modeling	Increases in social initiations and responses	Adequate
Nikopoulos and Keenan (2003)	MBD of video modeling	Improvements in reciprocal play and latency to social initiations	Strong
Nikopoulos and Keenan (2004)	MBD of video modeling	Decreases in latency to social initiations and increases in reciprocal play	Adequate
Nikopoulos and Keenan (2007)	Multiple-treatment design of video modeling	Improvements in social initiations and appropriate play for four of seven subjects	Adequate
Simpson et al. (2004)	MBD of embedded video and computer-based instruction	Improvements in sharing, following directions, and greetings	Strong

package on four children with autism in an integrated classroom. Each day, certain peers and targets were singled out as "leaders" whom the rest of the students imitated. The authors reported significant increases in imitation for targets and peers, but only small or absent concomitant increases in target social initiations. Because the intervention was implemented only at naturally occurring times throughout the day (as opposed to a systematic schedule), the setting may have lacked sufficient structure to evoke increases in other social behavior.

In such a structured setting, Ingersoll and Schreibman (2006) used reciprocal imitation training (RIT) with five children with autism. RIT is a naturalistic intervention capitalizing on contingent imitation and child motivation. This treatment is systematically applied to provide frequent learning opportunities, but also occurs within the context of natural play sessions to facilitate generalization. The application of RIT in this context led to universal gains in imitation skills and generalization to new materials, settings, and therapists in four of the five participants. The intervention's use of contingent imitation is a nice addition to this treatment because it shapes the prerequisite skill of recognizing imitation in another person before attempting to train an imitation response. Unlike Garfinkle and Schwartz (2002) these authors also recorded ancillary gains in other social skills (JA and pretend play), making this the first study to experimentally demonstrate the relationship between imitation training and the acquisition of these more complex social behaviors. Additional support for RIT was provided by Ingersoll, Lewis, and Kroman (2007) in a study to teach higher-order social skills, such as descriptive gestures.

Video Modeling

Video modeling (VM) involves a competent confederate performing a targeted skill on videotape; this video is shown repeatedly to a subject, who is then given the opportunity to perform the task in a real life setting. VM has several advantages over in vivo modeling. First, attentional difficulties can be addressed by emphasizing the salient features of the desired task. Second, video presentation is conducive to frequent repetition. Third, it capitalizes upon motivation; children who characteristically display a lack of inherent desire to engage in learning activities will often enjoy and may even request their VM tapes.

The use of VM has recently extended to complex behavior as researchers have

begun to use these procedures to target social skills. Much of this research focuses on increasing social initiations, a skill which may be especially difficult for children with ASDs because it requires a spontaneous effort, rather than a response to a cue from another person. Nikopoulos and Keenan (2003) did the first systematic investigation of VM to teach social initiations in seven children with autism spectrum disorders. Four of the participants acquired the social initiation response and maintained these skills at 1- and 2-month follow-up assessments. Those that successfully initiated also demonstrated generalization across experimenters, settings and stimuli. Although these findings are encouraging, it is unclear why the performance across subjects was inconsistent. The authors speculate that the students' disruptive behaviors interfered with their ability to attend to the video; they also suggest that the participants were not well matched on language ability. A clear link between language and performance on VM tasks has not been identified in the literature, but the relationship between language and imitation may be strong enough to affect a child's performance on such tasks.

There is another possibility that Nikopolous and Keenan fail to address – the effect of the type of model. It is unclear why the authors included three models (a peer, an unfamiliar adult, and a familiar adult), assigned one model to each child, and then neglected to discuss the differences between the groups. Of the three participants who did not acquire social initiation, two were assigned the peer model and one was assigned the unfamiliar adult. These are interesting findings, considering the research in favor of using peer models in videos and in in vivo imitation training. A more systematic evaluation of the effects of model type on skills acquisition would have been warranted in this study and is a direction for future research.

In a follow-up study (Nikopoulos and Keenan 2004), peers were used exclusively in the videotapes. This time the authors found consistent decreases in latency to social initiations in three children with autism following a VM intervention. Follow-up probes indicated robust effects at 1 and 3 months. The results in this study may have been more consistent across participants because they were matched in autism severity ratings, whereas the children in the 2003 study had varied profiles. Taken together, these two studies suggest that participant characteristics may play an important moderating role on the effects of VM interventions.

Video self modeling (VSM) is another approach in which the child acts as the appropriate model in the video. During these sequences, the child is either prompted by an adult to complete the action successfully or a "perfect" action is spliced from many imperfect tapings. A meta-analysis of VSM suggested that it is an effective strategy to address social-communication skills and functional skills in children with autism (Bellini and Akullian 2007), however because the skills in these studies were not targeted in naturalistic settings, generalization was limited. Bellini et al. (2007) explored the social validity of VSM by measuring social outcomes directed toward peers in a preschool classroom, rather than adults in a clinical setting. VSM was used to successfully teach social engagement to two children with autism; these skills maintained after the removal of the intervention.

A recent study showed that VM can also be used to teach complex social sequences to children with autism (Nikopoulos and Keenan 2007). In this study, three children were presented with a video of a peer engaging in a behavior sequence that included a social initiation (e.g., "Let's play") and subsequent object manipulation (e.g., picking up a ball). The participants demonstrated expected increases in social initiations and also engaged in more reciprocal play, peer imitation, and less isolated object manipulation. These results were generalized across peers and maintained at 1 and 2 months. It is noteworthy that the skills were acquired without external prompts or reinforcement during the intervention phase, indicating that in an intrinsically motivating setting (i.e., watching a video) spontaneous imitation may be more likely to occur.

Little research has examined the effects of VM on social cognitions (e.g., recognizing emotions or inferring another's mental state). These higher-order social behaviors emerge in typically developing children around the preschool age and are often impaired in children with autism. To address this question, Charlop-Christy and Daneshvar (2003) used video models to teach three participants perspective-taking (the ability to predict another person's behavior based on their inferred mental state). The children were tested on a classic perspective-taking task and then shown videos of familiar adults performing the task correctly. All three participants demonstrated increases in the percentage of correct responding following the intervention phase as well as generalization across test materials. However, it is difficult to say whether the children learned perspective-taking or a rote response to a familiar task. More convincing evidence for actual acquisition would come from generalization across perspective-taking *tasks*, rather than *stimuli*. While the evidence in favor of VM to teach advanced social skills is not yet convincing, there is a foundation to warrant further research in this area. Because internal behavior cannot be observed, researchers must rely on contrived tests to measure its emergence and development. The merit of future studies will depend on the use of multiple measures of social behavior and the combination of these measures with socially significant, behavioral outcomes (e.g., peer interactions).

Comparisons of VM with in vivo modeling have suggested that these procedures are equally efficacious. Gena et al. (2005) taught affective responding to three children with ASD through in vivo and VM, in a counterbalanced multiple-baseline design. High rates of acquisition were observed across subjects and no significant differences between the interventions emerged.

Only one study has attempted to systematically compare VM to another treatment in a group design. Kroeger et al. (2007) assigned 27 children with autism to receive either a direct teaching package or a group social skills package over the course of 5 weeks. The treatments were identical except that the direct teaching group watched videos of peers modeling appropriate social behavior for half of the session and received primary reinforcement for participating in the VM curriculum. Both groups improved on their scores of prosocial behavior, but the direct teaching group demonstrated significantly more gains than the play activities group. While this study provides encouraging support for intervention based on video modeling, there are several methodological limitations that detract from its results. First, random assignment was not used, due to scheduling difficulties. Second, the direct teaching package incorporated elements of group instruction, VM, and reinforcement. Because a component analysis was not conducted, it is impossible to determine the necessary aspects of the intervention.

It is also important to note that, while the VM literature is methodologically strong in general (e.g., Charlop-Christy and Daneshvar 2003; Maione and Mirenda 2006; Nikopoulos and Keenan 2003, 2004), some studies are less rigorous in their experimental design. One recurrent design flaw is the reliance on a two-tier multiple baseline design rather than the three demonstrations required for experimental control (e.g., Bellini et al. 2007; Nikopoulos and Keenan 2007).

A frequently raised concern in the literature is that the contrived nature of VM clips may lead to poorer generalization outcomes, especially across settings (Elksnin and Elksnin 1998). However, recent improvements in technology have resulted in the use of more naturalistic VM procedures. One group of researchers used computer-based VM to improve social skills in a classroom setting (Simpson et al. 2004). Four elementary-aged children with autism were shown video clips of three different appropriate skills (compliance, sharing, and greeting) at naturally occurring opportunities throughout the day. The computer-based instruction made it possible to show the video discretely in the context of the actual social situation, thereby enhancing the salience of the targeted skill and reducing the amount of time spent outside the classroom. All four students demonstrated increases in unprompted engagement of social skills; these outcomes were assessed in the natural environment, another strength of this study. The authors note that the students in this study already had these social skills in their repertoires; therefore the study demonstrated *increases* in skills but not necessarily skill *acquisition*. Maintenance data were not collected, so it cannot be determined if social engagement would persist in the absence of the intervention. Despite these limitations, the potential replication of the effects of computer-based VM and its extension to other learners are promising areas of future research.

PEER TRAINING

Early social skills teaching approaches using adults as mediators of treatment were criticized for not being representative of contingencies in the natural environment and for a lack of generalization (DiSalvo and Oswald 2002). This section focuses on using peers to teach social skills to address these concerns and is limited to the approaches with the most empirical support: peer buddies, peer networks, pivotal response training, and peer initiation training. A summary of these interventions can be found in Table 6.3.

Peer Buddies

The peer buddy model pairs a child with autism with a typically developing peer who is instructed to play and interact with the target child throughout the day. Laushey and Heflin (2000) had teachers instruct targets and peers to "stay with your buddy" and "talk to your buddy" without any other formal training. By merely increasing the amount of time the buddies spent together, they found an increase in the percentage of appropriate social initiations and responses by the children with autism. A brief withdrawal of the peer buddy system reversed the effects, thereby strengthening evidence for a relation between the intervention and positive outcome.

In a more sophisticated design, Roeyers randomized 85 children with autism to either a peer buddy group or a control group (Roeyers 1996). The buddies were provided with brief training on reacting to aggressive behavior, getting the attention of a target child, and general education about autism. Following a brief intervention, the targets demonstrated increased prosocial behavior, social responsiveness, and interaction duration; small increases in initiations were also observed. Although the control group showed minimal gains, the treatment group's outcomes were significantly above and beyond these changes. One of Roeyers' interesting findings was that both the children with autism and the peer buddies generalized these responses to untrained members of the classroom, which may be beneficial from a cost-effectiveness perspective. Generalization across peers is a major strength of these programs and is a recurring phenomenon in much of the peer-training literature.

Peer Networks

Peer networks develop social support for children with autism by offering group instruction to established peer groups, and are comparable to the peer buddy approach, except that training is provided at a group level. The literature in this area has demonstrated that providing peer groups with social interaction strategies (e.g., initiating and responding to conversation, providing clear instructions, giving compliments), general information about autism, and reinforcement strategies has been effective in improving their social interactions with classmates with ASD (Garrison-Harrell et al. 1997; Haring and Breen 1992).

Pivotal Response Training

Pivotal response training (PRT) is a naturalistic approach to teaching social skills that capitalizes on child motivation and promotes generalization that has been effective in teaching JA, imitation, and play skills (Whalen et al. 2006). Based on the success with adult therapists, Pierce and Schreibman (1995) taught typically developing peers to use PRT techniques with two children with autism. Both targets showed increases in social skills, including engagement, imitation, and JA. In 1997 the authors published their replication of this study with multiple peers and reported similar findings, as well as generalization of skills to untrained peers. The benefits of PRT were extended to a natural setting in a study by Harper et al. (2008). Peers were taught to use the motivational techniques described in the PRT manual to improve the social interactions (e.g., initiations, turn-taking, gaining attention) of classmates with

TABLE 6.3   Summaries and ratings for studies targeting peer training

Study	Design	Outcome	Rating
Garrison-Harrell et al. (1997)	MBD of a peer network	Increases in frequency and duration of social interactions	Adequate
Goldstein et al. (1992)	Reversal design of a peer-mediated intervention	Increases in social behavior of peers and targets directed toward each other	Adequate
Haring and Breen (1992)	MBD of a peer-mediated social network	Increases in number of interactions and target responses to social bids	Adequate
Haring and Lovinger (1989)	ABAC design of peer awareness training	Increases in peer initiations, targets responding, and interaction duration	Adequate
Harper et al. (2008)	MBD of peer-mediated pivotal response training	Increases in target initiations, social bids, and turn-taking exchanges	Adequate
Kamps et al. (2002)	Group comparison of peer-training interventions	Increases in frequency and duration of social interactions for targets and peers	Weak
Laushey and Heflin (2000)	Reversal design of peer tutors	Increases in targets' social skills	Strong
Lee et al. (2007)	MBD of peer initiation training	Increases in social interactions for peers and targets; decreases in target stereotypy	Strong
Owen-DeSchryver et al. (2008)	MBD of peer initiation training	Increases in peer initiations and target responses and initiations	Adequate
Pierce and Schreibman (1995)	MBD of peer-mediated pivotal response training	Increases in social engagement between targets and peers	Adequate
Pierce and Schreibman (1997)	MBD of peer-mediated pivotal response training	Increases in engagement and initiation between targets and peers	Adequate
Roeyers (1996)	Randomized trial of peer training	Increases in frequency of initiations, responsiveness, and interaction duration; decrease in target self-stimulatory behavior	Strong
Yang et al. (2003)	AB design of peer training	Increases in engagement and appropriate play	Weak

ASD at recess. The social gains observed in this study extend support for the efficacy of PRT in clinical settings.

Peer Initiation Training

Peer initiation training (PIT) is done individually and is more skills-based than the other approaches. Peers learn specific techniques for initiating and sustaining social interaction with targets; this may occur with or without basic education on autism. For example, Lee et al. (2007) taught peers in an inclusion classroom how to interact with targets by sharing, suggesting concrete play ideas, providing assistance, and being affectionate. This training increased the social engagement of two children with autism in their classroom. Similar findings have been reported in larger samples. Goldstein et al. (1992) intervened with five targets and ten peers in a classroom setting with a skills-training package to target attending, commenting, responding, and delivering prompts. Following training, four of the five targets increased in their rate of social interaction; the remaining student showed similar increases after one booster session.

These two studies tracked responding to social interactions as their outcome measure, but initiation is a more stringent test of an intervention's efficacy. A recent study (Owen-DeSchryver et al. 2008) provided initiation training to the peers of three targets in a general education classroom; the peers received a rationale for being friends with the targets, a discussion about the targets' strengths and weaknesses, and strategies to engage their friends in play. Universal increases in responding to social interactions were observed, and two of the three targets also increased their initiations.

These findings support the use of PIT in schools in which the teachers and peers are well trained by a research team. Barry and colleagues were interested in PIT from an effectiveness standpoint and looked at PIT outcomes outside school (Barry et al. 2003). An 8-week group intervention was provided to peers in a non-clinic setting; each week the peers received training and then engaged in play sessions with children with autism from the community. Some small, but not significant increases in the targets' social behavior were observed. The failure of PIT to generalize to a non-clinic setting may be due to several factors (e.g., limited familiarity, few naturally occurring opportunities to engage, potential inadequate treatment integrity). Overall, the use of peer training procedures in non-classroom settings is an under-researched area. These interventions are potentially useful for targets who are not enrolled in inclusive classrooms, and effectiveness studies are necessary to determine the ways in which they can benefit from peer-mediated treatments.

Potential Limitations to the Research

In synthesizing the body of research on peer training techniques, several issues come to light. There is some evidence that participant characteristics may moderate the effects of peer training interventions. For example, Goldstein and their colleagues (1992) included reports of composite scores on a battery of social and cognitive tests and found more progress in students with verbal ability than in preverbal children.

Intervention characteristics may also play an important role in treatment outcome. Sasso et al. (1998) examined both the effects of the number of buddies and the conditions of the interaction on target outcome and found main effects for the success of dyads over triads and for cooperative interactions (children playing a game together) over instructional conditions (peer teaching the game to a target). These results contrast with those of Kamps et al. (2002) who reported that learning groups in which peer buddies tutored targets on academic skills led to greater social interactions than social skills groups.

The potential moderating effects of participant and intervention variables are problematic to the existing literature because they are not systematically addressed – and are sometimes not even discussed. Until research controls for pre-intervention subject and treatment differences, we cannot know for whom peer training is best suited and under what conditions. In addition, we know little about which elements of existing interventions are essential to affect behavior change. Component analyses to identify these "active ingredients" would be helpful, especially when evaluating combination treatments or comparing multiple approaches.

Another question in the peer training research is whether social-based treatments have convincing specificity. Some studies suggest that social skills do not need to be explicitly targeted to exact social gains. For example, Kamps et al. (1994) introduced a class-wide peer tutoring intervention to teach reading skills and reported improved social interactions with targets during free play. These findings are consistent with the Kamps et al. (2002) study, as described above. Additional comparisons of socially focused treatments with instructional treatments are needed to clarify this relationship.

Early in the history of peer training research, Haring and Lovinger (1989) suggested that despite the efficacy of peer training models, they might not be as efficient as social skills treatment directed to the children with autism. They compared a training package for peers (including an autism awareness activity and reinforcement strategies) with a training package for targets (including teaching initiations and appropriate play behavior). The targets' social skills did not respond to an initial peer training intervention, but gains were observed when the skills were taught explicitly suggesting that peer training alone may not always be a sufficient intervention. Unfortunately the authors did not run a counterbalanced group, which would have clarified whether the explicit target training would have worked on its own or whether the combination treatment was necessary. Although these limitations need to be addressed, they do not significantly undermine the efficacy of peer training procedures and there is strong evidence for the continued use of peer-mediated interventions in general education environments.

SOCIAL STORIES

Social Stories (Gray 2000) are widely used by teachers and parents attempting to alter the social behaviors of children with ASDs. In spite of the popularity and face validity of this method, it has limited empirical support for teaching social skills (e.g., Reynhout and Carter 2006). Social Stories have been reported as helpful when used in combination with other techniques (e.g., Thiemann and Goldstein 2001) but, without a systematic dismantling of these teaching packages, it is not possible to know to what extent, if any, Social Stories have an impact on learners. Table 6.4 summarizes the research.

Although Gray (2000) describes very specific guidelines for creating the stories and presenting them to students, those addressing social skills have been widely adapted in research projects. Population characteristics also vary (i.e., from children with comorbid cognitive impairments to learners in the average or above-average range of intelligence). The time between when the child hears the story and the opportunity for a social interaction also varies considerably, with some children

TABLE 6.4   Summaries and ratings for studies on Social Stories

Study	Design	Outcome	Rating
Barry and Burlew (2004)	MBD of Social Stories for appropriate play	Improvements in appropriate play with toys and peers	Weak
Chan and O'Reilly (2008)	MBD of treatment package including Social Stories	Improvements in behavior for one subject, variable response in another subject	Weak
Delano and Snell (2006)	MBD of social stories	Increases in seeking attention, initiations, and commenting	Strong
Hutchins and Prelock (2006)	AB design of Social Stories and Comic Strip Conversations	Gains in target skill by one of two subjects	Weak
Norris and Dattilo (1999)	AB design of Social Stories	Some improvements in social interactions in one subject	Weak
Sansosti and Powell-Smith (2006)	MBD of Social Stories	Increases in social engagement for two of three subjects	Weak
Scattone (2008)	MBD of video modeling and Social Stories	Increases in eye contact but not smiling or initiations	Weak
Scattone et al. (2006)	MBD of Social Stories for social skills	Modest improvements in behavior for one of three subjects and greater improvement for a second	Weak
Quirmbach et al. (2009)	Group comparison of two Social Story formats and one control condition	Rapid acquisition of social game-playing behaviors for participants with either Social Story format but not in control condition	Adequate

hearing the stories at home before school and others hearing them just before the target event.

The weakest studies, from a design perspective, used an AB design. For example, Hutchins and Prelock (2006) employed an AB strategy of baseline followed by intervention, with parents as the teachers for two children on the autism spectrum. Based solely on parental report, one child made gains in acquisition of the target skill and the other did not. Designs of this kind which do not involve the repeated introduction of the independent variable are not sufficient to allow one to demonstrate that the intervention was effective. Among other limits, there were no demonstrations of treatment fidelity, independent observations by naïve observers, or measures of maintenance of change.

Norris and Dattilo (1999) brought somewhat more rigor to their research, but were also limited by their use of an AB design. The effects of three Social Stories on the appropriate and inappropriate social interactions of an 8-year-old girl with autism were examined in this study. Rates of socially appropriate behaviors remained low after the stories were introduced and there was no decrease in intervals of no social interaction. Her socially inappropriate behavior was variable during baseline and demonstrated considerable variability throughout the course of treatment.

For children, choosing activities and toys during peer interactions is an important social behavior. Barry and Burlew (2004) examined the value of Social Stories for teaching appropriate play to two children with "severe" autism. The authors applied a multiple component instructional package, including Social Stories; verbal, gestural and physical prompts; and offering verbal praise for appropriate behavior. However, a lack of component analysis created a threat to the internal validity of the study, as there is no way to determine the specific contribution of Social Stories to the outcome. In addition, a multiple baseline design was conducted across two children and not the necessary minimum of three people to demonstrate the impact of the treatment.

Scattone et al. (2006) attempted to control for some of the variation in previous studies of story content and presentation method by following Gray's rules carefully and avoiding the use of additional instructional procedures. In a multiple baseline design across participants, each of three high-functioning boys with ASD used a personalized Social Story for a targeted social behavior. Although the baseline measures for all three boys were low and stable, response to intervention was variable. One child showed no change after the introduction of his Social Story, a second made modest but clear changes, and the third child showed large changes. Unfortunately, the unintended teacher use of verbal prompts created a threat to the internal validity of the study.

Sansosti and Powell-Smith (2006) employed a multiple base design across three high-functioning, elementary-aged boys with Asperger syndrome to evaluate the duration of social engagement. The parents applied the treatment procedure at home and social behavior was observed at school. For two of the boys the baseline data reflected good to excellent stability, and they both showed clear treatment effects and continued maintenance of behavior. The third child never achieved a stable baseline, nor was his behavior during treatment stable. As a result, it was not possible for the authors to demonstrate consistent changes across the three participants.

Social Stories and VM were both provided to a boy with Asperger syndrome in a study using multiple treatment techniques across the behaviors of eye contact, smiling, and social initiations (Scattone 2008). The treatments were associated with large gains in eye contact, small changes in smiling, and modest gains in initiations. Unfortunately, these data do not allow us to draw any conclusions about the relative benefits of Social Stories, as video modeling alone has shown beneficial effects for teaching social skills and the effects of the two procedures were not examined separately.

Chan and O'Reilly (2008) made Social Stories part of a treatment package that also included role plays. A multiple baseline across three behaviors revealed clear effects for one participant and a more variable response in a second. The lack of consistent response is problematic and, again, the combination of Social Stories and role plays makes it impossible to ascertain whether Social Stories alone would have had a beneficial impact.

The strongest study we reviewed (Delano and Snell 2006) used Social Stories to teach appropriate social engagement and decrease inappropriate social engagement in three young boys with autism in a multiple probe design. The authors also collected data on the target skills of seeking attention, initiating comments, initiating requests and making contingent comments. The study attempted to improve upon Thiemann and Goldstein's study (2001) by assessing the use of Social Stories in isolation. Following low, stable baselines, each boy in succession showed a clear response to the introduction of treatment. However, as the reading of the story was faded over time, their level of engagement declined. A possible threat to internal validity in this study was the physical presence of training peers during the Social Stories intervention. It is impossible to know how this exposure may have altered the peers' behavior, making them more receptive and responsive to bids from the child with autism. In spite of this issue, it is important to note that the authors paid detailed attention to experimental design, included measures of both maintenance and generalization, reported on fidelity checks, and used well-trained observers to collect data. Therefore, this investigation represents the best single subject study we reviewed on Social Stories.

The only group design study we reviewed was conducted by Quirmbach and their colleagues (2009) who used a pre-test/post-test repeated measures randomized control group design with 45 children with ASD aged from 7 to 14 years. They explored the benefits of two different formats of Social Stories (the standard format or a directive format) to teach participants to greet an adult, invite him to play a game, ask which game the adult preferred and accept the adult's selection. The randomly assigned control group heard a story of comparable length unrelated to the targeted social skills. Both the standard and directive story formats were equally effective in motivating the children to apply the skills during interactions with the adult research assistant and both groups were superior in performance to the control group. A very important finding was that for the children with ASD, a Verbal Comprehension Index of 68 or higher on the WISC-IV (Wechsler 2003) was associated with benefits from these Social Stories, which were not accompanied by pictures. There were significant limitations to this study. Although the intervention was effective, it was brief: follow-up for maintenance occurred 1 week after the training and it is impossible to know how the children would have performed over an extended time. Another concern is that, while a useful set of skills was taught with the Social Stories, the skills were not assessed with peers but with an adult research assistant. To measure social validity, age-appropriate peers need to be part of future studies. In addition, multiple raters were involved in data collection but there was no report of inter-rater reliability figures, nor were fidelity checks done to document that the procedures used in reading the stories and responding during the game sessions were consistent from one child and condition to the next. There was also no description of the actual procedures used to assign participants randomly to conditions. These concerns aside, Quirmbach et al. (2009) took an important step toward bringing greater rigor to the research on using Social Stories to teach social skills.

Based on the studies by Delano and Snell (2006) and Quirmbach et al. (2009), our overall description of the research on Social Stories is that for teaching social skills this method falls into the category of "emerging findings awaiting replication." There is a pressing need for additional studies that isolate the use of Social Stories as a single intervention to determine to what extent this method is, in and of itself, effective and, if it is not, whether it enhances the potency of other procedures when included in a treatment package. We need to know to what extent these skills are used appropriately with peers over time.

Teaching Social Skills and Social Cognition in Groups

There are two major aspects to being socially effective. One is social cognition, or the ability to interpret the feelings and intent of another person based on such cues as facial expression, body posture and gesture, and the ability to realize that one's own knowledge may not be shared by others. In addition to social cognition, one needs a broad array of specific social skills for addressing the myriad interactions we encounter. Because people with ASD experience challenges in both social cognition and social skills, some social skills groups have focused on each area or a blend of these two areas. Table 6.5 summarizes this work.

Teaching social skills in groups seems inherently appropriate as the fundamental goal of teaching social skills is to increase social interactions. We discussed above the use of peers as models and playmates for very young children on the autism spectrum. There is a smaller body of work on teaching social skills to groups, older children, adolescents or adults of participants all of whom are on the autism spectrum. Two early studies (Mesibov 1984; Williams 1989) and one more recent study (Mishna and Muskat 1998) relied on anecdotal reports or very limited data and are not discussed in depth here. A summary of these findings can be found in Table 6.5.

Theory of Mind

The term "theory of mind" (ToM) describes the ability to recognize that one person's knowledge may conflict with the knowledge of another. Research on ToM highlights the challenges for people on the autism spectrum in making these determinations. There is a large body of work on ToM and how people on the spectrum respond to ToM tasks as compared to typically developing peers or those who have an intellectual deficit (Baron-Cohen et al. 1985, 1986; Leslie and Frith 1988). Ozonoff and Miller (1995) argue that this ToM deficit makes many commercial social skills programs inappropriate for a person on the autism spectrum and they explored the extent to which it would be possible to teach ToM skills to this population. Their participants were five adolescents with autism in a treatment group and four in a control group, none of whom had an intellectual disability. The treatment group received 7 weeks of training in basic social skills including conversation behavior, selecting topics of interest, reading nonverbal signals, listening, and giving compliments. The next 7 weeks of treatment focused on perspective taking and other TOM skills. The five boys in the treatment group demonstrated post-treatment gains on TOM tasks while the control group showed little or no change. However, parent and teacher ratings failed to identify any changes in social skills post-treatment. Thus, while the boys may have learned to respond more accurately to the structured tests, their parents and teachers did not see behavioral changes in daily life. The small sample size, failure to demonstrate socially meaningful change, and lack of direct observational data were among the weak points of this early study.

The relationship among ToM, executive function, and facial expression recognition has also been evaluated. Solomon et al. (2004) used laboratory tests and parental ratings to evaluate the impact of a 20-week social skills group for nine children and a concurrent psycho-educational group for parents, as compared to a wait list control group. They found significant changes in the laboratory-based tasks of facial expression recognition and problem solving in the treatment group compared to the controls. Although this study included a control group and random assignment to conditions, it was limited in that there were no direct measures of social behavior. Additionally, the laboratory-based context of most of the data makes it impossible to know to what extent these changes might be related to behavioral changes in a naturalistic setting.

In a more recent study Gevers et al. (2006) offered a group experience to 18 children diagnosed with PDD-NOS. Participants attended 21 weekly sessions of an hour each, which focused on ToM; parents attended five sessions on ToM. This study lacked both a control group and direct behavioral observations. Providing both parent and child training at the same time was also a source of threat to internal validity.

TABLE 6.5   Summaries and ratings for studies on group and social cognition treatments

Study	Design	Outcome	Rating
Barnhill et al. (2002)	Group design of social skills group	Very modest changes in social behavior	Weak
Bauminger (2002)	Group design of CBT and social skills training	Improvements in social-interpersonal problem solving and affective repertoire	Weak
Bauminger (2007a)	Group design of group instruction for social skills	Improvements in social skills	Weak
Bauminger (2007b)	Group design of individual instruction for social skills	Improvements in social skills	Weak
Crooke et al. (2008)	Group design of social cognition-based group intervention	Improvements in social skills	Weak
Gevers et al. (2006)	Group design of social skills group for children and parents	Improvement in cognitive tasks; parental reports of improved social behavior	Weak
Le Goff (2004) and LeGoff and Sherman (2006)	Group design and long-term outcomes of LEGO therapy	Increases in appropriate social interactions; improvements in autistic symptoms	Adequate
Lopata et al. (2006)	Group design of social skills group versus blended behavioral and social skills package	Overall improvements in social skills, no change in adaptability, and an increase in atypical behavior; no between-group differences	Weak
Owens et al. (2008)	Group design of LEGO therapy versus Social Use of Language programme and a no-treatment control	Improvements in autism-specific social interaction scores and decreases in maladaptive behavior for both intervention groups, with greater gains in the LEGO group	Strong
Ozonoff and Miller (1995)	Group design of social-cognition versus treatment as usual	Gains in some theory of mind tasks, but not in daily life	Weak
Solomon et al. (2004)	Group design of social skills group and concurrent psycho-education for parents	Improvements in facial expression recognition and problem solving	Weak
Tse et al. (2007)	Group design of CBT and social skills blend	Increases in social competence	Weak
Turner-Brown et al. (2008)	Group design of social-cognitive blended package versus treatment as usual	Trend toward improvements in social cognition, but no statistically significant changes in behavior	Weak

Turner-Brown et al. (2008) blended social cognition skills and social interaction skills in a pilot study with 11 adults with high-functioning autism. They divided the participants into two groups, with six enrolled in a group experience and five receiving treatment as usual. The curriculum was based on a previously developed program for teaching social comprehension or skills to people with schizophrenia, which the authors modified to address the needs of people with ASD. Although significant changes were observed in the social cognition components of the program, there were no statistically meaningful changes in the application of social skills. The small sample size, inability to make random assignment to the two groups, and the lack of data collection in natural settings were significant limits of this study. This pilot study suggested it was possible to modify social cognitions, but it remains unclear to what extent these cognitions generalize to social behavior.

Cognitive-Behavioral Therapy

A number of studies have employed cognitive behavioral techniques to teach social skills to young people in group settings (see Chapter 7). In a study with 46 adolescents diagnosed with Asperger syndrome or high-functioning autistic disorder, Tse et al. (2007) reported that small-group social skills training blending psychoeducational and experiential components resulted in statistically significant gains in social competence. Six separate groups were run over time but no control condition was included. In addition, results were based on participant and parental ratings; the lack of objective data on naturalistic functioning limits the validity of these findings. Crooke et al. (2008) describe an 8-week, 60-min group treatment for six boys with Asperger syndrome or high-functioning autistic disorder using a social cognition approach. The data were presented for each boy using bar graphs, instead of the standard line graphs. A nonparametric Wilcoxon Signed Rank test was performed and indicated significant changes from pre to post. However, the absence of a control group and the use of a non-traditional format for presenting SSED data make it impossible to evaluate the impact of treatment.

In another study of the value of cognitive-behavioral therapy (CBT) for improving social skills, Lopata et al. (2006) offered a summer program for 21 6-to-13-year-old boys with Asperger syndrome. One group received social skills instruction in isolation. A second group received an additional behavioral treatment consisting of a point system for appropriate social behavior and for following rules and directions, and a response cost for failing to engage in these behaviors. Three standardized scales were used to measure behavior pre- and post-treatment, but no direct observations of behavior were coded. Although parents rated their children as having made gains following treatment, the staff members gave more variable ratings, reporting improvement in social skills, but no significant change in adaptability, and an increase in atypical behavior. As is the case for several other studies on this topic, the lack of objective data creates a threat to the internal validity of the study. No significant differences emerged between the conditions. Although this study lacked an untreated comparison group and we cannot conclude that the camp experience led to changes, the presence of a comparison group makes it a rare study in this domain.

Webb et al. (2004) taught high-functioning teens with ASDs social skills including sharing ideas, complementing others, offering help or encouragement, making recommendations nicely, and exercising self-control. They used several self-report measures of change and relied on role plays to assess social behavior before and after treatment, as well selecting two participants for multiple probes of each of the five behaviors. However, taking role play data from the teens about a specific skill to represent the group as a whole was a relatively weak measure of behavior change. The only other measure, the pre–post assessment of the groups on each skill, was also weak because there was no control group against which to compare performance. The study could have been methodologically stronger had it included either a control group and a larger sample or a true multiple baseline design.

An AB design was used to examine appropriate social behavior in 7-to-9-year-old children with ASDs in general education classrooms (Yang et al. 2003). Four children received social skills instruction in small groups and their social behavior in the classroom was tracked through daily teacher ratings. Two other children who did not participate in the group were tracked for comparison purposes. The baseline data for the children varied greatly; in addition, there was no evidence of immediate change with the onset of treatment in three of the four participants. Rather, performance remained highly variable across the 64 weeks of treatment. Although a trend analysis found small-to-medium effects for the experimental children over time, the changes are difficult to see visually and hence not very meaningful in terms of impact on the learners.

In a study looking at paralanguage social skills, such as recognizing affect in others, Barnhill et al. (2002), enrolled eight adolescent boys and one adolescent girl in a group-based intervention. Eight sessions included a 1-h discussion of specific topics of recognizing and responding to facial expressions, followed by 2–3 h of in vivo practice during a recreational activity. A small sample size, diagnostically mixed group, and lack of a control group make it difficult to interpret the findings.

Bauminger (2002) adopted a cognitive behavioral approach to create a 7-month social skills curriculum for a group of 15 high-functioning youths on the autism spectrum. In this study, social cognition included abilities such as being able to "read" another person, understanding the meaning of their verbal and nonverbal communication, and inferring the mental states of others (i.e., theory of mind). Bauminger (2002) argues that high-functioning children on the autism spectrum need to both understand social rules and norms and process the social information that is available in their interactions. Her training program involved teaching social–interpersonal problem-solving and improving the child's affective repertoire by increasing awareness of feelings in himself or herself and in others. Although the children showed gains in social skills, the absence of a control group makes it impossible to demonstrate convincingly that the intervention was the active ingredient of change. Two more recent studies by Bauminger (2007a, b) addressed group instruction in social skills and suffered from a similar lack of a control group. One of these studies (Bauminger 2007b) evaluated a group format for teaching social skills and the other (Bauminger 2007a) used an individual format for teaching social skills to 19 children. Both studies reported benefits for the participants. In spite of their design flaws, the investigations by Bauminger are the best set of studies to date, in that they used highly sophisticated methods to assess skills, train the students, and gather data. The addition of an appropriate control group to her methods provides a good template for high-quality future research.

LEGO® Therapy

Of more recent interest is the use of LEGO play as a medium for individual and group instruction to teach social skills. LEGO therapy aims to provide a setting in which children work in dyads or groups toward a common goal. Each child is assigned a specific role: the "engineer" directs the action; the "supplier" locates the appropriate pieces; and the "builder" assembles the structure. Each of these jobs is essential to the completion of the task and the children rotate through them. Because multiple examples of verbal and nonverbal communication (e.g., including joint attention, eye contact, and perspective-taking) are required among children to successfully finish the activity, this treatment approach strongly emphasizes social skills. One aspect of LEGO therapy that is highlighted in the literature is its ability to capitalize on child impetus and interest; in particular, the structure of the task and inherent qualities of the materials are considered highly motivating for children with ASD. A small set of studies has begun to explore the efficacy of the LEGO approach and the characteristics of those who are likely to benefit from this treatment.

The first description of LEGO therapy was published by LeGoff in 2004. In this study, the efficacy of treatment was evaluated with a repeated-measures design with seven groups of children (47 participants in total). Following completion of an initial 3- or 6-month wait list, the children were provided with weekly individual and group LEGO therapy over the course of 12–24 weeks. Participants therefore served as their own wait-list control group. Intervention effects were assessed using both behavioral observations (i.e., social competence; duration of social interaction) and the Gilliam Autism Rating Scale (GARS). The results indicated significant gains in all three outcome measures from wait-list control to treatment and no changes associated with maturation. It was also found that less significant language impairments pre-treatment predicted greater gains following the intervention.

These initial findings are encouraging, but the limitations of the research should be noted. First, although the increases in the duration of social interaction achieved statistical significance, the absolute change measured was 15 s. It is unclear whether this constitutes a "clinically significant" difference and measures of social validity are necessary supplements to evaluate changes in social behavior. Second, measurement issues compromised the integrity of the data collection. Coders were not blind to the purposes of the study and did not achieve high reliability.

Similar concerns extend to the follow-up study (LeGoff and Sherman 2006), in which 3-year outcome data from the original participants were presented with the addition of an alternative-treatment control group. More significant social gains were demonstrated in the LEGO group versus the comparison group and these benefits maintained over time. Verbal ability predicted treatment response, an effect that was more potent for the LEGO therapy group than the control group. Again, coders (i.e., the first author and parents) were not blind and the authors acknowledge that greater exposure to the children in the LEGO group may have influenced subjective progress ratings.

These first two studies provide important preliminary support for LEGO therapy as a social skills intervention but are limited in their comparisons to wait-list or no-treatment control groups. To address this gap, a recent study evaluated the relative efficacy of the LEGO approach, the Social Use of Language Programme (SULP), and a no-treatment control group (Owens et al. 2008). In contrast to LEGO therapy, SULP uses a more structured, curricular approach to teaching social skills by focusing particularly on perspective-taking and adult modeling. While the inclusion of an alternative treatment group contributes to the strength of the design, it is important to note the SULP does not qualify as an evidence-based intervention. Owens, Granader, and their colleagues replicated the previous findings of social gains and extended the results by demonstrating significant decreases in inappropriate behavior. Behavioral gains were observed in both treatment groups; social gains were observed in the LEGO therapy groups only. In addition, social validity measures indicated parent satisfaction and child enjoyment.

The current research on LEGO therapy suggests that it is a viable, cost- and time-effective intervention for teaching social skills to children with autism. However, there are several limitations to the approach as well as areas in need of future research. Although the therapy is intended to be applicable for individuals with varying language functioning, it appears to be best suited for children with mild language deficits. In fact, eligibility criteria set out by Owens et al. (2008) focused specifically on participants with an IQ of 70 or greater. More research is needed on the success of the LEGO approach with more significantly impaired individuals.

The experimental designs employed (i.e., repeated measures with wait-list control, group comparison without random assignment, group comparison with quasi-random assignment) limit the internal validity of the results. While these designs are sufficient for preliminary research, they need to be extended to include more gold-standard methodologies, such as RCTs that include evidence-based treatment comparisons. The outcome measures employed include both behavioral observation and report measures. The behavioral social variables are well-operationalized and appear to capture a measure of clinical significance. However, the limited psychometric properties of the GARS suggest that this tool might not be indicated to evaluate behavior change in a research setting. Future studies that include measures such as the ADOS or

the ADI to evaluate the efficacy of LEGO therapy would be of interest.

Finally, the research thus far does not provide information on the unique treatment components that are responsible for behavior change. For example, both the use of group therapy alone (Owens et al. 2008) and a combination with individual therapy (LeGoff 2004; Legoff and Sherman 2006) were associated with treatment gains. By comparing it to SULP, Owens and their colleagues (2008) provided some evidence that the motivating materials and goal-directed group aims are active ingredients in LEGO therapy. However, it is unclear what specific elements (e.g., materials, child motivation, structure, or agency) are responsible for the observed gains. Component analyses that address these various characteristics are necessary in the future for identifying relevant mechanisms of change.

Overall, the research on teaching social skills in group settings is disappointing. Although some studies showed encouraging clinical outcomes, methodological concerns (e.g., the lack of control groups or rigorous SSED), along with the limited number of studies that examined behavior beyond the laboratory, used participants who clearly met diagnostic criteria, and used fidelity checks of treatment implementation, and employed naïve observers to code data highlight the need for high quality research in this domain. Of exception are the recent studies on LEGO therapy that are of sufficient quality to suggest that group-based social skills intervention is a promising area of research. However, the presence of multiple "weak" studies does not yet warrant a label of evidence-based practice for teaching social skills in groups. It is a domain that should take high priority and more rigorous group studies on LEGO therapy and on the Bauminger model supplemented with a control group would provide a valuable starting point for such research.

Conclusion

The research with SSED on social skills clearly demonstrates the efficacy of many of these interventions with children with ASD but, even with sound methodologies and compelling data, these studies offer us little insight into the *relative* efficacy of such treatments compared to other approaches. Some notable exceptions have been highlighted (e.g., Kasari et al. 2006; Roeyers 1996), but they are few and require replication. It is also challenging to pinpoint the exact pre-treatment participant characteristics that may moderate or predict the effects of these interventions. As mentioned above, the language ability of the children in the study by Nikopoulos and Keenan (2003) may have contributed to their variability in skill acquisition; unfortunately small sample sizes and a lack of randomized group assignment makes it impossible to test for these relations in a SSED. This limitation was also discussed in relation to much of the peer training literature (Goldstein et al. 1992; Kamps et al. 2002; Sasso et al. 1998). Future research on social skills should take advantage of group designs to explore some of these potential predictors and compare these interventions to other established treatments.

The inclusion of older learners with autism is also a necessary dimension to future research. As is common in much of the autism literature many of the studies on social skills focused mainly on preschool-aged children, with some minimal inclusion of children in elementary school (e.g., Simpson et al. 2004). In typically developing children social skills, undergo a critical period during the preschool years, so it is understandable that researchers target this population. However, the success of social interventions with elementary-aged students suggests that the window of opportunity to teach these skills may not be necessarily closed.

TABLE 6.6   Status of treatment approaches to teaching social skills

Treatment approach	Status
Joint attention	Established
Imitation	Established
Peer training	Promising
Social Stories	Promising
Social skills and cognition groups	Promising

Social skills deficits have been shown to negatively influence relationships of older learners with their peers in inclusion settings, and middle- and high-school-aged students may still benefit from ongoing social development. The need for more research on older adolescents and adults is also compelling. Replications of established interventions with these populations could be clinically significant, and would add to the external validity of these treatments.

In conclusion, many interventions based on social skills have a strong or emerging evidence base, particularly models targeting joint attention, imitation, and peer training (see Table 6.6). Other areas (e.g., Social Stories and teaching older learners social skills in groups), while clinically in wide use, have little high-quality empirical support.

References

APA. (2000). *Diagnostic and statistical manual of mental disorders*, (4th ed. – text revision). Washington, DC: American Psychiatric Association.

Barnhill, G. P., Cook, K. T., Tebbenkamp, K., & Smith Myles, B. (2002). The effectiveness of social skills intervention targeting nonverbal communication for adolescents with Asperger syndrome and related pervasive developmental disorders. *Focus on Autism and Other Developmental Disabilities, 17*, 112–118.

Baron-Cohen, S., Leslie, A. M., & Frith, U. (1985). Does the autistic child have a "theory of mind?". *Cognition, 21*, 37–46.

Baron-Cohen, S., Leslie, A. M., & Frith, U. (1986). Mechanical, behavioral and intentional understanding of picture stories in autistic children. *British Journal of Developmental Psychology, 4*, 113–125.

Barry, L. M., & Burlew, S. B. (2004). Using Social Stories to teach choice and play skills to children with autism. *Focus on Autism and Other Developmental Disabilities, 19*, 45–51.

Barry, T. D., Klinger, L. G., Lee, J. M., Palardy, N., Gilmore, T., & Bodin, S. D. (2003). Examining the effectiveness of an outpatient clinic-based social skills group of high-functioning children with autism. *Journal of Autism and Developmental Disorders, 33*, 685–701.

Bauminger, N. (2002). The facilitation of social-emotional understanding and social interaction in high-functioning children with autism: Intervention outcomes. *Journal of Autism and Developmental Disorders, 32*, 283–298.

Bauminger, N. (2007a). Brief report: Individual social-multi-modal intervention for HFASD. *Journal of Autism and Developmental Disorders, 37*, 1593–1604.

Bauminger, N. (2007b). Brief report: Group social-multi-modal intervention for HFASD. *Journal of Autism and Developmental Disorders, 37*, 1605–1615.

Bellini, S., & Akullian, J. (2007). A meta-analysis of video modeling and video self-modeling interventions for children and adolescents with autism spectrum disorders. *Exceptional Children, 73*, 264–287.

Bellini, S., Akullian, J., & Hopf, A. (2007). Increasing social engagement in young children with autism spectrum disorders using video self modeling. *School Psychology Review, 36*, 80–90.

Chan, J. M., & O'Reilly, M. F. (2008). A Social Stories™ intervention package for students with autism in inclusive classroom settings. *Journal of Applied Behavior Analysis, 41*, 405–409.

Charlop-Christy, M. H., & Daneshvar, S. (2003). Using video modeling to teach perspective taking to children with autism. *Journal of Positive Behavior Interventions, 5*(1), 12.

Crooke, P. J., Hendrix, R. E., & Rachman, J. Y. (2008). Brief report: Measuring the effectiveness of teaching social thinking to children with Asperger syndrome (AS) and high functioning autism (HFA). *Journal of Autism and Developmental Disorders, 38*, 581–591.

Delano, M., & Snell, M. E. (2006). The effects of social stories on the social engagement of children with autism. *Journal of Positive Behavior Interventions, 8*, 29–42.

DiSalvo, C. A., & Oswald, D. P. (2002). Peer-mediated interventions to increase the social interaction of children with autism: Consideration of peer expectations. *Focus on Autism and Other Developmental Disabilities, 17*, 198–207.

Elksnin, L. K., & Elksnin, N. (1998). Teaching social skills to students with learning and behavior problems. *Intervention in School and Clinic, 33*, 131–140.

Garfinkle, A. N., & Schwartz, I. S. (2002). Peer imitation: Increasing social interactions in children with autism and other developmental disabilities in inclusive preschool classrooms. *Topics in Early Childhood Special Education, 22*(1), 26–38.

Garrison-Harrel, L., Kamps, D., & Kravits, T. (1997). The effects of peer networks on social-communicative behaviors for students with autism. *Focus on Autism and Other Developmental Disabilities, 12*, 241–255.

Gena, A., Couloura, S., & Kymissis, E. (2005). Modifying the affective behavior of preschoolers with autism using in-vivo or video modeling and reinforcement contingencies. *Journal of Autism and Developmental Disorders, 35*(5), 545–556.

Gevers, C., Clifford, P., Mager, M., & Boer, F. (2006). Brief report: A Theory-of-Mind-based social-cognition training program for school-aged children with pervasive developmental disorders: An open study of its effectiveness. *Journal of Autism and Developmental Disorders, 36*, 567–571.

Goldstein, H., Kaczmarek, L., Pennington, R., & Shafer, K. (1992). Peer-mediated intervention: Attending to, commenting on, and acknowledging the behavior of preschoolers with autism. *Journal of Applied Behavior Analysis, 25*, 289–305.

Gray, C. (2000). *The new Social Story book*. Arlington: Future Horizons.

Haring, T. G., & Breen, C. G. (1992). A peer-mediated social network intervention to enhance the social integration of person with moderate and severe disabilities. *Journal of Applied Behavior Analysis, 25*, 319–333.

Haring, T. G., & Lovinger, L. (1989). Promoting social interaction through teaching generalized play initiation responses to preschool children with autism. *Journal of the Association for Persons with Severe Handicaps, 14*, 58–67.

Harper, C. B., Symon, J. B. G., & Frea, W. D. (2008). Recess is time-in: Using peers to improve social skills of children with autism. *Journal of Autism and Developmental Disorders, 38*, 815–826.

Hutchins, T. L., & Prelock, P. A. (2006). Using social stories and comic strip conversations to promote socially valid outcomes for children with autism. *Seminars in Speech and Language, 27*, 47–59.

Hwang, B., & Hughes, C. (2000). Increasing early social-communicative skills of preverbal preschool children with autism through social interactive training. *Journal of the Association for Persons with Severe Handicaps, 25,* 18–28.

Ingersoll, B., & Schreibman, L. (2006). Teaching reciprocal imitation skills to young children with autism using a naturalistic behavioral approach: Effects on language, pretend play, and joint attention. *Journal of Autism and Developmental Disorders, 36*(4), 487–505.

Ingersoll, B., Lewis, E., & Kroman, E. (2007). Teaching the imitation and spontaneous use of descriptive gestures in young children with autism using a naturalistic behavioral intervention. *Journal of Autism and Developmental Disorders, 37,* 1446–1456.

Jahr, E., Eldevik, S., & Eikeseth, S. (2000). Teaching children with autism to initiate and sustain cooperative play. *Research in Developmental Disabilities, 21*(2), 151–169.

Kamps, D. M., Barbetta, P. M., Leonard, B. R., & Delquadri, J. (1994). Classwide peer tutoring: An integration strategy to improve reading skills and promote peer interactions among students with autism and general education peers. *Journal of Applied Behavior Analysis, 27,* 49–61.

Kamps, D., Royer, J., Dugan, E., Kravits, T., Gonzalez-Lopez, A., et al. (2002). Peer training to facilitate social interaction for elementary students with autism and their peers. *Exceptional Children, 68,* 173–187.

Kasari, C., Freeman, S., & Paparella, T. (2006). Joint attention and symbolic play in young children with autism: A randomized controlled intervention study. *Journal of Child Psychology and Psychiatry, 47*(6), 611–620.

Kroeger, K. A., Schultz, J. R., & Newsom, C. (2007). A comparison of two group-delivered social skills programs for young children with autism. *Journal of Autism and Developmental Disorders, 37,* 808–817.

Laushey, K. M., & Heflin, L. J. (2000). Enhancing social skills of kindergarten children with autism through the training of multiple peers as tutors. *Journal of Autism and Developmental Disorders, 30,* 183–193.

Lee, S., Odom, S. L., & Loftin, R. (2007). Social engagement with peers and stereotypic behavior of children with autism. *Journal of Positive Behavior Interventions, 9,* 67–79.

LeGoff, D. B. (2004). Use of LEGO as a therapeutic medium for improving social competence. *Journal of Autism and Developmental Disorders, 34,* 557–571.

LeGoff, D. B., & Sherman, M. (2006). Long-term outcome of social skills intervention based on interactive LEGO play. *Autism, 10,* 317–329.

Leslie, A. M., & Frith, U. (1988). Autistic children's understanding of seeing, knowing, and believing. *British Journal of Developmental Psychology, 6,* 315–324.

Lopata, C., Thomeer, M. L., Volker, M. A., & Nida, R. E. (2006). Effectiveness of a cognitive-behavioral treatment on the social behaviors of children with Asperger disorder. *Focus on Autism and Other Developmental Disabilities, 21,* 237–244.

Maione, L., & Mirenda, P. (2006). Effects of video modeling and video feedback on peer-directed social language skills of a child with autism. *Journal of Positive Behavior Interventions, 8*(2), 106–118.

Martins, M., & Harris, S. (2006). Teaching children with autism to respond to joint attention initiations. *Child & Family Behavior Therapy, 28*(1), 51–68.

McGrath, A. M., Bosch, S., Sullivan, C. L., & Fuqua, R. W. (2003). Training reciprocal social interactions between preschoolers and a child diagnosed with autism. *Journal of Positive Behavior Interventions, 5,* 47–54.

Mesibov, G. B. (1984). Social skills training with verbal autistic adolescents and adults: A program model. *Journal of Autism and Developmental Disorders, 14,* 395–404.

Mishna, F., & Muskat, B. (1998). Group therapy for boys with features of Asperger syndrome and concurrent learning disabilities: Finding a peer group. *Journal of Child and Adolescent Group Therapy, 8,* 97–114.

Nikopoulos, C. K., & Keenan, M. (2003). Promoting social initiation in children with autism using video modeling. *Behavioral Interventions, 18*(2), 87–108.

Nikopoulos, C. K., & Keenan, M. (2004). Effects of video modeling on social initiations by children with autism. *Journal of Applied Behavior Analysis, 37,* 93–96.

Nikopoulos, C. K., & Keenan, M. (2007). Using video modeling to teach complex social sequences to children with autism. *Journal of Autism and Developmental Disorders, 37,* 678–693.

Norris, C., & Dattilo, J. (1999). Evaluating effects of a Social Story on a young girl with autism. *Focus on Autism and Other Developmental Disabilities, 14,* 180–186.

Owen-DeSchryver, J. S., Carr, E. G., Cale, S. I., & Blakeley-Smith, A. (2008). Promoting social interactions between students with autism spectrum disorders and their peers in inclusive school settings. *Focus on Autism and Other Developmental Disabilities, 23,* 15–28.

Owens, G., Granader, Y., Humphrey, A., & Baron-Cohen, S. (2008). LEGO therapy and the social use of language programme: An evaluation of two social skills interventions for children with high functioning autism and Asperger syndrome. *Journal of Autism and Developmental Disorders, 38*, 1944–1957.

Ozonoff, S., & Miller, J. N. (1995). Teaching theory of mind: A new approach to social skills training for individuals with autism. *Journal of Autism and Developmental Disorders, 25*, 405–433.

Pierce, K., & Schreibman, L. (1995). Increasing complex social behaviors in children with autism: Effects of peer-implemented pivotal response training. *Journal of Applied Behavior Analysis, 28*, 285–295.

Pierce, K., & Schreibman, L. (1997). Multiple peer use of pivotal response training to increase social behaviors of classmates with autism: Results from trained and untrained peers. *Journal of Applied Behavior Analysis, 30*, 157–160.

Quirmbach, L. M., Lincoln, A. J., Feinberg-Gizzo, M. J., Ingersoll, B. R., & Andrews, S. M. (2009). Social Stories: Mechanisms of effectiveness in increasing game play skills in children diagnosed with autism spectrum disorder using a pretest posttest repeated measures randomized control design. *Journal of Autism and Developmental Disorders, 39*, 299–321.

Reichow, B., Volkmar, F. R., & Cicchetti, D. V. (2008). Development of an evaluative method for determining the strength of research evidence in autism. *Journal of Autism and Developmental Disorders, 38*, 1311–1319.

Reynhout, G., and Carter, M. (2006) Social Stories™ for children with disabilites. *Journal of Autism and Developmental Disorders, 36*:445–469.

Rocha, M. L., Schreibman, L., & Stahmer, A. C. (2007). Effectiveness of training parents to teach joint attention in children with autism. *Journal of Early Intervention, 29*(2), 154–172.

Roeyers, H. (1996). The influence of nonhandicapped peers on the social interactions of children with a pervasive developmental disorder. *Journal of Autism and Developmental Disorders, 26*, 303–320.

Sansosti, F. J., & Powell-Smith, K. A. (2006). Using social stories to improve the social behavior of children with Asperger syndrome. *Journal of Positive Behavior Interventions, 8*(1), 43–57.

Sasso, G. M., Mundschenk, N. A., Melloy, K. J., & Casey, S. D. (1998). A comparison of the effects of organismic and setting variables on the social interaction behavior of children with developmental disabilities and autism. *Focus on Autism and Other Developmental Disabilities, 13*, 2–17.

Scattone, D. (2008). Enhancing the conversation skills of a boy with Asperger's disorder through Social Stories and video modeling. *Journal of Autism and Developmental Disorders, 38*, 395–400.

Scattone, D., Tingstrom, D. H., & Wilczynski, S. M. (2006). Increasing appropriate social interactions of children with autism spectrum disorders using Social Stories™. *Focus on Autism and Other Developmental Disabilities, 21*(4), 211–222.

Simpson, A., Langone, J., & Ayres, K. (2004). Embedded video and computer based instruction to improve social skills for students with autism. *Education and Training in Developmental Disabilities, 29*, 240–252.

Solomon, M., Goodlin-Jones, B. L., & Adler, T. (2004). A social adjustment enhancement intervention for high functioning autism, Asperger's syndrome, and pervasive developmental disorder, NOS. *Journal of Autism and Developmental Disorders, 34*, 649–668.

Thiemann, S., & Goldstein, H. (2001). Social stories, written text cues, and video feedback: Effects on social communication of children with autism. *Journal of Applied Behavior Analysis, 34*, 425–446.

Tse, J., Strulovitch, J., Tagalakis, V., Meng, L., & Fombonne, E. (2007). Social skills training of adolescents with Asperger syndrome and high-functioning autism. *Journal of Autism and Developmental Disorders, 37*(10), 1960–1968.

Turner-Brown, L. M., Perry, T. P., Dichter, G. S., Bodfish, J. W., & Penn, D. (2008). Brief report: Feasibility of social cognition and interaction training for adults with high functioning autism. *Journal of Autism and Developmental Disorders, 38*, 1777–1784.

Webb, B. J., Miller, S. P., Pierce, T. B., Strawser, S., & Jones, W. P. (2004). Effects of social skill instruction for high-functioning adolescents with autism spectrum disorders. *Focus on Autism and Other Developmental Disabilities, 19*, 53–62.

Wechsler, D. (2003). *Wechsler intelligence scales for children* (4th ed.). San Antonio: The Psychological Corporation.

Whalen, C., & Shreibman, L. (2003). Joint attention training for children with autism using behavior modification procedures. *Journal of Child Psychology and Psychiatry, 44*, 456–468.

Whalen, C., Schreibman, L., & Ingersoll, B. (2006). The collateral effects of joint attention training on social initiations, positive affect, imitation, and spontaneous speech for young children with autism. *Journal of Autism and Developmental Disorders, 36*(5), 655–664.

Williams, T. I. (1989). A social skills group for autistic children. *Journal of Autism and Developmental Disorders, 19*, 143–155.

Yang, N. K., Schaller, J. L., Huang, T. A., Wang, M. H., & Tsai, S. F. (2003). Enhancing appropriate social behaviors for children with autism in general education classrooms: An analysis of six cases. *Education and Training in Developmental Disabilities, 38*, 405–416.

Yang, T., Wolfberg, P. J., Wu, S., & Hwu, P. (2003). Supporting children on the autism spectrum in peer play at home and school: Piloting the Integrated Play Groups model in Taiwan. *Autism: The International Journal of Research and Practice, 7*(4), 437–453.

Zercher, C., Hunt, P., Schuler, A., & Webster, J. (2001). Increasing joint attention, play and language through peer supported play. *Autism, 5*(4), 374–398.

CHAPTER 7

Cognitive Behavioral Therapy in High-Functioning Autism: Review and Recommendations for Treatment Development

Jeffrey J. Wood, Cori Fujii, and Patricia Renno

ABBREVIATIONS

ADHD	Attention deficit hyperactivity disorder
ADI-R	Autism diagnostic interview – revised
ADOS	Autism diagnostic observation schedule
ASDs	Autism spectrum disorders
CARS	Childhood Autism Rating Scale
CBT	Cognitive behavioral therapy
CGI	Clinical global improvement
DSM-IV-TR	Diagnostic and Statistical Manual of Mental Disorders 4th edition
NIMH	National Institutes of Mental Health
OCD	Obsessive – compulsive disorder
ODD	Oppositional defiant disorder
PCIT	Parent – child interaction therapy
PDD-NOS	Pervasive developmental disorder not otherwise specified
RCT	Randomized control trial
RUPP	Research Units on Pediatric Psychopharmacology
SRS	Social Responsiveness Scale
SSED	Single subject experimental design
SST	Social skills training

INTRODUCTION

Individuals with autism spectrum disorders (ASDs) who have acquired functional communication strategies – particularly more cognitively able individuals at or beyond the elementary school age group – may be candidates for talk-based therapies similar to those employed with children and adults with mental health disorders,

B. Reichow et al. (eds.), *Evidence-Based Practices and Treatments for Children with Autism*,
DOI 10.1007/978-1-4419-6975-0_7, © Springer Science+Business Media, LLC 2011

such as anxiety (e.g., cognitive behavioral therapy, CBT). While talk-based therapies are widely used in community settings for school-aged youth and adults with ASD (Hess et al. 2008), the evidence base for using many such treatments is surprisingly weak. Compared to other types of intervention in autism (e.g., applied behavior analysis for young children) and interventions for other types of neurodevelopmental disorder (e.g., attention deficit/hyperactivity disorder, ADHD), there are very few well-designed studies of CBT and other talk-based therapies for individuals with autism. Of those studies that have been conducted, results are mixed, requiring a careful comparative analysis of the extant treatment literature to distinguish potentially promising practices from those that are less promising. This chapter endeavors to provide such an analysis and, in so doing, to draw preliminary conclusions about worthwhile practices currently available for implementation, as well as to identify directions for further development of treatment techniques.

We begin by defining the parameters of CBT and related talk-based therapies as distinguished from other behavioral interventions for individuals with ASD. CBT treatments are based upon cognitive science models of behavior, emotion, and thought; contemporary CBT treatments have been particularly influenced by the memory retrieval competition model (Brewin 2006). Conceptualized in information-processing terms, CBT aims to promote *retrievable memories* of adaptive responses that can successfully compete with and suppress memories of previously learned maladaptive responses evoked under "real world" conditions outside the therapy office. CBT methods used to achieve this are psychoeducation (learning about the nature of one's mental health condition), Socratic questioning and collaborative discussions to build up awareness of thought and emotion and to teach thought- and behavior-based coping skills, and behavioral experimentation, in which alternative responses to challenging situations are attempted in real-world settings and then reflected upon in structured discussions in order to build up potent memories of adaptive patterns of thought and behavior for future use in similar (not necessarily identical) situations.

A fundamental difference between CBT and strictly behavioral treatments (e.g., operant or classical conditioning-based models) is the conceptualization of mechanisms of change and complementary intervention techniques. While purely behavioral interventions assume that largely automatic (and unobservable) learning processes (e.g., extinction; associative learning; modeling) promote behavioral change and symptom remission, CBT-based models seek to promote changes in thinking and volitional behavior (e.g., identifying and challenging maladaptive interpretations of social situations) that are adaptable to multiple situational contexts. A simple example of phobia treatment illustrates differences between CBT and purely behavioral approaches: in the former, catastrophic beliefs about a feared stimulus would be identified and challenged to build up to facing the phobic stimulus and, after habituation occurs, the therapy would promote the development of principles for thinking about the feared stimulus differently to build a benign memory schema of the stimulus that could compete with and suppress the fearful schema that the patient had prior to treatment (Wood and McLeod 2008). The need for such competition stems from the cognitive science finding that prior memory schemata cannot be "deleted" and are often prone to return and override insufficiently developed alternative (adaptive) schemata. In contrast, a purely behavioral approach would involve gradual exposure to a feared stimulus to achieve extinction of the conditioned (fearful) response with no emphasis on related thoughts; and when fear and avoidance were eliminated in one setting, the procedure might be repeated in several other settings in an effort to achieve generalization (Brewin 2006). Clearly, the putative learning processes and corresponding techniques used to promote change differ significantly in these two types of treatment (further description of CBT technique is given below, in "Enhancing CBT Treatments for ASD Symptoms").

It is important to note that while differentiation between CBT and non-CBT interventions can be made easily at a conceptual level, there can be some ambiguity in this distinction in practice because treatments used in many clinical trials are often summarized so succinctly that it is difficult to ascertain how much emphasis is given to cognitive behavioral techniques. Also, the simple fact that language is used as an element of treatment, for example, clearly does not distinguish CBT from other autism interventions; many non-CBT interventions, such as applied behavior analysis, joint attention training, or imitation training, often use substantial amounts of therapist-initiated speech during the interventions, with the goal of eliciting target verbal or nonverbal behaviors during the therapy sessions (e.g., coordinated eye gaze, commenting, and pointing). One factor that differentiates CBT and related mental health therapies from other autism interventions is the way in which speech and language are used during treatment. As noted above, in CBT and related therapies, verbal communication between therapist and patient is partly used as a means to identify and challenge specific thoughts, such as realistic versus irrational beliefs. Another factor that often differentiates CBT and related mental health therapies from other behavioral treatments in autism is that the explicit goals of treatment are often in the domains of psychiatric symptomatology in the former.

Two methodological factors that often differentiate clinical trials of CBT in autism from other behavioral interventions in autism are the types of outcome measures used to document efficacy and the age groups included in the interventions. In defining desirable study features for research intended to establish efficacious treatments, Chambless and Hollon (1998) noted that it was important that valid and reliable measures of symptom counts or diagnostic status, preferably including those rated by an evaluator blind to treatment status and study hypotheses, be used as primary outcome measures. Of the small number of controlled trials of CBT for individuals with ASD, most have included this kind of measure. Many of these have focused on comorbid mental health features, such as anxiety (Chalfant et al. 2007), and one of these trials utilized a parent-rated measure of core autism symptoms that is norm-referenced and used in the diagnosis of ASD (Wood et al. 2009a). In comparison, many treatment studies of other behavioral interventions for autism, such as variants of applied behavioral analysis, have often utilized:

- Observational measures with high specificity to the treatment (e.g., imitation) that have good external validity and often evidence of inter-rater reliability but rarely have evidence of concurrent or convergent validity from psychometric studies and have unknown utility as measures of ASD diagnostic status or symptomatology
- Direct measures of receptive and expressive language with good psychometric properties that nonetheless are not specific to core autism symptoms per se (but rather, measure diagnostically nonspecific aspects of language acquisition and proficiency)
- General measures of intellectual ability that do not reflect core autism symptoms
- Nonspecific measures of social skills or social adjustment that are not typically used in the evidence-based assessment of ASD

The distinctions in choice of outcome measures in clinical trials of CBT versus other behavioral interventions in ASD do not necessarily reflect fundamental differences between these treatments, although it is possible that measure selection (or publication of specific outcomes illustrating significant treatment effects) indirectly indicates the putative domains most likely affected by differing interventions.

Second, most studies of non-CBT social awareness interventions have been conducted with toddlers or preschoolers with ASD (see Chap. 6), whereas almost all studies of interventions described as "CBT" or "mental health interventions" for ASD have been with elementary school children or older individuals. Interestingly, some of the interventions designated as CBT with an emphasis on social skills outcomes (Bauminger 2002) have utilized intervention methods similar to some social awareness training procedures used with preschoolers (Ingersoll et al. 2007), which raises the question of whether a false dichotomy has indeed been established and that terms such as CBT have at times been used to describe interventions for older individuals that are similar in content to interventions with different names that have been used with young children. Traditionally, CBT and other forms of psychotherapy for mental health disorders have been studied primarily with school-aged children and older individuals. Maintaining this tradition in the field of autism treatment may be sensible for descriptive purposes, but the potential overlap between such therapies and those with different names used with younger children with ASD should be acknowledged.

Given the overlapping nature of goals and methods of CBT and other behavioral interventions for ASD, as well as the pragmatic value of minimizing overlap in the review of studies with other chapters in this book, we focus forthwith on interventions that use verbally mediated language to discuss an individual's thoughts, problems, and solutions (not merely for modeling or prompting), that are conducted with school-aged children or older, and that attempt to reduce the symptomatology of a mental disorder, including ASD or a comorbid mental health problem, as measured by diagnostically specific outcome assessments. We also consider other interventions that are explicitly described as "CBT" by the treatment developers, even if they do not meet all of these three criteria, for the sake of comparison.

PSYCHIATRIC COMORBIDITY IN ASD

The majority of the clinical trials reviewed in this article focused on psychiatric comorbidity (e.g., anxiety), as opposed to core autism symptoms, as the primary target of treatment and outcomes assessment. Hence, a brief overview of psychiatric comorbidity among youths with ASD is now given. Numerous descriptive studies of comorbidity in more or less representative samples of youths with ASD have been conducted over the past decade and conclusions are relatively homogeneous: in general, there are very high rates of comorbid disorders in youth on the autism spectrum, well exceeding typically developing youth as well as youth with other (serious) mental health conditions such as conduct disorder (de Bruin et al. 2007; Green et al. 2000; Russell and Sofronoff 2005; Sukhodolsky et al. 2007). Social anxiety in particular occurs at higher rates in youths with ASD than in the typically developing population, with results from a number of studies indicating 20–57% of children and adolescents with high functioning ASD exhibit clinically relevant symptoms of social anxiety (Kuusikko et al. 2008; Muris et al. 1998; Simonoff et al. 2008), as compared to 1–5% in typically developing youth. Depressive disorders often increase significantly in adolescence among youths with ASD, and attention deficit and disruptive behavior disorder profiles are also very common in youth on the autism spectrum. Comorbidity in ASD is not without its controversies. For example, the latest version of the *Diagnostic and Statistical Manual of Mental Disorders* (DSM-IV-TR; APA 2000) prohibits a comorbid diagnosis of ADHD among those with an ASD, whereas the earlier version did not (APA 1994).

The most common hypotheses about psychiatric comorbidity in ASD have been that there may be a common genetic linkage between ASD and other psychiatric disorders, increasing the risk of each; that the stresses caused by having an ASD (e.g., social rejection, sensory overresponsiveness, confusion in light of communication challenges) overwhelm coping skills and induce emotional and behavioral disorders; or that core autism symptoms are sometimes "counted as" aspects of a comorbid disorder that has phenotypically similar features (Baron-Cohen 1989; Bellini 2006; Gadow et al. 2008; Gillott et al. 2001; Groden et al. 2006). For example, the social avoidance characterizing many youth on the spectrum – stemming from low social motivation and restricted interests – could be mistaken for social anxiety, which also can manifest, in part, as social avoidance. Although this is an important point in terms of psychiatric nosology, it may have less import in the realm of treatment. This is because symptom reduction is likely to be helpful whether the symptoms ultimately reflect a separate psychiatric disorder or are simply a manifestation of autism that is causing adaptive difficulties.

Linkages between comorbid psychiatric symptomatology and functional problems in youths with ASD are both self-evident and empirically documented. For example, a very hyperactive child is going to have greater adaptational challenges in a classroom than one who is not, all other things being equal. A depressed child preoccupied with unpleasant thoughts will have a lower quality of daily life than one who is not. A growing body of research has demonstrated links between high anxiety in ASD and a number of functional impairments, such as poor social responsiveness and other social skill deficits (Bellini 2004; Sukhodolsky et al. 2008) and increased ASD symptom severity (Ben-Sasson et al. 2008; Kelly et al. 2008). In short, whether comorbid symptoms and disorders are entirely distinct from an individual's core autism spectrum disorder or not, there is clearly a relationship between the presence of such symptoms and more overall impairment and distress in affected youth, underscoring the importance of treatments that can relieve such symptoms.

A Review of CBT and Related Mental Health Treatments in ASD

This section is organized around treatment studies for (a) comorbid anxiety and mood problems; (b) comorbid disruptive behavior problems; and (c) core autism symptoms (as well as nonspecific social problems). In each subsection, the nature of the problem (e.g., anxiety) and relevance to individuals with autism is discussed, the extant treatment literature is reviewed, and each study is abstracted in tabular format and rated according to the criteria for strong, adequate or weak research methodology described in Chap. 2.

Anxiety and Mood Disturbance

Anxiety disorders are common among youth and adults with ASD, as noted above (de Bruin et al. 2007; Green et al.

2000; Klin et al. 2005; Leyfer et al. 2006; Muris et al. 1998). Among the more common anxiety disorders in the DSM-IV-TR (APA 2000) are generalized anxiety disorder, typified by disabling worry; separation anxiety disorder, characterized by intense fear of separating from caregivers; obsessive–compulsive disorder (OCD), involving repeated intrusive thoughts and rituals; and social phobia, characterized by a fear of humiliation and corresponding avoidance of specific social situations. A recent survey conducted by the National Autistic Society found that anxiety was the second most highly cited problem reported by parents of children with ASD (Mills and Wing 2005). Often, additional comorbid disorders coincide with anxiety disorders in the ASD population (e.g., oppositional defiant disorder, ODD), resulting in complex and severe clinical presentations (de Bruin et al. 2007; Klin et al. 2005; Muris et al. 1998).

CBT is a well-supported treatment modality for otherwise typically developing youth with anxiety disorders (Walkup et al. 2008). Some promising research on adapted CBT for youths with ASD and comorbid anxiety disorders has emerged in recent years. Sofronoff et al. (2005) evaluated two variants of a 6-week CBT program in group-therapy format that focused on emotion recognition and cognitive restructuring for children with Asperger syndrome. Parent-report measures showed declines in child anxiety symptoms in the CBT groups as compared to a wait-list group; however, participating children did not necessarily meet criteria for an anxiety disorder at pre-treatment. Similarly, in 12- and 16-week group-therapy CBT interventions for comorbid anxiety and ASD in children, Chalfant et al. (2007) found that anxiety outcomes were superior for the immediate treatment group relative to the wait-list arm. However, noteworthy limitations of these studies were that the study therapists, rather than independent

evaluators blind to treatment assignment, administered the post-treatment diagnostic interviews; and that treatment fidelity was not assessed. Reaven et al. (2009) studied 33 children (aged 8–14 years) with ASD and comorbid anxiety disorders, assigning them (using a nonrandomized assignment paradigm) to immediate treatment in group-therapy format CBT or a wait-list. Outcome measures were child- and parent-reported anxiety symptoms using psychometrically sound questionnaires. Youth in the immediate treatment group improved more than the wait-list group on parent-reported symptoms, but not child-reported symptoms. This may have been attributable to low pre-treatment child-report symptom scores.

In one study adhering to Chambless and Hollon's (1998) suggested research methodology for clinical trials research (Wood et al. 2009b), 40 children aged 7–11 years were randomized to either 16 sessions of a manualized, individualized CBT program plus two school consultation sessions or to a waiting list. CBT in this study incorporated coping skills training (e.g., identifying "calm" thoughts) and in-vivo exposure elements (facing fears hierarchically) as well as significant parent- and teacher-training components to ensure that new behaviors and ideas were practiced in school and home settings rather than just in therapy sessions. The program incorporated various motivational elements (e.g., use of children's special interests as examples of concepts; use of a comprehensive reward system during sessions and at home) to maintain engagement and to promote the recall of adaptive responses over maladaptive counterparts. Participating children had an average of 4.18 psychiatric disorders at intake. Despite the high level of comorbidity, children randomized to CBT had primary outcomes comparable to those of other studies treating childhood anxiety in typically developing patients (Barrett et al. 1996; Wood et al. 2006), with large effect sizes for most outcome measures; remission of all anxiety disorders for over half of the children by post-treatment or follow-up; and a high rate of positive treatment response on the Clinical Global Impressions – Improvement scale (CGI-I) (78.5% from intent-to-treat analyses). As with the Reaven et al. (2009) study, child-reported anxiety did not differ significantly from pre-treatment to follow-up; however, a floor effect was expected, as baseline levels were low and decreased with treatment.

Collectively, these studies and other pilot work using case studies or AB designs (Lehmkuhl et al. 2008; Ooi et al. 2008; Sze and Wood 2007, 2008) indicate that CBT is a promising modality for anxiety in the ASD population. Although CBT was a general treatment approach used in each of these studies, with a focus on challenging irrational fearful beliefs and developing rational beliefs as a common treatment element, other elements of treatment varied widely. It should be noted that one of the more influential clinical trials of CBT for pediatric anxiety disorders in typically developing children and youth (Kendall et al. 1997) convincingly demonstrated that the *cognitive* intervention aspects of the treatment (e.g., challenging irrational beliefs) alone – when not paired with in vivo exposure elements – do not appear to be even modestly effective in reducing children's anxiety levels. However, the CBT programs evaluated for individuals with ASD and high anxiety varied widely with regard to the emphasis placed on in vivo exposure relative to less active treatment elements (e.g., cartooning, role-playing). At the extremes of the continuum, the Wood et al. (2009b) RCT involved in vivo exposure at home on a daily basis for the majority of the 16-session treatment, which spanned 4–5 months for most youth; whereas the Sofronoff et al. (2005) six-session treatment focused entirely on a series of creative anxiety management skills tailored for youths with ASD but

with no explicit in vivo exposure elements. Some (but not all) CBT trials conducted with typically developing children and youth with anxiety disorders (Barrett et al. 1996; Barrett 1998; Wood et al. 2006) have found that including parent training in the intervention leads to superior intervention effects as compared to exclusively child-focused treatments. Many of the group design studies for youths with ASD and high anxiety included concurrent child- and parent-intervention components. Sofronoff et al. (2005) included two active treatment groups – one with child-only treatment and one with concurrent child- and parent-treatment – and found some evidence suggesting that combined child and parent treatment was more effective than solely working with the children at both post-treatment and the follow-up assessment. This is an impressive finding given the relatively brief duration of this treatment.

The majority of the treatment programs studied in group design studies used a group-therapy treatment format with a structured sequence of sessions for all participants. In comparison, the Wood et al. (2009b) study used an individual therapy format with modular design (Chorpita et al. 2004) in which individual treatment components were selected by the therapist and supervisor on a session-by-session basis using a clinical algorithm matching the client's presenting characteristics and most pressing clinical needs with corresponding treatment elements. As an example, a child who was socially isolated at school would receive a social coaching module, in which social approach behaviors are broken down into steps, anxious beliefs about each step are discussed and rationalized, and then steps are practiced in various real-world settings such as parks and school playgrounds repeatedly until a sufficiently advanced level of the skill (e.g., joining recess games) is evidenced consistently. The same child would also be a candidate for the peer buddy module in which select peers at school would be trained to invite and include the target child in games and conversations to reduce the level of difficulty for the targeted social behaviors. No clinical trials thus far have compared the relative efficacy of structured group-format CBT interventions with individually administered, modularized interventions of this kind and it will be important to determine whether the more complex and clinically challenging modular approach is indeed necessary.

White and Roberson-Nay (2009) have suggested that social anxiety may be related specifically to social loneliness (vs. emotional loneliness) and could possibly mediate the child's level of involvement in activities with peers. This potential link between anxiety and social engagement has led to the investigation of the effects of social skills interventions on anxiety outcomes in youths with ASD in an interesting recent trial. Cotugno (2009) examined the effectiveness of a 30-week social skills group intervention for 18 children (ages 7–11) diagnosed with ASD. Children were split into older (ages 10–11 years) and younger (ages 7–9 years) groups. Cotugno employed a peer-based group model within a cognitive-developmental framework, using a combination of group therapy, cognitive-behavioral, and social skill instruction techniques in order to address the social competency needs and concerns of the children with ASD. In addition, the intervention took into account which one of five predetermined stages of group development the children were in, with each stage specifying the processes and sets of behaviors necessary to pass through to the next stage. Each stage focused on different elements of group formation and cohesion while fostering relationships between group members. Measures of anxiety at post-treatment showed that both the younger and older groups of children showed significant improvements in parent ratings of anxiety; however the younger group showed a greater positive shift than the older group. The results of this study provide some support for the relationship between social skills and anxiety, and give some evidence to the positive effects of a social skills intervention on anxiety in children with ASD. However, Cotugno did not use an evidence-based measure of anxiety, instead using two items from the MGH YouthCare Social Competency/Social Skill Development Scale that focused on the child's level of stress and anxiety management. Further research examining the link between social skills training and anxiety should include additional anxiety measures in order to gain a better understanding of the nature of this relationship.

Table 7.1 presents a summary of the characteristics of the CBT interventions that have been evaluated in previous studies of individuals with ASD and concurrent anxiety and mood problems. It should be noted that although the research methodology was less sophisticated in the majority of the studies in this group, of those with stronger methods, treatment outcomes were promising.

Disruptive Behavior Problems

Children with ASD often present with comorbid disruptive behavior disorders such as ADHD or ODD (de Bruin et al. 2007; Klin et al. 2005; Muris et al. 1998). As noted above, DSM-IV-TR (APA 2000) rules out the concurrent diagnosis of ADHD when an ASD is diagnosed, but there is a controversy over whether or not this exclusion should be continued in future versions of the DSM. Some researchers have found evidence suggesting that a comorbid diagnosis of ADHD should be allowed due to the clinically distinct representation of ADHD in children with autism compared with children that are diagnosed with only one of these disorders (Goldstein and Schwebach 2004; Reiersen and Todd 2008;

TABLE 7.1   Clinical trials and case studies of treatments for anxiety in individuals with ASD

Study	Participants	Study type	Method	Primary outcome measures	Quality of study methods[a]	Outcomes
Cardaciotto and Herbert (2004)	• $N=1$ • 23-year-old male • Diagnosed with Asperger syndrome and social anxiety disorder	• Case study	• Manual • No treatment fidelity measure • 14 weekly sessions • Individual CBT	• Self-report measure of social phobia symptoms • Clinician's rating of impairment	• Weak	• Self-report measures of social phobia symptoms within normal limits (40th percentile) • Clinician rating of impairment was "very much improved"
Chalfant et al. (2007)	• $N=47$ • 8–13 years old • 34 males	• Randomized controlled trial (wait-list control)	• Manual • No treatment fidelity measure • Twelve 2-h sessions • Group CBT • Parent and child groups	• Semi-structured diagnostic psychiatric interview for anxiety disorders • Parent- and child-report measures of child anxiety	• Adequate	• Significantly more subjects in the immediate treatment condition no longer met criteria for any anxiety disorder, compared to the wait-list condition • Self-report measures had significant group x time interactions
Cotugno (2009)	• $N=18$ • 7–11 years old • Diagnosed with ASD	• Open trial	• No manual • No treatment fidelity measure • 30 weekly 1-h sessions • Group social skills training	• Teacher-report measure of social-behavioral adjustment • Parent-report measure of social competency and social skill development	• Weak	• Significant increase in positive social behavior • Significant increase in school adjustment • Significant improvement in stress and anxiety management and flexibility with transitions

(Continued)

TABLE 7.1 (Continued)

Study	Participants	Study type	Method	Primary outcome measures	Quality of study methods[a]	Outcomes
Lehmkuhl et al. (2008)	• N = 1 • 12-year-old male • Diagnosed with high-functioning autism and obsessive–compulsive disorder	• Case study	• Manual • No treatment fidelity measure • 10 sessions of 50 min • Individual CBT	• Semi-structured diagnostic psychiatric interview for obsessive–compulsive disorder • Child-report measure of obsessive–compulsive disorder	• Weak	• Post-treatment OCD score within normal limits based on interview • Post-treatment OCD within normal limits on self-report • Both treatment gains maintained at the 3-month follow-up
Ooi et al. (2008)	• N = 6 • 9–13 years old • Diagnosed with ASD	• Open trial	• Manual • No treatment fidelity measure • 16 sessions of 90 min • Group CBT	• Parent- and child-report measures of child anxiety	• Weak	• No statistically significant findings
Reaven et al. (2009)	• N = 33 • 8–14 years old • 26 males • Diagnosed with ASD and anxiety disorders	• Group • Comparison without random assignment	• Manual • Fidelity checklists • 12 sessions of 90 min • Group CBT • Parent and child groups	• Parent- and child-report measures of child anxiety	• Adequate	• Significant decrease in severity of • Anxiety in the immediate treatment group versus wait-list group on parent report of anxiety symptoms

Study	Participants	Design	Treatment	Measures	Fidelity	Results
Reaven and Hepburn (2003)	• $N=1$ • 7-year-old female • Diagnosed with Asperger syndrome and obsessive–compulsive disorder	• Case study	• Manual • No treatment fidelity measure • 14 sessions • CBT • Medication	• Semi-structured diagnostic psychiatric interview for obsessive–compulsive disorder	• Weak	• Lowered OCD score by the end of treatment • Most of the original symptoms remitted
Sofronoff et al. (2005)	• $N=71$ • 10–12 years old • 62 males • Non-standardized report of high anxiety	• Randomized controlled trial	• Manual • Fidelity checklists; 25% sessions videotaped and coded for fidelity • Weekly supervision • Six 2-h sessions • Three groups (child; child and parent; wait-list)	• Parent-report measures of child anxiety and social worries	• Adequate	• Parent report of anxiety yielded a main effect of time and a time x group interaction (both treatment groups better than wait-list; combined group with greatest improvements)
Sze and Wood (2007)	• $N=1$ • 11-year-old female • Diagnosed with high-functioning autism and three anxiety disorders	• Case study	• Manual • No treatment fidelity measure • Weekly therapist supervision • 16 sessions of 90 min • Family CBT	• Semi-structured diagnostic psychiatric interview for anxiety disorders	• Weak	• No longer met criteria for separation anxiety, generalized anxiety, or obsessive–compulsive disorder after treatment

(Continued)

TABLE 7.1 (Continued)

Study	Participants	Study type	Method	Primary outcome measures	Quality of study methods[a]	Outcomes
Sze and Wood (2008)	• N = 1 • 10-year-old male • Diagnosed with Asperger Disorder and two anxiety disorders	• Case study	• Manual • No treatment fidelity measure • Weekly therapist supervision • 16 sessions of 90 min • Family CBT	• Semi-structured diagnostic psychiatric interview for anxiety disorders • Clinician's rating of impairment • Parent-report measure on child anxiety symptoms	• Weak	• No longer met criteria for generalized anxiety or social phobia after treatment • Clinician rating of impairment "very much improved" • Shifted from clinically significant to normal on parent measure of anxiety (lowered ~1 SD)
Wood et al. (2009b)	• N = 40 • 7–11 years old • 27 males • Diagnosed with ASD and an anxiety disorder	• Randomized controlled trial (wait-list control)	• Manual • Fidelity assessed • Weekly therapist supervision • 16 sessions of 90 min • Family CBT	• Semi-structured diagnostic psychiatric interview for anxiety disorders • Clinician's rating of impairment	• Strong	• 64% in the immediate treatment condition no longer met criteria for an anxiety disorder • 92% of immediate treatment group showed a positive treatment outcome based on clinician's rating

[a]The quality was assessed using the criteria described by Reichow (Chap. 2)

Koyama et al. 2006). Others have found that individuals with ASD and ADHD scored similarly on several measures assessing these disorders, making it difficult to differentiate between the two (Hattori et al. 2006). The presence of disruptive behavior problems in many children with ASD has led researchers to investigate various interventions targeting these behaviors.

Parent–Child Interaction Therapy (PCIT) is a well-supported intervention model for typically developing children with externalizing disorders. A pilot study for the use of PCIT for externalizing disorders for children with comorbid ASD has yielded promising findings (Solomon et al. 2008). In this study, 19 male participants, aged 5–12 years were randomly assigned to an immediate treatment or wait-list condition, matched by age, cognitive level, and behavioral symptoms. Treatment consisted of 12 weeks of modified PCIT in which the parents were trained by therapists in child-directed interaction for 6 weeks and in parent-directed interaction for 6 weeks. During the child-directed interaction sessions, parents were coached by therapists to praise and reinforce appropriate behaviors and ignore inappropriate behaviors. In the parent-directed interaction sessions, parents were trained to give clear, simple commands and consistently reinforce child compliance. Areas of the treatment that were adapted especially for children with ASD were prohibiting children from talking excessively about special interests, redirecting children's attention, and giving praise for children's initiations of interactions. On parent reports of behavioral problems and atypicality, several group by time interaction effects emerged, showing a statistically significant difference between the immediate treatment and wait-list conditions at post-treatment. Other scales of externalizing behavior did not differ between groups, but main effects of time were generally evident, showing a decrease in both groups. The limitations to

this study included only assessing problem behaviors through parent reports, a small sample size, and no formal measure of treatment fidelity.

In a randomized controlled trial of CBT conducted by Sofronoff et al. (2007), 45 children (aged 10–14 years) diagnosed with Asperger Syndrome and initially rated as high in anger were assigned to either a 6-week immediate intervention group or a wait-list group. Treatment consisted of 6 weekly 2-h sessions for both child and parent. The manualized therapy sessions focused on exploring positive and negative emotions, cognitions related to coping with anger, Social Stories to promote emotion management, and designing individualized coping plans for anger management. There was a significant reduction in the number of parent-reported anger episodes after treatment in the immediate intervention group, with gains maintained 6 weeks after treatment completion. Qualitative interviews conducted with participants' teachers post-treatment revealed participants' use of strategies they had learned through the program to manage their anger within their classroom. One methodological weakness in this study was that no diagnostic criteria or operational definition of an externalizing disorder was used for case selection at pre-treatment. In addition, all outcome measures were parent-report, with the exception of the qualitative interviews with teachers.

Other types of structured mental health treatments for youth with externalizing disorders and ASD that have been explored include multimodal approaches and mindfulness training. In a case study of a multimodal treatment for a 9-year-old boy diagnosed with PDD-NOS and externalizing behavior problems, a manualized behavioral treatment summer camp program, medication, behavioral parent training, and school consultations were employed for 4 years (Wymbs et al. 2005). According to the case description, the combined therapy was successful in promoting some prosocial behaviors and reducing targeted problem behaviors in the participant. Mindfulness training has also been explored as a potential treatment for children with externalizing disorders. In one study by Bögels et al. (2008), 14 children aged 11–18 years with externalizing problems (four of whom had an ASD diagnosis and ten of whom had other diagnoses) completed eight group sessions of adapted mindfulness-based cognitive therapy. Parents also received eight group training sessions. Unfortunately results were not broken down by entry diagnosis so it is impossible to determine how effective this treatment was in ASD per se. Nonetheless, overall results showed significant improvement on child reports of externalizing behaviors and inattention; parent reports, on the other hand, showed few changes on the key study outcomes of disruptive behavior. These effects were maintained at an 8-week follow-up. As with other studies of disruptive behavior treatments in ASD, this study had its weaknesses, including a small sample size, a lack of a randomized experimental design, and no teacher report measures.

On the whole, there have been relatively few studies in this area and only two of the four studies reviewed achieved a methodological rating of even Adequate (see Table 7.2) according to the criteria described by Reichow et al. (2008). The modification of PCIT by Solomon et al. (2008) is especially promising as it is based upon a well-established behavioral intervention for externalizing disorders in otherwise typically developing children that has yielded large effect sizes and good maintenance of treatment effects in disruptive behavior disorders. The modifications for ASD made by Solomon, Ono and their colleagues were thoughtful and appropriate. The methodology of PCIT resembles that of many applications of applied behavior analysis for ASD, so it is unclear whether this intervention would offer anything above and beyond what children receiving good quality ABA would already be getting. However, this is an empirical question that could easily be tested. The intervention by Sofronoff et al. (2007) was developed specifically for ASD and takes a more cognitively based approach to anger management than the largely behavioral PCIT approach. Although this study had the weakness of not enumerating cases with a specific diagnostic algorithm, the intervention methods are unique and may be a basis for further treatment development. As with the anxiety trial (Sofronoff et al. 2005), it is impressive that significant results were attained after only six treatment sessions. Finally, while the study by Bögels et al. (2008) was not specific to ASD and thus does not offer specific guidance about applicability to autism and related conditions, the success that mindful awareness training has had with adult patients in large, structured clinical trials suggests that it could be a promising technique to address not only the behavior problems sometimes associated with ASD, but also the inattention that is a nearly ubiquitous feature of ASD, whether or not an ADHD diagnosis is specifically present.

Autism Symptoms and Social Impairment

A key goal in the field of autism treatment research is the discovery of methods that reduce or eliminate the primary symptoms of ASD (McDougle et al. 2005). Core autism symptoms are wide-ranging and multifaceted, spanning from specific social communication impairments such as deviant eye gaze, to language eccentricities such as echolalia, to repetitive behaviors such as stereotypies. A common finding is that individuals on the autism spectrum with categorically lower levels of ASD symptoms (e.g., those meeting criteria for PDD-NOS and not autism per se) have better overall

TABLE 7.2 Clinical trials and case studies of treatments for disruptive behavior in individuals with autism spectrum disorder (ASD)

Study	Participants	Study type	Method	Primary outcome measures	Quality of study methods[a]	Outcomes
Bögels et al. (2008)	• N = 14 • 11–18 years olds • 8 males • Primary diagnosis of ADHD, ODD/CD, or ASD	• Open trial (within subject wait-list)	• Manual • No treatment fidelity measure • Weekly therapist supervision • 8 weekly sessions of 90 min • Child and parent groups	• Child personal goals • Parent goals for child • Parent personal goals	• Weak	• Significant differences on personal goals from pre- to post-treatment for goals • Gains were maintained at the 8-week follow-up
Sofronoff et al. (2007)	• N = 45 • 10–14 year olds • 43 males • Diagnosis of ASD • Caseness determined by reports of high levels of anger	• Randomized controlled trial (wait-list control)	• Manual • Weekly therapist supervision, weekly therapist checklist, and 25% of sessions were videotaped • 6 weekly sessions of 2 h • Child and parent groups	• Parent-report measure of child anger • Parent-report measure of relationship with authority subscale	• Adequate	• Parent report of child anger showed a main effect of time for the immediate treatment group • Relationship with authority subscale had a significant time × group interaction
Solomon, Ono, et al. (2008)	• N = 19 • 5–12 year olds • All male • Diagnosed with ASD • High levels of disruptive behavior	• Randomized controlled trial (wait-list control)	• PCIT manual • No treatment fidelity measure • Two phases (six sessions each): child-directed interaction and parent-directed interaction • Group supervision	• Parent-report measures of child conduct problems, behaviors, and emotions	• Adequate	• Parent reports of conduct problems and atypicality yielded a group × time interaction • Several scales reflecting externalizing behavior had nonsignificant group differences as well

(Continued)

TABLE 7.2   (Continued)

Study	Participants	Study type	Method	Primary outcome measures	Quality of study methods[a]	Outcomes
Wymbs et al. (2005)	• N = 1 • 9-year-old male • Diagnosed with PDD-NOS and ADHD	• Case study (4 years)	• Manual • No treatment fidelity measure • Multimodal behavioral and medical treatment	• Rate of teasing • Peer nominations	• Weak	• Rates of teasing decreased during treatment • Mixed results with regard to peer • Nominations (some increase in positive nominations, but also some increase in negative nominations)

[a]The quality was assessed using the criteria described by Reichow et al. (2008)

prognoses than those with categorically higher levels (e.g., those meeting full DSM-IV criteria for autistic disorder) (Helt et al. 2008). Logically, interventions need to reduce core autism symptoms as much as possible to improve prognosis. Evidence of such change should be documented in clinical trials by using as outcome measures those "gold standard," evidence-based assessments of core autism symptoms that are used to diagnose autism and determine symptom severity. Such assessments include, for example, the Autism Diagnostic Observation Schedule (ADOS; Lord et al. 1999), Autism Diagnostic Interview – Revised (ADI-R; Le Couteur et al. 2003), and the Childhood Autism Rating Scale (CARS; Schopler et al. 1998). Use of such measures would parallel those evidence-based, symptom-count and diagnostic measures used in studies of the treatment of comorbid psychiatric disorders in ASD, such as anxiety disorders (Chalfant et al. 2007), in which the same instruments used to diagnose the disorder – rather than features associated with the disorder, such as social maladjustment or cognitive bias – are employed as primary outcome measures, following contemporary methodological best practices for clinical trials (Chambless and Hollon 1998).

Despite the clear rationale for using such evidence-based measures of core autism symptoms as primary outcomes in ASD behavioral intervention research, these types of assessment have rarely been used in clinical trials, whether in studies of applied behavior analysis, social awareness interventions, or CBT or mental health interventions for autism. This trend is, in part, related to the tradition in studies of applied behavior analysis to employ single subject experimental designs (SSED), such as multiple baseline designs and reversal designs to evaluate treatment effects on observable target symptoms. While such measures frequently index specific core autism symptoms (e.g., presence of

observed stereotypies), such measures are not used in the evidence-based diagnosis of ASD and thus cannot be construed as indicators of the overall severity of an individual's autism-spectrum symptom profile at post-treatment (e.g., even with stereotypies completely eliminated through a behavioral treatment, many other ASD symptoms can remain present which may maintain a bleak prognosis based on actuarial prediction were a broader, evidence-based assessment of autism to be administered). Seemingly, many of the classic SSED trials have been conducted to demonstrate the *capacity* of an intervention approach to markedly affect the expression of specific autism symptoms or related problems (e.g., poor adaptive skills). Due to the nature of SSEDs – specifically, the need for many repeated measures – trials using this design have generally not utilized broad measures of ASD symptoms as outcome measures, and even group design studies of treatments that might affect core autism symptom domains have typically not reported using evidence-based measures of autistic disorder (e.g., the ADOS), opting instead to employ nonspecific measures of, for example, social skills (e.g., as measured by the Social Skills Rating Scale). The handful of studies of CBT and related mental health interventions that have endeavored to address social communication deficits in autism have generally followed this pattern.

Bauminger (2002, 2007a, b) has conducted three open trials (AB designs without a control group) of CBT for school-aged children with ASD focusing on remediating a variety of social deficits. The intervention approach taken has been sophisticated and responsive to findings from basic research in autism. For example, Bauminger (2002) cites contemporary research suggesting that deficits in social initiations and understanding of complex emotional cues in social situations account for more of the deficit in social adjustment, such as friendship quality, among high-functioning children with autism than do the effects of low social motivation or aversive social behavior (Sigman and Ruskin 1999). She also notes that core deficits in areas such as theory of mind skills – particularly in their application to social behavior – are considered critical social cognition targets for effective interventions to address. Finally, among the observable aspects of typical social behavior among high-functioning children with ASD in naturalistic settings, Bauminger (2002) notes that reduced frequency of social play (as opposed to, for example, solitary play or disengagement) is a distinguishing feature of many children on the spectrum that requires direct attention in intervention programs. The CBT interventions in the Bauminger (2002, 2007a, b) trials flow from this basic research by matching treatment goals to the pivotal areas identified in these studies. All three trials yielded evidence of improvement (although causal effects cannot be confirmed with the open nature of the studies) in social outcomes, again with some interesting variability. Each trial used excellent observational measurement paradigms, although, as with most other studies of interventions for ASD, evidence-based diagnostic measures of core ASD symptoms were not included in the assessment battery.

Bauminger (2002) references cognitive behavioral theory, noting that a CBT intervention for autistic social deficits must make the assumption that (sometimes maladaptive) cognition guides interpersonal behavior in youths with ASD; and that, therefore, (adaptive) alterations to cognitive structures can make a positive impact on interpersonal behavior. In this study, several elements were notable: children's classroom teachers were responsible for an intervention taking 3 h per week over 7 months conducted at school and which relied heavily on guiding a dyad consisting of the target child and a typically developing peer through a series of 13 social skill lessons (e.g., cooperating) that were to be practiced at recess, on the phone, on playdates, and so forth ($N = 15$; aged 8–17 years old). Parents were also asked to support children in learning and implementing these social skills. The intervention was presented by the teacher to the dyad, allowing for individualization (e.g., by having pairs of children choose activities that they both liked). After intervention, children approximately doubled their number of observed positive social interchanges with peers in naturalistic observations at school – particularly eye contact, expressions of interest in others, and talking about their own experiences. They were more likely to initiate positive interactions than they were to respond positively to peers' initiations to them. Teachers also rated children as improved in certain positive social skills on the Social Skills Rating Scale.

Bauminger (2007a) replicated these treatment and assessment procedures and included several additional assessment measures in an open trial of CBT for 19 youths with ASD, aged 7–11 years old. In this trial, the observational measure yielded slightly different outcomes. As before, there were significant pre- to post-treatment improvements in observed positive social behavior, but this time the specific social skills affected were initiating and responding to others with eye contact and sharing. There was a corresponding reduction of "low-level" social behaviors (e.g., repetitive behaviors). There was also a main effect of response type in which initiating social communication was more frequent than responding to it. However, children's self-reports of loneliness, social acceptance, and other aspects of self-worth did not change from pre- to post-treatment. A 4-month follow-up assessment provided evidence of maintenance of treatment effects. In short, this study was a successful replication of the 2002 trial, with similar limitations (e.g., no control group) but with a slightly different pattern of improvement in specific social behaviors and evidence of durability of the treatment effect over a modest follow-up period. Clearly, this treatment model is promising and merits more thorough evaluation in a randomized trial.

A group-therapy CBT treatment (with between three and six children per group, at least half of whom were typically developing) with many commonalities with the Bauminger (2002) intervention but focusing more on within-group interaction as a vehicle for learning, was also evaluated by Bauminger (2007b). Again, an AB design was used ($N=26$) and, in addition to playground observations, a classic theory-of-mind task and a sorting task tapping executive functioning were administered as outcome measures. Interestingly, while there was substantial improvement in social behaviors amongst the therapy group members while interacting during the sessions from pre- to post-treatment, this effect did not generalize to the playground setting, in which no significant improvement was found in social behaviors over the course of the 7-month interval from baseline to post-treatment. However, there was evidence of improvement in both theory-of-mind abilities and executive functioning. While the former finding seems to flow from the emphasis placed on understanding others' perspectives in the intervention curriculum, the impact of the treatment on youths' sorting ability and concept formation in the executive functioning task is less easily explained and offers an intriguing path for further exploration in controlled trials. Overall, this study paralleled the results of most group-therapy-based "social skills interventions" (Rao et al. 2008), which generally improve social behaviors within the immediate group but fail to find a generalization effect in the child's social relationships outside the therapy program. Since Bauminger essentially adapted the therapeutic concepts and methods from her more individually oriented CBT interventions (2002, 2007a) for this group-therapy

trial, it is worth considering whether there is more merit in individually oriented social interventions in autism (if, as Bauminger notes, the child's ecological influences are addressed through the individual intervention), as compared to group-based interventions, than has traditionally been assumed.

Lopata et al. (2006) conducted a randomized controlled group design study of an ASD intervention designated as "CBT" focused on improving social communication and social adaptive functioning. This study compared two versions of a 6-week, 5 days per week summer treatment program: intensive CBT emphasizing social skills training and the same CBT focusing on social skills training combined with behavioral management strategies. Twenty-one children participated, most of whom were randomly assigned to a condition. Impressively, the 6-h day was pre-programmed with repeated social skills training and practice opportunities, using a structured program plan to guide specific activities (e.g., starting conversations). Primary foci were social deficits characteristics of ASD; emotion recognition; and awareness of and engagement in interests other than one's own. Some attention to intervention fidelity was given. A nonspecific measure of outcome, the Behavior Assessment System for Children, was administered to teachers and parents at pre- and post-treatment. On three of the subscales reflecting social behavior, there were relatively consistent improvements from pre- to post-treatment for both treatment groups, with a few exceptions. The groups did not differ on any measure, precluding any causal implications from being drawn about the impact of either condition. Of potential note, the mean teacher ratings at pre-treatment were all in the normal range (the average score was within 5 or 6 T-score points of the population mean on all three subscales, suggesting teacher raters were not aware of the full spectrum of symptoms sometimes displayed by the participants). Pre–post effect sizes were generally in the small to medium range. Given the unclear implications about the impact of the intervention per se, as well as the expense of about 180 h of treatment per student, it is difficult to draw conclusions about this treatment program, but the authors must be commended for attempting a large-scale behavioral intervention for school-aged children with ASD in a camp format – a modality that has had considerable success in the treatment of ADHD (Pelham et al. 2000).

In the other randomized controlled trial in this group of studies, Wood et al. (2009a) compared nine children with ASD (aged 7–11 years) randomized to CBT with 10 children randomized to a wait-list condition. The CBT treatment was as described in the Wood et al. (2009b) clinical trial for children with ASD and comorbid anxiety disorders. The CBT program emphasized in vivo exposure supported by parent training and school consultation to promote emotion regulation and social communication skills. Parents of the final 19 participants in the Wood et al. (2009b) study completed a standardized autism symptom checklist at baseline, post-treatment/post-wait-list, and 3-month follow-up assessments. The Social Responsive Scale (SRS) covers all the broad autism spectrum symptom domains found in higher-functioning individuals and has acceptable sensitivity and specificity for the prediction of ASD diagnoses (Constantino and Gruber 2005). There was a statistically significant difference between the CBT group and the wait-list group at post-treatment/post-wait-list on total parent-reported autism symptoms on the SRS, with a medium to large effect size. Treatment gains were maintained at 3-month follow-up. Of course, this study was limited by a small sample and reliance on parent reports of symptomatology, which are vulnerable to bias. Evidence-based assessments of core autism symptoms based on independent evaluators' ratings and direct observations of children's behavior (e.g., the ADOS) will need to be employed in future studies of such CBT programs to more convincingly determine their potential for reducing the expression and severity of core autism symptoms.

Table 7.3 presents a summary of CBT interventions evaluated in studies of individuals with ASD that have focused on addressing autism symptoms and social deficits. In this small group of studies, substantial variability in treatment methods, research design, and outcome measurement foci was again in evidence. As noted, the programs utilized summer camp, school, or clinic settings; relied on individual versus group treatment modalities; ranged from 16 weekly, 90-min sessions to 180 h of therapeutic camp activities compressed into 6 weeks; were more or less closely tied to CBT theory as well as basic research in autism; and used primary outcome measures ranging from questionnaire measures of nonspecific symptom domains, to behavioral observations of social initiation and responsiveness during recess, to parent reports of core autism symptoms on a validated, normed instrument. Common characteristics among the programs are that they relied on social ecological models of development and behavior change by directly intervening with peers, teachers, and parents; made efforts to promote adaptive social behavior within the children's peer milieus; and emphasized development of social cognitive skills such as perspective taking. There was some evidence of symptom improvement in each trial, although effect sizes varied widely, and evidence-based research methodology was variably employed. Some general conclusions may be drawn: CBT that emphasizes direct experiences in the child's social milieu and that is closely linked with conceptual training on others' perspectives and emotional states – especially when presented in an individualized format in a high-dose, high-density fashion in the middle-childhood

TABLE 7.3   Clinical trials and case studies of treatments for autism symptoms and social problems in individuals with autism spectrum disorder (ASD)

Study	Participants	Study type	Method	Primary outcome measures	Quality of study methods[a]	Outcomes
Bauminger (2002)	• N=15 • 8–17 years old • 11 males diagnosed with ASD	• Open trial	• Manual • No treatment fidelity measure • Individual supervision 1–2 times/month • 3 h/week for 7 months • Involved child's main teacher, parent, and typical peer	• Behavioral observations at school • Child measure of emotion recognition, experience and understanding	• Weak	• Increased positive social behavior at school • Increase in identification and knowledge of specific emotions, including those that require perspective taking
Bauminger (2007a)	• N=19 • 7–11 years old • 18 males • Diagnosed with ASD	• Open trial	• Manual • No treatment fidelity measure • Individual supervision 1–2 times/month • 3 h/week for 7 months • Involved child's main teacher, parent, and typical peer	• Teacher-report of child social skills • School observation of child social behaviors	• Weak	• Significantly higher scores on the teacher-report measure of social skills • Significant increases in positive social behavior (eye contact, sharing)
Bauminger (2007b)	• N=26 • Mean age: 8 years • 24 males • Diagnosed with ASD	• Open trial	• Manual • No treatment fidelity measure • Individual supervision 1–2 times/month • 2 weekly sessions for 7 months • Teacher-led small social skills groups (typical and ASD students)	• School observation of child social behaviors	• Weak	• Group social behaviors improved within the treatment groups • Group social behaviors during observations at recess did not improve

(Continued)

TABLE 7.3 (Continued)

Study	Participants	Study type	Method	Primary outcome measures	Quality of study methods[a]	Outcomes
Cashin (2008)	• $N=1$ • 13-year-old male • Diagnosed with Asperger syndrome	• Case study	• No manual • No treatment fidelity measure • Narrative therapy (unclear on number of sessions)	• Number of intense anger outbursts per month	• Weak	• Lowered intense anger outbursts to once per month
Lopata et al. (2006)	• $N=21$ • 6–13 years old • All male • Diagnosed with ASD	• Randomized controlled trial	• Manual • No treatment fidelity measure • Summer camp: 6 h per day, 5 days per week for 6 weeks • Two groups: social skills training and social skills training with behavioral supports	• Parent- and teacher-report of behavior on three scales: social skills, adaptability, and atypicality	• Adequate	• No group differences at post-treatment • For both groups, parent and teacher behavior reports showed significant increase in the social skills domain • Parent behavior report showed a decrease in odd or unusual behavior • Teacher behavior report showed an increase in odd or unusual behavior
Lord (1996)	• $N=1$ • 19-year-old male • Diagnosed with Autism	• Case study	• No manual • No treatment fidelity measure • CBT medication	• Number of violent outbursts and aggressive behaviors	• Weak	• Some decrease in aggressive behaviors
Wood et al. (2009a)	• $N=19$ • 7–11 years old • 16 males • Diagnosed with ASD and an anxiety disorder	• Randomized controlled trial (wait-list control)	• Manual • Fidelity check • Weekly individual supervision • 16 sessions of 90 min • Family CBT	• Parent report of core autism symptoms	• Adequate	• Significant group difference in ASD symptoms post-treatment (lower ASD symptoms in immediate treatment group)

[a]The quality was assessed using the criteria described by Reichow et al. (2008).

(and possibly adolescent) age-group – appears to be a promising practice for addressing at least some core autism symptoms and improving social adjustment in high-functioning youths with ASD. However, the extant evidence is quite preliminary and does not yet meet the guidelines of Chambless and Hollon (1998) even for "possible efficacy" due to the research methods employed; the outcomes were not of such a large magnitude to suggest that there is no room for improvement in these treatment methods.

CBT in Autism Treatment: Future Directions

A number of conceptually derived treatment manuals have been developed for individuals with ASD that employ cognitive behavioral strategies and related mental health treatment methods. However, many questions remain. Even the most methodologically sophisticated of the clinical trials in this group of studies does not provide the level of definitive support that exists in other pediatric psychopathology treatment domains, such as anxiety disorders or conduct problems. For example, rigorous multi-site trials of CBT have been conducted for several other types of childhood disorder in which active and pill placebo control conditions have been employed, offering strong support for certain manual-based CBT treatment programs (POTS Study Group 2004; Walkup et al. 2008). The methods employed in these studies should serve as models for investigations of the most promising CBT programs for individuals with ASD.

Before initiating large clinical trials, however, further treatment refinement and pilot testing is probably advisable – particularly for CBT treatments targeting the core autism symptom domains. ASD is a clinically challenging domain of psychopathology and, given the shortcomings of seemingly pragmatic and sensible interventions such as social skills training (SST) in affecting social adjustment among school-aged youths with ASD (Rao et al. 2008), focused attention must be given to developing robust methods that overcome the generalization and maintenance problems exemplified in most research of the SST modality. Although not successful as an intervention modality itself, this body of research does constitute an important corpus that offers some cues about steps to take in developing other treatment modalities focusing on the social communication domain in ASD: it calls into question the utility of learning paradigms for group social skills that are not tailored to the individual's symptom presentation and individual differences; it suggests that the use of hypothetical scenarios and role plays may be insufficient for generalization and maintenance to occur; and it suggests that measurement strategies need both to address directly the extent of generalization and maintenance and to assess core autism symptoms with validated measurement instruments rather than only measures of nonspecific areas of social adjustment or narrow indices of social behavior in naturalistic contexts such as amount of eye contact during playground time at school.

Need for Evidence-Based Assessment of Core Autism Symptoms as Primary Clinical Outcomes

With regard to the latter point, a brief review of best practice recommendations for evidence-based assessment in behavioral clinical trials (Chambless and Hollon 1998; Reichow et al. 2008) suggests that many clinical trials focusing on the treatment of core autism symptoms are found wanting (see Chap. 14, which addresses this point in greater detail). From the perspective of evidence-based treatment and assessment, a treatment's ultimate goal is to achieve a clinically meaningful reduction of symptoms of a disorder or clinical remission of the disorder (as defined categorically). To test the effects of an intervention on such outcomes, psychometrically reliable and valid measures administered by an independent evaluator blind to the patient's treatment condition and the study hypotheses are viewed as the gold standard.

Table 7.4 gives a sample of evidence-based assessment measures that have at least some evidence of adequate psychometric properties in the ASD youth population. Measures specific to core autism symptoms as well as psychiatric comorbidity and administered by independent evaluators as well as rated by children and parents are noted. Although not all have been administered as outcome measures in extant clinical trials in ASD, each of these measures appears to have promise for such use. There are two issues to bear in mind in considering use of these measures for clinical trials research. First, measures administered by independent evaluators (such as psychiatric interview schedules) often require specific training and certification and therefore generally add to the cost of a trial. Second, we harbor some reservations about extant child self-report measures using a paper and pencil format in ASD, including the two measures noted in Table 7.4 (i.e., the Multidimensional Anxiety Scale for Children (MASC; March 1998) and the Loneliness Rating Scale (Asher et al. 1984)), due to the cognitive demands of such measures; we believe that more effort is probably needed to refine and validate such measures in the ASD youth population.

Enhancing CBT Treatments for ASD Symptoms

In light of the contemporary principles for CBT development noted in the introduction, we offer four recommendations for enhancing the efficacy of CBT interventions in autism that could potentially build towards more robust treatment models with the capacity to reduce core autism symptoms in affected high-functioning individuals. Our experiences in developing and testing CBT treatments for children with ASD (Wood et al. 2009a, b) and other psychiatric disorders (Wood et al. 2006), as well as the panoply of evidence-based practices that are available for the treatment of a wide variety of childhood mental health conditions (Kazdin and Weisz 2003) have informed these recommendations.

As a general principle, in developing CBT treatment methods for children with ASD, target goals (e.g., social skill development and generalization) need to be matched with procedures for enhancing memory retrieval. For example, to promote reciprocal conversation skills, the encoding specificity principle from basic memory research suggests that skill learning should occur in the actual settings where conversational deficits are exhibited, rather than in simulated social situations such as therapy settings, as is often done in traditional social skills training. As a second example, research on levels of processing in human memory has demonstrated that deep semantic processing – rather than rote memorization – increases the chance of the retrieval of a target memory (e.g., for a social skill). To promote deep semantic processing of new concepts, Socratic questions (questions that incorporate hints of the correct answer) can be posed by the therapist to encourage children to put accurate answers in their own words. The combination of repeated in vivo rehearsal of social skills in real-world settings coupled with Socratic discussions about the positive effects of such skills may promote deep semantic processing and increase the memory retrieval of the targeted skills in naturalistic contexts while helping to suppress memories of habitual maladaptive responses such as social avoidance (Sze and Wood 2007, 2008; Wood et al. 2009a, b).

TABLE 7.4   Promising evidence-based assessment measures for clinical trials for individuals with autism spectrum disorder (ASD)

Measure type	Scale	Domains assessed	Acceptable psychometric properties in ASD?	Used as outcome in clinical trials?
Independent evaluator-rated measures	Autism Diagnostic Observa-tion Schedule (ADOS) (Lord et al. 1999)	Core autism symptoms	Well established	Dawson et al. (2009)
	Autism Diagnostic Interview – Revised (ADI-R) (Lord et al. 1994)	Core autism symptoms	Well established	No
	Anxiety Disorders Interview Schedule for DSM-IV (Silverman and Albano 1996)	Comorbid psychiatric disorders	Preliminary evidence (Wood et al. 2009a, b)	Wood et al. (2009a, b)
	Children's Yale-Brown Obsessive–Compulsive Scale – Modified for Pervasive Developmental Disorders (CYBOCS-PDD) (Scahill et al. 2006)	Repetitive behaviors	Some evidence (Scahill et al. 2006)	King et al. (2009)
	Live school observational ratings	Peer social engagement and appropriateness	Yes	Bauminger (2002)
	Classroom sociometric/ social network ratings	Social acceptance	Yes (Chamber-lin et al. 2007)	Frankel et al. (2007)
Child-rated scales	Multidimensional Anxiety Scale for Children (MASC; March 1998)	Anxiety	Some evidence (Bellini 2004)	Wood et al. (2009b)
	Loneliness Rating Scale (Asher et al. 1984)	Loneliness	Some evidence (Bauminger and Kasari 2000)	Bauminger (2007a)
Parent-rated scales	Social Responsiveness Scale (SRS; Constantino and Gruber 2005)	Core autism symptoms	Well established	Wood et al. (2009a)
	Child Symptom Inventory-4 (CSI-4; Gadow and Sprafkin 2002)	Comorbid psychiatric symptoms	Yes (Gadow and Sprafkin 2002)	Gadow et al. (2007)

Recommendation 1: Use Verbally Mediated Methods That Can Promote Conceptual Development and Generalization

A key critique of strictly behavioral intervention methods (e.g., operant conditioning) is that no explicit verbally mediated concept is produced by the intervention (Brewin 2006). A simple example is illustrative: A child is taught to compliment peers at school about the toys they have and the games they are playing (e.g., "Cool dinosaur!"). However, when with parents, who do not play with toys, the child has no basis for giving compliments because no conceptual principle has been taught and no contingencies have been set up in the home environment. Arguably, if the child had developed concepts about others' perspectives, and the impact of others' perspectives on how they treat the child, the tendency of compliments to positively affect others' perspectives, and principles for adapting compliments appropriately across settings accompanied by behavioral experimentation involving "playing detective" to see if specific compliments "work" in various social situations by paying attention to changes in others' facial expression and tone of voice (a naturalistic reinforcer that also attunes children to key sources of information about others' mental states), then an appropriate adaptation of the social skill across settings could more easily be derived. Generally, the development of accurate, language-mediated concepts pertaining to various life situations that can yield adaptive behavioral (and emotional) responses is a key goal of CBT that differentiates it from purely behavioral therapies that do not promote explicit cognitive formulations (Brewin 2006).

Socratic questioning provides enough information in the question to guide individuals towards correct types of answer while still eliciting sufficient thinking and reflection to promote insight and avoid the pitfalls of superficial rote learning (e.g., immediately before entering a playground interaction: "If you offered her a turn, what is a nice thought she might have about you…? …Like, 'Bea is…?' …oh, a good friend? So she would like you being so friendly to her?") All skill development and practice efforts in CBT should be supported by guided conversations in which the therapist or caregiver uses Socratic questioning to promote conceptual development and perspective taking. The immediacy of such planning helps ensure the affected individual remembers what to say when initiating the interaction moments later, and allows therapists or caregivers to check in soon after the interaction has transpired to discuss whether the planned behavior had the intended effect (e.g., elicited friendly responses) and why it did or did not. The linkage between engaging in immediate behaviors in naturalistic contexts and deep semantic processing of the rationale should lead to enhanced memory formation and retrieval. Thus, rather than using a stimulus–response paradigm to elicit social behaviors without facilitating comprehension, as has been criticized in other intervention methods in ASD such as facilitated communication, this cognitively based approach teaches principles of social interaction through hands-on experience and verbal discussions to promote accuracy of social cognition (presupposing, as noted in Bauminger (2002), that inaccurate social cognition in ASD accounts for part of the core social deficits). High-functioning, school-age children with ASD generally have sufficient language capacity to engage in and benefit from such conversations, although visual aides (e.g., writing concepts or drawing supporting pictures), incentives, and good humor are also helpful in ensuring active participation (Sofronoff et al. 2005; Sze and Wood 2007, 2008).

Recommendation 2: Adapt the CBT Concepts of Graded Hierarchies and In vivo Exposures to Form a Core Treatment Plan Based Around Explicit, Objective Goals for Individuals with ASD

Many CBT programs for child anxiety disorders use graded hierarchies as the basis of the treatment plan (Kendall 1994). Traditionally, such hierarchies have focused on feared situations and involve small incremental steps that guide children towards proficiency in new target behaviors. A hierarchy for a specific phobia might be getting close to a phobic object and observing it until anxiety is low and touching or holding the phobic object until anxiety recedes.

Directly facing feared situations in this manner is known as "in vivo exposure." Hierarchies for more complex anxiety disorders (e.g., separation anxiety disorder) may have 20 or more steps spanning multiple situations and exposures. Although hierarchies are naturally useful in organizing classical conditioning procedures in the treatment of anxiety, we have found that incorporating non-anxiety-related goals, such as friendship building, self-help skills acquisition, and compliance with caregivers, into the hierarchy effectively organizes all target behaviors into a single, integrated treatment plan for schoolchildren with ASD (Wood et al. 2009a, b).

Core ASD symptoms and comorbid problems may be organized, sequenced, and prioritized via the hierarchy. In hierarchy-based treatment plans in CBT, ultimate goals are set forth in behavioral and observable terms (e.g., engage in appropriate peer play 100% of the time during recess), which permits the delineation of specific tasks that the child can engage in to build up to ultimate goals (e.g., "play handball each day at recess for 5 min while keeping hands and feet to self" – an early task building up to consistent appropriate social participation during unstructured playtime). The transformation of ultimate goals into a series of increasingly challenging behavioral tasks is an important therapeutic technique that is similar to task analysis, helping individuals learn components of a skill sequentially, and slowly develop tolerance for activities that may initially be frustrating. Such learning procedures enhance long-term retention and mastery (Brewin 2006). The hierarchy-based approach does not assume that a set amount of therapeutic time will be sufficient for improvement of a specific problem area but rather sets specific goals that *should* be achieved by an individual prior to therapy termination (hence, calling for an individualized treatment approach that responds to the individual's progress from session to session).

Hierarchy goals focus primarily on behaviors outside the therapy room, with an emphasis on selecting situations where dysfunction actually manifests – such as school – to promote generalization (Bauminger 2002). For example, rather than merely focusing on the patient's ability to pose conversational questions to the therapist in a session (as part of the ultimate goal of achieving appropriate reciprocal social interactions), such questions would be practiced in a wide variety of social settings with different partners (e.g., with familiar and novel peers and staff at school, at playgrounds, in the waiting room, etc.) to promote generalization. A combination of cognitive and behavioral strategies as well as parent and teacher support are needed to achieve success with such assignments.

During hierarchy development, goals and steps (often entailing in vivo exposures) are refined and rated (methods for hierarchy development are discussed in detail elsewhere; e.g., see the work of Wood and McLeod (2008)). *Difficulty ratings* are an important feature of CBT rarely employed in other therapeutic paradigms; using a scale (e.g., 0–10), each subgoal is rated by the patient (and parent, as appropriate) in terms of "how hard would it be to do" or "how anxious would it make you?" These ratings help guide the ordering of therapeutic tasks in terms of what to address first. Knowledge of the perceived difficulty of the planned behavioral tasks can be the difference between making slow, steady progress and stalling permanently on a step that the patient is not ready to take.

CBT usually begins with fairly easy tasks from the hierarchy to ensure early success. Over the arc of treatment, the affected individual addresses goals and exposure tasks at an increasingly challenging level of difficulty until target skills are mastered. The leverage and motivation provided by the reward system (see Recommendation 4), carefully nurtured rapport with the therapist (e.g., as maintained by using special interests as examples and metaphors, as in the work of Sze and Wood (2007, 2008)), and activation of the individual's pride through success and praise generally drive progress during hierarchy-based tasks.

Recommendation 3: Social Skills Can Be Developed by Individuals with ASD but Are Most Likely to Be Generalized and Maintained through In vivo Exposure

Core ASD deficits in both verbal (e.g., off-topic responding and one-sided conversations) and nonverbal (e.g., poor body boundaries and poor eye contact) aspects of communication often underlie poor peer relationships among individuals with ASD (Barnhill et al. 2002). Traditional social skills training for youths with ASD often focuses on learning new skills in hypothetical situations by interacting with children or adult collaborators in a therapy room (e.g., "imagine a child steps on your toe while you are in the lunch line ..."). The encoding specificity principle in cognitive science suggests that treatment must go beyond these hypothetical situations and emphasizes practicing new social skills in the actual settings where problems are experienced. In CBT, appropriate social skills (e.g., positive entry behavior) and coping skills (e.g., relaxation and suppression of urges to act inappropriately) can be practiced in small steps in such settings and expanded until mastery is achieved. Hence, generalization and maintenance of social skills are naturally programmed into in vivo exposures.

One method for promoting successful in vivo social exposures is parent-training on social coaching, a technique used to provide children with information about social situations and etiquette that can lead to positive, reinforcing social experiences (Sze and Wood 2008; Wood et al. 2009a). In social coaching, caregivers (parents, aides or teachers) prompt the child to engage in specific social behaviors (verbal and nonverbal) immediately preceding actual social interactions (i.e., moments before, rather than hours or days before). Rather than a purely behavioral (priming) technique, Socratic questioning is used before and after each interaction, as noted above (i.e., incorporating the child in the formation of each social plan and challenging him or her each time to think through the "why" question – "why would these behaviors be useful?").

In social coaching, social behaviors are taught by reinforcing a series of successive approximations of specific conversational skills under real-world conditions, allowing for encoding specificity (that is, increasing the chance a target behavior will be recalled and reproduced in the future by teaching it in environments where it is desirable to use (Brewin 2006) and natural reinforcement (i.e., from positive peer and other responses). Initial target social behaviors can include basic greetings, farewells, and compliments. For example, a parent might coach her daughter to greet various family members appropriately upon their homecoming each day. This can then be expanded to a variety of other settings where social interactions occur (e.g., interactions with family friends and playdates with peers). Once initial elements of conversations are mastered, social coaching can be used to help children carry on longer appropriate conversations by prompting them to use specific skills after the initial greetings, such as relevant questions about the partner's interests (sometimes referred to as "playing detective" (Frankel and Myatt 2003)) and "me-too" disclosures in response to the partner's conversational topics that show social commonality and maintain focus on the topic. One-on-one aides and other school professionals who have ready access to the child's social situations can be trained in social coaching as well (Wood et al. 2009a). Although caregivers primarily deliver this intervention, a therapist can develop the initial set of social tasks and the social coaching procedure with the child in settings such as parks, playgrounds, and at recess. After the child and therapist have developed a comfortable routine, parents and relevant school caregivers can be included in these sessions for the purpose of modeling and transfer of control (in which the therapist has the caregiver take over the therapist's role and receive feedback and coaching from the therapist as needed). One critical social situation that caregivers ultimately must support effectively is playdate-hosting, an activity that, with corresponding Socratic discussions, has the potential to enhance perspective taking and reciprocity.

This intervention approach can be seamlessly and naturally incorporated into families' daily routines and carried out in high doses indefinitely for little or no cost. Research on young children with autism suggests that high-dosage, long-term behavioral interventions (Koegel et al. 2003; Lovaas and Smith 2003) are often necessary for large improvements. Although high-functioning, school-age children are often less clinically impaired than the younger participants in studies of early, intensive behavioral interventions, they are still treatment-resistant (Rao et al. 2008) and likely need a high dose of social intervention to move them towards typicality. In short, using CBT for the development of social skills is likely to be effective if hierarchical in vivo exposure is emphasized, appropriate preparations are made to help the child develop skills to handle specific in vivo social tasks and gain increasingly sophisticated schemas of social situations, and a high-dose, caregiver-mediated approach is taken.

Recommendation 4: Use a Comprehensive Reward or Incentive System Throughout CBT, Employing the Most Motivating Reinforcers Available

Deficits in children's motivation related to ASD (Koegel and Egel 1979; Koegel and Mentis 1985) necessitate a comprehensive reward or incentive program, a core element of efficacious treatments for ASD and disruptive behavior disorders (Webster-Stratton and Reid 2003). Specific tasks and goals delineated in the hierarchy (see Recommendation 2) can provide target behaviors to include on the rewards chart each week (e.g., "Each day, call a student from class and ask for the homework assignment politely – 1 point"). Our experience suggests that between three and five daily target behaviors can be on the rewards chart at any given time, including school-related behaviors (more than five simultaneous goals is confusing for most children and, hence, counterproductive) (see Wood and McLeod 2008). When highly desired activities are leveraged through such a system, children are more likely to engage fully in therapeutic tasks and homework, greatly assisting in CBT progress (Sze and Wood 2007, 2008). In contrast with typical applied behavior analysis principles, which advocate a gradually increasing use of contingency management, we have found that for most school-aged youths with ASD in our clinical trials beginning the program by making key motivating privileges, activities, and items (e.g., access to electronics or materials related to special interests (Attwood 2003)) contingent on the child's successful completion of daily therapeutic goals is a much more efficient and unambiguous method that often propels early progress in therapy and, subjectively, appears to enhance treatment expectancies and optimism in most family members at the critical early alliance formation period of CBT (Chiu et al. 2009). In sum, these procedures are an indispensable core "behavioral" method in CBT for children. When used to encourage children to learn skills (e.g., prosocial communication) we have found that there is rarely a need to continue such extrinsic motivators indefinitely – just until the skills have been mastered and have become intrinsically motivating (i.e., by yielding natural positive consequences such as enjoyable peer interactions). This is potentially evidenced by the maintenance of treatment effects on core ASD symptoms in the pilot RCT by Wood et al. (2009a) showing that social responsiveness scores were maintained or improved 3 months after treatment was terminated.

Conclusion

A number of promising CBT intervention programs have been developed for school-aged children, adolescents, and, to a lesser extent, adults with high-functioning autism spectrum disorders. In no case is the evidence base definitive in its support of these programs at present, in no small part due to the methodological limitations of the existing studies (e.g., small sample sizes, lack of random assignment, no evidence of treatment fidelity, failure to use evidence-based, diagnostic measures of ASD symptoms and failure to use diagnoses as primary outcome measures). This is not necessarily reflective of the weakness of the programs themselves but it leaves questions about the efficacy and strength of effects unanswered at the present time. Some clues about the clinical significance of the interventions can be attained by calculating effect sizes from the available data and, interestingly, effects ranged from small to large depending on the study and outcome measure in question. While potentially encouraging, effect sizes generated from studies with methodological weaknesses cannot be treated as definitive. In short, many of the programs reviewed above show potential merit for addressing autism and its comorbidities but require further evaluation to determine the breadth and depth of clinical efficacy in this treatment-resistant population. In the meantime, practitioners would be encouraged to adopt practices from this body of research that show evidence of strong effects in studies using more robust research designs.

Because of the inherent difficulties in the treatment of individuals with ASD and the history of limited success in theoretically derived interventions for affected school-aged youths and adults (Rao et al. 2008), clinicians in research and practice settings are encouraged to further develop the CBT intervention practices tested in the extant clinical trials reviewed in this chapter. Incorporating principles of learning and memory retrieval from contemporary cognitive science, as well as from research in autism (Bauminger 2002), offers a key avenue for the refinement and expansion of current CBT treatment methods. Devising robust methods for promoting the understanding and encoding of social concepts so that therapeutically induced memories are retrieved in novel situations that challenge individuals with autism, rather than the habitual maladaptive social responses that characterize this spectrum of disorders, will require ongoing treatment development efforts, careful pilot testing, and above all else, clinical imagination.

References

APA. (1994). *Diagnostic and statistical manual of mental disorders* (4th ed. – text revision). Washington, DC: American Psychiatric Association.

APA. (2000). *Diagnostic and statistical manual of mental disorders* (4th ed. – text revision). Washington, DC: American Psychiatric Association.

Asher, S. R., Hymel, S., & Renshaw, P. D. (1984). Loneliness in children. *Child Development, 55*(4), 1456–1464.

Attwood, T. (2003). Frame work for behavioral interventions. *Child and Adolescent Psychiatric Clinics of North America, 12*, 65–86.

Barnhill, G. P., Cook, K. T., Tebbenkamp, K., & Smith Myles, B. (2002). The effectiveness of social skills intervention targeting nonverbal communication for adolescents with Asperger syndrome and related pervasive developmental disorders. *Focus on Autism and Other Developmental Disabilities, 17*, 112–118.

Baron-Cohen, S. (1989). Do autistic children have obsessions and compulsions? *The British Journal of Clinical Psychology, 28*(3), 193–200.

Barrett, P. M. (1998). Evaluation of cognitive-behavioral group treatments for childhood anxiety disorders. *Journal of Clinical Child Psychology, 27,* 459–468.

Barrett, P. M., Dadds, M. R., & Rapee, R. M. (1996). Family treatment of childhood anxiety: A controlled trial. *Journal of Consulting and Clinical Psychology, 64,* 333–342.

Bauminger, N. (2002). The facilitation of social-emotional understanding and social interaction in high-functioning children with autism: Intervention outcomes. *Journal of Autism and Developmental Disorders, 32,* 283–298.

Bauminger, N. (2007a). Brief report: Individual social-multi-modal intervention for HFASD. *Journal of Autism and Developmental Disorders, 37,* 1593–1604.

Bauminger, N. (2007b). Brief report: Group social-multi-modal intervention for HFASD. *Journal of Autism and Developmental Disorders, 37,* 1605–1615.

Bauminger, N., & Kasari, C. (2000). Loneliness and friendship in high-functioning children with autism. *Child Development, 71,* 447–456.

Bellini, S. (2004). Social skill deficits and anxiety in high-functioning adolescents with autism spectrum disorders. *Focus on Autism and Other Developmental Disabilities, 19,* 78–86.

Bellini, S. (2006). The development of social anxiety in adolescents with autism spectrum disorders. *Focus on Autism and Other Developmental Disabilities, 21,* 138–145.

Ben-Sasson, A., Cermak, S. A., Orsmond, G. I., Tager-Flusberg, H., Kadlec, M. B., & Carter, A. S. (2008). Sensory clusters of toddlers with autism spectrum disorders: Differences in affective symptoms. *Journal of Child Psychology and Psychiatry, 49,* 817–817.

Bögels, S., Hoogstad, B., van Dun, L., de Schutter, S., & Restifo, K. (2008). Mindfulness training for adolescents with externalizing disorders and their parents. *Behavioural and Cognitive Psychotherapy, 36,* 193–209.

Brewin, C. R. (2006). Understanding cognitive behaviour therapy: A retrieval competition account. *Behaviour Research and Therapy, 44,* 765–784.

Cardaciotto, L., & Herbert, J. D. (2004). Cognitive behavior therapy for social anxiety disorder in the context of Asperger's Syndrome: A single subject report. *Cognitive and Behavioral Practice, 11,* 75–81.

Cashin, A. (2008). Narrative therapy. A sychotherapeutic approach in the treatment of adolescents with Asperger's disorder. *Journal of Child and Adolescent Psychiatric Nursing, 21(1),* 48–56.

Chalfant, A. M., Rapee, R., & Carroll, L. (2007). Treating anxiety disorders in children with high functioning autism spectrum disorders: A controlled trial. *Journal of Autism and Developmental Disorders, 37,* 1842–1857.

Chamberlin, B., Kasari, C., & Rotheram-Fuller, E. (2007). Involvement or isolation? The social networks of children with autism in regular classrooms. *Journal of Autism and Developmental Disorders, 37*(2), 230–242.

Chambless, D. L., & Hollon, S. D. (1998). Defining empirically supported therapies. *Journal of Consulting and Clinical Psychology, 66,* 7–18.

Chiu, A. W., McLeod, B. D., Har, K., & Wood, J. J. (2009). Child-therapist alliance and clinical outcomes in cognitive behavioral therapy for child anxiety disorders. *Journal of Child Psychology and Psychiatry, 50,* 751–758.

Chorpita, B. F., Taylor, A. A., Francis, S. E., Moffitt, C., & Austin, A. A. (2004). Efficacy of modular cognitive behavior therapy for childhood anxiety disorders. *Behavior Therapy, 35,* 263–287.

Constantino, J. N., & Gruber, C. P. (2005). *the social responsiveness scale (SRS) manual.* Los Angeles: Western Psychological Services.

Cotugno, A. J. (2009). Social competence and social skills training and intervention for children with autism spectrum disorders. *Journal of Autism and Developmental Disorders, 39,* 1268–1277.

Dawson, G., Rogers, S., Munson, J., Smith, M., Winter, J., et al. (2009). Randomized, controlled trial of an intervention for toddlers with autism: The early start Denver model. *Pediatrics, 125*(1), e17–23.

de Bruin, E. I., Ferdinand, R. F., Meester, S., de Nijs, P. F., & Verheij, F. (2007). High rates of psychiatric comorbidity in PDD-NOS. *Journal of Autism and Developmental Disorders, 37,* 877–886.

Frankel, F., & Myatt, R. (2003). *Children's friendship training.* New York: Brunner-Routledge.

Frankel, F., Myatt, R., & Feinberg, D. (2007). Parent-assisted friendship training for children with autism spectrum disorders: Effects of psychotropic medication. *Child Psychiatry and Human Development, 37*(4), 337–346.

Gadow, K. D., & Sprafkin, J. (2002). *Child symptom inventory-4 screening and norms manual.* Stony Brook, NY: Checkmate Plus.

Gadow, K. D., Sverd, J., Nolan, E. E., Sprafkin, J., & Schneider, J. (2007). Immediate-release methylphenidate for ADHD in children with comorbid chronic multiple tic disorder. *Journal of the American Academy of Child and Adolescent Psychiatry, 46,* 840–848.

Gadow, K. D., Roohi, J., DeVincent, C. J., & Hatch-well, E. (2008). Association of ADHD, tics, and anxiety with dopamine transporter (*DAT1*) genotype in autism spectrum disorder. *Journal of Child Psychology and Psychiatry, 49*, 1331–1338.

Gillott, A., Furniss, F., & Walter, A. (2001). Anxiety in high-functioning children with autism. *Autism, 5*(3), 277–286.

Goldstein, S., & Schwebach, A. J. (2004). The comorbidity of pervasive developmental disorder and attention deficit hyperactivity disorder: Results of a retrospective chart review. *Journal of Autism and Developmental Disorders, 34*, 329–339.

Green, J., Gilchrist, A., Burton, D., & Cox, A. (2000). Social and psychiatric functioning in adolescents with Asperger syndrome compared with conduct disorder. *Journal of Autism and Developmental Disorders, 30*, 279–293.

Groden, J., Baron, M. G., & Groden, G. (2006). Assessment and coping strategies. In M. G. Baron, J. Groden, G. Groden, & L. P. Lipsitt (Eds.), *Stress and coping in autism* (pp. 15–41). Oxford: Oxford University Press.

Hattori, J., Ogino, T., Abiru, K., Nakano, K., Oka, M., & Ohtsuka, Y. (2006). Are pervasive developmental disorders and attention-deficit/hyperactivity disorder distinct disorders? *Brain & Development, 28*, 371–374.

Helt, M., Kelley, E., Kinsbourne, M., Pandey, J., Boorstein, H., et al. (2008). Can children with autism recover? If so, how? *Neuropsychology Review, 18*, 339–366.

Hess, K. L., Morrier, M. J., Heflin, L. J., & Ivey, M. L. (2008). Autism treatment survey: Services received by children with autism spectrum disorders in public school classrooms. *Journal of Autism and Developmental Disorders, 38*, 961–971.

Ingersoll, B., Lewis, E., & Kroman, E. (2007). Teaching the imitation and spontaneous use of descriptive gestures in young children with autism using a naturalistic behavioral intervention. *Journal of Autism and Developmental Disorders, 37*, 1446–1456.

Kazdin, A. E., & Weisz, J. R. (Eds.). (2003). *Evidence-based psychotherapies for children and adolescents.* New York: Guilford.

Kelly, A. B., Garnett, M. S., Attwood, T., & Peterson, C. (2008). Autism spectrum symptomatology in children: The impact of family and peer relationships. *Journal of Abnormal Child Psychology, 36*, 1069–1081.

Kendall, P. C. (1994). Treating anxiety disorders in children: Results of a randomized clinical trial. *Journal of Consulting and Clinical Psychology, 62*, 100–110.

Kendall, P. C., Flannery-Schroeder, E., Panichelli-Mindel, S. M., Southam-Gerow, M., Henin, A., & Warman, M. (1997). Therapy for youths with anxiety disorders: A second randomized clinical trial. *Journal of Consulting and Clinical Psychology, 65*(6), 366–380.

King, B. H., Hollander, E., Sikich, L., McCracken, J. T., Scahill, L., et al. (2009). Lack of efficacy of citalopram in children with autism spectrum disorders and high levels of repetitive behavior: Citalopram ineffective in children with autism. *Archives of General Psychiatry, 66*, 583–590.

Klin, A., Pauls, R., Schultz, R., & Volkmar, F. (2005). Three diagnostic approaches to Asperger syndrome: Implications for research. *Journal of Autism and Developmental Disorders, 35*, 221–234.

Koegel, R. L., & Egel, A. L. (1979). Motivating autistic children. *Journal of Abnormal Psychology, 88*, 418–426.

Koegel, R. L., & Mentis, M. (1985). Motivation in childhood autism: Can they or won't they? *Journal of Child Psychology and Psychiatry, 26*, 185–191.

Koegel, R. L., Koegel, L. K., & Brookman, L. I. (2003). Empirically supported pivotal response interventions for children with autism. In A. E. Kazdin & J. R. Weisz (Eds.), *Evidence-based psychotherapies for children and adolescents.* New York: Guilford.

Koyama, T., Tachimori, H., Osada, H., & Kurita, H. (2006). Cognitive and symptom profiles in high functioning pervasive developmental disorder not otherwise specified and attention deficit/hyperactivity disorder. *Journal of Autism and Developmental Disorders, 36*, 373–380.

Kuusikko, S., Pollock-Wurman, R., Jussila, K., Carter, A. S., Mattila, M., Ebeling, H., et al. (2008). Social anxiety in high-functioning children and adolescents with autism and Asperger syndrome. *Journal of Autism and Developmental Disorders, 39*(9), 1697–1709.

Le Couteur, A., Lord, C., & Rutter, M. (2003). *The autism diagnostic interview revised.* Los Angeles: Western Psychological Services.

Lehmkuhl, H. D., Storch, E. A., Bodfish, J. W., & Geffken, G. R. (2008). Brief report: Exposure and response prevention for obsessive compulsive disorder in a 12 year-old with autism. *Journal of Autism and Developmental Disorders, 38*, 977–981.

Leyfer, O. T., Folstein, S. E., Bacalman, S., Davis, N. O., Dinh, E., et al. (2006). Comorbid psychiatric disorders in children with autism: Interview development and rates of disorders. *Journal of Autism and Developmental Disorders, 36*, 849–861.

Lopata, C., Thomeer, M. L., Volker, M. A., & Nida, R. E. (2006). Effectiveness of a cognitive-behavioral treatment on the social behaviors of children with Asperger disorder. *Focus on Autism and Other Developmental Disabilities, 21*, 237–244.

Lord, C. (1996). Treatment of a high-functioning adolescent with autism: A cognitive-behavioral approach. In M. A. Reinecke & F. M. Dattilio (Eds.), *Cognitive therapy with children and adolescents: A casebook for clinical practice* (pp. 394–404). New York: Guilford.

Lord, C., Rutter, M., & Le Couteur, A. (1994). Autism diagnostic interview – Revised: A revised version of a diagnostic interview for caregivers of individuals with possible pervasive developmental disorders. *Journal of Autism and Developmental Disorders, 24*(5), 659–685.

Lord, C., Rutter, M., DiLavore, P. C., & Risi, S. (1999). *Autism diagnostic observation schedule*. Los Angeles: Western Psychological Services.

Lovaas, O. I., & Smith, T. (2003). Early and intensive behavioral intervention in autism. In A. E. Kazdin & J. R. Weisz (Eds.), *Evidence-based psychotherapies for children and adolescents* (pp. 325–340). New York: Guilford.

March, J. (1998). *Manual for the multidimensional anxiety scale for children*. Toronto: Multi-Health Systems.

McDougle, C. J., Scahill, L., Aman, M. G., McCracken, J. T., Tierney, E., et al. (2005). Risperidone for the core symptom domains of autism: Results from the RUPP Autism Network study. *The American Journal of Psychiatry, 162*, 1142–1148.

Mills, R., & Wing, L. (2005). Researching interventions in ASD and priorities for research: Surveying the membership of the NAS. Paper presented at the annual meeting of the National Autistic Society, London

Muris, P., Steerneman, P., Merckelbach, H., Holdrinet, I., & Meesters, C. (1998). Comorbid anxiety symptoms in children with pervasive developmental disorders. *Journal of Anxiety Disorders, 12*, 387–393.

Ooi, Y. P., Larn, C. M., Sung, M., Tan, W. T. S., Goh, T. J., et al. (2008). Effects of cognitive-behavioural therapy on anxiety for children with high-functioning autistic spectrum disorders. *Singapore Medical Journal, 49*, 215–220.

Pelham, W. E., Gnagy, E. M., Greiner, A. R., Hoza, B., Hinshaw, S. P., et al. (2000). Behavioral versus behavioral and pharmacological treatment in ADHD children attending a summer treatment program. *Journal of Abnormal Child Psychology, 28*, 507–525.

POTS Study Group. (2004). Cognitive-behavior therapy, sertraline, and their combination for children and adolescents with obsessive-compulsive disorder: The Pediatric OCD Treatment Study (POTS) randomized controlled trial. *Journal of the American Medical Association, 292*, 1969–1976.

Rao, P. A., Beidel, B. C., & Murray, M. J. (2008). Social skills interventions for children with Asperger's syndrome or high-functioning autism: a review and recommendations. *Journal of Autism and Developmental Disorders, 38*, 353–361.

Reaven, J., & Hepburn, S. L. (2003). Cognitive-behavioral treatment of obsessive-compulsive disorder in a child with Asperger syndrome: A case report. *Autism, 7*(2), 145–165.

Reaven, J. A., Blakeley-Smith, A., Nichols, S., Dasari, M., Flanigan, E., & Hepburn, S. (2009). Cognitive-behavioral group treatment for anxiety symptoms in children with high-functioning autism spectrum disorders: A pilot study. *Focus on Autism and Other Developmental Disabilities, 24*, 27–37.

Reichow, B., Volkmar, F. R., & Cicchetti, D. V. (2008). Development of an evaluative method for determining the strength of research evidence in autism. *Journal of Autism and Developmental Disorders, 38*, 1311–1319.

Reiersen, A. M., & Todd, R. D. (2008). Co-occurrence of ADHD and autism spectrum disorders: Phenomenology and treatment. *Expert Review of Neurotherapeutics, 8*, 657–669.

Russell, E., & Sofronoff, K. (2005). Anxiety and social worries in children with Asperger disorder. *The Australian and New Zealand Journal of Psychiatry, 39*(7), 633–638.

Scahill, L., McDougle, C. J., Williams, S. K., Dimitropoulos, A., Aman, M. G., McCracken, J., et al. (2006). Children's Yale-Brown obsessive compulsive scale modified for pervasive developmental disorders. *Journal of the American Academy of Child and Adolescent Psychiatry, 45*, 1114–1123.

Schopler, E., Reichler, R. J., & Renner, B. R. (1998). *The childhood autism rating scale (CARS)*. Los Angeles, CA: Western Psychological Services.

Sigman, M., &Ruskin, E. (1999). Continuity and change in the social competence of children with autism, Down syndrome, and developmental delays. *Monographs of the Society for Research in Child Development, 64*(1), v–114.

Silverman, W. K., & Albano, A. M. (1996). *The anxiety disorders interview schedule for DSM-IV-TR – child and parent versions*. San Antonio, TX: Graywind.

Simonoff, E., Pickles, A., Charman, T., Chandler, S., Loucas, T., & Baird, G. (2008). Psychiatric disorders in children with autism spectrum disorders: Prevalence, comorbidity, and associated factors in a population-derived sample. *Journal of the American Academy of Child and Adolescent Psychiatry, 47*(8), 921–929.

Sofronoff, K., Attwood, T., & Hinton, S. (2005). A randomised controlled trial of CBT intervention for anxiety in children with Asperger syndrome. *Journal of Child Psychology and Psychiatry, 46,* 1152–1160.

Sofronoff, K., Attwood, T., Hinton, S., & Levin, I. (2007). A randomized controlled trail of a cognitive behavioural intervention for anger management in children diagnosed with Asperger syndrome. *Journal of Autism and Developmental Disorders, 37,* 1203–1214.

Solomon, M., Ono, M., Timmer, S., & Goodlin-Jones, B. (2008). The effectiveness of parent child interaction therapy for families of children on the spectrum. *Journal of Autism and Development Disorders,* 38, 1767–1776.

Solomon, M., Ozonoff, S., Carter, C., & Caplan, R. (2008). Formal thought disorder and the autism spectrum: Relationship with symptoms, executive control, and anxiety. *Journal of Autism and Development Disorders, 38,* 1474–1474.

Sukhodolsky, D. G., & Scahill, L.(2007). Disruptive behavior in persons with Tourette syndrome: Phenomenology, assessment, and treatment. In D. W. Woods, J. C. Piacentimi, & J. T. Walkup. (Eds). *Treating Tourette Syndrome and Tic Disorders,* (pp. 199–221). New York: Guilford.

Sukhodolsky, D. G., Scahill, L., Gadow, K. D., Arnold, L. E., Aman, M. G., et al. (2008). Parent-rated anxiety symptoms in children with pervasive developmental disorders: Frequency and association with core autism symptoms and cognitive functioning. *Journal of Abnormal Child Psychology, 36,* 117–117.

Sze, K., & Wood, J. (2007). Cognitive behavioral treatment of comorbid anxiety disorders and social difficulties in children with high-functioning autism: A case report. *Journal of Contemporary Psychotherapy, 37,* 133–143.

Sze, K. M., & Wood, J. J. (2008). Enhancing CBT for the treatment of autism spectrum disorders and concurrent anxiety: A case study. *Behavioural and Cognitive Psychotherapy, 36,* 403–409.

Walkup, J. T., Albano, A. M., Piacentini, J., Birmaher, B., Compton, S. N., et al. (2008). Cognitive behavioral therapy, sertraline, or a combination in childhood anxiety. *The New England Journal of Medicine, 359,* 2753–2766.

Webster-Stratton, C., & Reid, M. J. (2003). Treating conduct problems and strengthening social and emotional competence in young children: The Dina Dinosaur treatment program. *Journal of Emotional and Behavioral Disorders, 11,* 130–143.

White, S., & Roberson-Nay, R. (2009). Anxiety, social deficits, and loneliness in youth with autism spectrum disorders. *Journal of Autism and Developmental Disorders, 39,* 1006–1013.

Wood, J. J., & McLeod, B. M. (2008). *Child anxiety disorders: A treatment manual for practitioners.* New York: Norton.

Wood, J. J., Piacentini, J. C., Southam-Gerow, M., Chu, B. C., & Sigman, M. (2006). Family cognitive behavioural therapy for child anxiety disorders. *Journal of the American Academy of Child and Adolescent Psychiatry, 45,* 314–324.

Wood, J. J., Drahota, A., Sze, K., Van Dyke, M., Decker, K., et al. (2009). Brief report: Effects of cognitive behavioral therapy on parent-reported autism symptoms in school-age children with high-functioning autism. *Journal of Autism and Developmental Disorders, 39,* 1609–1612.

Wood, J. J., Drahota, A., Sze, K., Har, K., Chiu, A., & Langer, D. A. (2009). Cognitive behavioral therapy for anxiety in children with autism spectrum disorders: A randomized, controlled trial. *Journal of Child Psychology and Psychiatry, 50,* 224–234.

Wymbs, B. T., Robb, J. A., Chronis, A. M., Massetti, G. M., Fabiano, G. A., et al. (2005). Long-term, multimodal treatment of a child with Asperger's syndrome and comorbid disruptive behavior problems: A case illustration. *Cognitive and Behavioral Practice, 12,* 338–350.

Psychopharmacology in Children with PDD: Review of Current Evidence

Lawrence Scahill and Susan Griebell Boorin

ABBREVIATIONS

ADHD	Attention deficit hyperactivity disorder
CARS	Childhood Autism Rating Scale
CGI-I	Clinical global impression-Improvement
CYBOCS	Children's Yale-Brown Obsessive–Compulsive Scale
DSM-IV-TR	Diagnostic and Statistical Manual of Mental Disorders, 4th edition
FDA	Food and Drug Administration
HSQ	Home Situations Questionnaire
OCD	Obsessive–compulsive disorder
PDD	Pervasive developmental disorder
PDD-NOS	Pervasive developmental disorder, not otherwise specified
RUPP	Research Units on Pediatric Psychopharmacology
SSRI	Selective serotonin reuptake inhibitor
STAART	Studies to Advance Autism Research and Treatment

INTRODUCTION

Over the past 20 years, there has been an increase in the identification of children with autism and phenotypically related conditions, Asperger disorder, and pervasive developmental disorder not otherwise specified (PDD-NOS) (Fombonne 2005). This increased recognition has brought in its wake greater demand for interventions – educational, psychosocial and psychopharmacological. A look at the literature over the past 20 years shows a rather impressive list of medications that have been examined in children with pervasive developmental disorders (PDDs) – albeit with varying degrees of rigor. These include

B. Reichow et al. (eds.), *Evidence-Based Practices and Treatments for Children with Autism*,
DOI 10.1007/978-1-4419-6975-0_8, © Springer Science+Business Media, LLC 2011

antipsychotics, such as haloperidol and risperidone, alpha-2 agonists, such as clonidine and guanfacine, methylphenidate, antidepressants and the gastrointestinal hormone, secretin. In addition, medication such as fenfluramine, amantadine, and naltrexone has been examined in at least one study. To date, the best-studied medication in children with PDD is secretin, which has been examined in approximately 13 placebo-controlled trials (Levy and Hyman 2005). It has yet to show superiority to placebo. Although several medications have been evaluated for treatment of children with PDD, only a handful of trials have included more than 40 subjects. Over the past decade, however, evidence has emerged on the use of risperidone, the selective serotonin reuptake inhibitors (SSRIs), fluoxetine and citalopram, and methylphenidate in children with PDDs. Coincidently, these three classes of medication are also among the most commonly used in this population (Aman et al. 2003; Oswald and Sonenklar 2007; Mandell et al. 2008). This chapter reviews results from recently published reports mostly from federally-funded, multi-site randomized clinical trials. The review is organized according to target symptoms for medication intervention in children with PDDs, such as hyperactivity and impulsiveness, repetitive behavior, and the triad seriously maladaptive behavior: tantrums, aggression, and self-injury.

HYPERACTIVITY

Methylphenidate

Currently, the *Diagnostic and Statistical Manual of Mental Disorders* (DSM-IV-TR; APA 2000) advises against the use of the label attention deficit hyperactivity disorder (ADHD) in children with PDD. The rationale is simple: hyperactivity, impulsiveness, and distractibility in a child with PDD can be explained by the presence of PDD, thus, the ADHD label is unnecessary. However, hyperactivity, disruptive behavior and impulsive behavior are common complaints by parents of children with PDD. In addition, the surveys cited above show that hyperactivity is a common reason for using medications such as stimulants and alpha-2 agonists (clonidine and guanfacine) in children with PDD. Until recently, however, most trials involved small samples.

The Research Units on Pediatric Psychopharmacology Autism Network published the largest study on methylphenidate in children with PDD accompanied by hyperactivity (RUPP 2005a). The study of 72 children was designed to evaluate the efficacy and safety of multiple doses of methylphenidate and included a 2-month extension for children who showed a positive response. Based on prior studies, the investigators noted that children with PDD appear to have greater vulnerability to adverse effects of methylphenidate than typically developing children with ADHD. Therefore, the study was divided into three phases. First, there was a seven-day, test-dose period in which each child received two days on placebo and two days on each of the three dose levels of methylphenidate that would be used in the randomized crossover trial. During this seven-day test dose period, there was daily phone contact with the parent to review tolerability.

The dose strengths used in the study were described as *low*, *medium* and *high*. The low dose was approximately 0.15 mg/kg; the medium dose was approximately 0.25 mg/kg and the high dose was 0.5 mg/kg. The dosing schedule followed the pattern set by Multimodal Treatment Study of Children with ADHD Trial (MTA Cooperative Group 1999) with equal morning and noon doses and a 4 pm dose of approximately half the strength of the earlier doses. Thus, for a child weighing 22 kilos, the low dose was 2.5 mg three times daily; the medium dose was 5 mg in the morning, 5 mg at noon, and 2.5 mg at 4 pm; and the high dose 10, 10, and 5 mg at these same times. Compared to methylphenidate doses used in typically developing children, these dose levels are conservative and reflect the concern for adverse effects in this population. Children who tolerated all doses in the test dose period entered the 4-week, double-blind trial and received three doses of methylphenidate or placebo for 1 week each in random order. For safety reasons, there was an exception to this random sequence. Children who tolerated the low dose and the medium dose but not the high dose, were included in the randomized trial. However, they were not randomized to the high dose. Instead, they received 2 weeks of medium dose – under double-blind conditions. At the end of the 4-week, double-blind trial, the research team at each site used a systematic algorithm based on parent and teacher measures and clinician ratings to select the *best dose* for each subject. If the best dose was one of the three active doses, children were followed for 8 additional weeks at that dose in an open label trial (Posey et al. 2007).

Seventy-two children entered the trial; six did not tolerate the medication during the test week and were not included in the randomized, double-blind, placebo crossover trial. Thus, 66 children entered the randomized phase of the study. These children were approximately 7.5 years of age (range: 5–13.7 years); 59 were boys and 7 were girls. The eligibility criteria required children to be at least moderately hyperactive, have a mental age of at least 18 months, and have a diagnosis of PDD (autistic disorder, PDD-NOS, or Asperger disorder). Forty-seven (approximately 73%) of the children met criteria for autistic disorder, 14 met criteria for PDD-NOS, and five were diagnosed with Asperger disorder.

On the primary outcome measure, the hyperactivity subscale of the Aberrant Behavior Checklist (ABC), both parents and teachers rated the subjects in the severe range at baseline. The ABC is a standardized behavior rating scale that was developed for assessing treatment effects and behavior problems in people with developmental disabilities (Brown et al. 2002). All three doses of the medications were superior to placebo in reducing hyperactivity and impulsiveness as measured by the ABC hyperactivity subscale. The magnitude of benefit for methylphenidate in this population was considerably lower than what has been observed in typically developing children with ADHD (MTA Cooperative Group 1999). The magnitude of Cohen's d were 0.25 for the low dose, 0.20 for the medium dose and 0.48 for the high dose on teacher ratings; on parent ratings, the effect sizes were 0.29, 0.54, and 0.40 for low, medium and high doses, respectively. Subtracting out the effects of placebo, the percentage improvement over baseline ranged from 10% to 17% on parent ratings and 10% to 19% on teacher ratings. In general, parents reported slightly greater benefit than teachers. This pattern is the opposite of what is observed in stimulant trials of typically developing children with ADHD, in which teachers usually report greater benefits than parents. In addition to a lower magnitude and slightly different pattern of response than for typically developing children with ADHD, children in the RUPP Autism Network trial showed lower tolerability to methylphenidate. Thirteen of the original 72 children exited the trial due to adverse events. This figure of 18% is considerably higher than what is observed in typically developing children with ADHD treated with methylphenidate. Irritability was the most common adverse effect leading to early exit from the trial (RUPP 2005a).

In conclusion, at doses ranging from 12.5 to 25 mg per day (the medium dose level used in the trial), methylphenidate appears to be effective for 50–60% of children with a PDD accompanied by hyperactivity. The magnitude of improvement is approximately 20%, which is lower than is observed in typically developing children with ADHD. In this dose range (12.5 to 25 mg per day), methylphenidate is likely to be well tolerated by school-aged children with PDD. An effort to produce greater improvement by increasing the dose is likely to result in increased adverse effects.

Guanfacine

In a companion trial conducted with the RUPP methylphenidate trial, the investigators evaluated guanfacine in 25 children with PDD and hyperactivity (Scahill et al. 2006). The children entered this 8-week, open-label study by two pathways. During the screening phase of the methylphenidate trial, children who failed to show a positive response to methylphenidate were invited to enter directly into the open-label guanfacine trial. Children who exited the methylphenidate trial due to adverse effects or lack of efficacy were also invited to enter the guanfacine trial. The mean age of the sample was 9.0 years; 7 subjects met criteria for autistic disorder and 18 met criteria for PDD-NOS. Most of the subjects were boys ($N=23$). The baseline ABC hyperactivity subscale scores were slightly higher than the baseline for children who entered the methylphenidate trial. After 8 weeks of treatment, the parents rated the children as approximately 40% improved and teachers rated about 25% improvement (given open-label design, there was no correction for placebo). In addition to improvement in hyperactivity, guanfacine was also rated as showing improvement on the parent-rated irritability subscale of the ABC. The irritability subscale includes maladaptive behaviors such as tantrums, aggression and self-injury. However, this effect on irritability was only medium in magnitude. Gains in hyperactivity were also accompanied by improvement in attention as measured by the SNAP-IV, which provides separate scores for hyperactivity and inattention (Bussing et al. 2008).

The dosing of guanfacine in this population appears slightly different to what has been reported in children with Tourette syndrome (Horrigan and Barnhill 1995; Scahill et al. 2001). For example, in the study of children with Tourette syndrome by Scahill et al. (2001), the modal dose was 2.5 mg per day spread over three doses (e.g., 1 mg in the morning, 0.5 mg after school time, and 1 mg at bedtime). In this sample of children with PDD (which was slightly younger than the participants in the previous guanfacine trials), the medication was given in two doses and the modal dose was 1.5 mg per day (e.g., 0.5 mg in the morning and 1 mg at bedtime).

Handen et al. (2008) evaluated the efficacy and safety of guanfacine in 11 children (10 boys and 1 girl, age range 5–9 years) with developmental disabilities (PDD = 6; intellectual disability without PDD = 5) accompanied by symptoms of ADHD. Using a modified crossover design, subjects were randomly assigned to receive guanfacine for 4 weeks followed by a 1-week washout and then a week of placebo. Alternatively, subjects received a week of placebo followed by 4 weeks of guanfacine and then the 1-week washout. Adjusting for the effects of placebo, the mean change on the ABC hyperactivity subscale showed a 35% improvement, which was statistically significant. However, only five of the 11 subjects were classified as achieving a positive response. Guanfacine was administered three times daily (morning, noon, and late afternoon). The target dosage was 3 mg/day, which was tolerated by eight of the 11 subjects. The dose-limiting adverse effects included drowsiness, irritability, and enuresis. The rationale for this target dose was not mentioned and these results suggest that a more flexible dosing strategy is worth considering.

A new extended-release formulation of guanfacine has been developed and has shown superiority to placebo in a short-term trial conducted in typically developing children with ADHD (Biederman et al. 2008). This product has not been tested in children with PDD.

In conclusion, these pilot data from the guanfacine trials are encouraging, but more study is clearly needed. Guanfacine appears to be better tolerated than in the several small studies that have previously been done with clonidine in this population (Jaselskis et al. 1992). However, drowsiness, irritability and mid-sleep awakening were relatively common in these pilot guanfacine trials and may limit dose escalation. In many cases, these adverse effects can be managed by dose manipulation. In other cases, it may be necessary to discontinue the medication. As with methylphenidate, children with PDD appear to be more vulnerable to the adverse effects of guanfacine. Using the currently available immediate-release compound in young children, the dose typically starts with 0.25 mg at night or 0.5 mg at bedtime for older school-aged children. The dose range is likely to be between 1.5 to 3 mg/day given in two or three divided doses.

Repetitive Behavior

Selective serotonin reuptake inhibitors (SSRIs) have recently been reported to be the most common class of medications prescribed for children with PDD (Oswald and Sonenklar 2007; Mandell et al. 2008). The SSRIs available on the US market include citalopram, escitalopram, fluoxetine, fluvoxamine, paroxetine, sertraline, and clomipramine.

The tricyclic antidepressant clomipramine is considered a serotonin reuptake inhibitor because it is less selective. It was the first medication in this broad class of antidepressants to be evaluated in children and adults with pervasive developmental disorder (Scahill and Martin 2005). However, clomipramine has several drawbacks in this population, including the need for a cardiogram prior to medication, the need for periodic drug level monitoring, and the propensity to lower to seizure threshold, which is of concern in this population. Therefore, most of the attention in children with PDD has focused on the SSRIs.

Despite the common use of the SSRIs in this population, these drugs have not been well studied in children with PDD. The rationale for using the SSRIs in children with PDD stems, in part, from the observed benefits of these medications in children with obsessive–compulsive disorder (OCD). Indeed, several of the SSRIs, including fluoxetine, fluvoxamine, and sertraline, are approved for the treatment of OCD in children. Although the magnitude of the effect sizes for these medications in children with OCD is not large, they have consistently shown to superiority over placebo. Based on this observation and the observation that children with PDDs have preoccupations and repetitive behaviors, many clinicians and investigators have proposed that the SSRIs may be useful in this population as well. The questions concerning whether preoccupations and repetitive behavior in children with PDD are the same as unwanted thoughts (obsessions) and unwanted rituals (compulsions) in children with OCD remain unclear. Early open-label trials showed some promise for SSRIs in children with PDD. A recurring observation was the emergence of insomnia, agitation, impulsiveness and hyperactivity (Kolevzon et al. 2006; Scahill and Martin 2005).

Fluoxetine

The first placebo-controlled trial with an SSRI in children with PDD was conducted by Hollander et al. (2005). In that study, 39 children were enrolled in a crossover trial consisting of 8 weeks on fluoxetine or placebo followed by a washout and then crossover to the other treatment condition for 8 weeks. The mean age of the children was 10 and there were 30 boys and nine girls. A large number (90%) of the participants met criteria for autism; 10% were diagnosed with Asperger's disorder. The IQ showed a wide range from 30 to 132 but more than half had intellectual disability. The primary outcome measure was a version of the Children's Yale-Brown Obsessive Compulsive Scale (CYBOCS; Scahill et al. 2006) modified for children with PDD (Scahill et al. 1997). The CYBOCS-PDD differs from the CYBOCS in that the five obsessional items are not used. The score ranges from zero to 20 for the five compulsion items (time spent, interference, distress, resistance, and degree of control). In the study by Hollander et al. (2005), the range of scores on the CYBOCS-PDD was from eight to 18, suggesting that the sample included children with mild to severe repetitive behavior. Liquid fluoxetine was started at a low dose of 2.5 mg and increased gradually over the first several weeks. In the first arm of the trial (when half of the children were treated with fluoxetine and the other half of the children received placebo), both groups started the study with a score of approximately 13 on the CYBOCS-PDD and showed a modest change from baseline (10% improvement in the fluoxetine group compared to 4% improvement in the placebo group; the magnitude of the effect size was approximately $d=0.25$). When data from both phases of the crossover trial were evaluated, the investigators reported a significant improvement for fluoxetine compared to placebo. However, the effect size was small.

Using a conservative dose adjustment approach, the investigators were able to show that it is possible to avoid the commonly reported activation effects of SSRIs in children with PDD. Indeed, anxiety and insomnia appeared to be more common in the placebo condition compared to the fluoxetine condition; agitation occurred in 46% of children while on fluoxetine compared to 44% during the placebo phase. In conclusion, this study showed that fluoxetine showed a small effect compared to placebo, but was well tolerated when administered in a slow upward fashion.

The results of this trial stand in stark contrast to a recent press released by the Neuropharm Group (2009). This pharmaceutical company launched a pivotal trial with a new formulation of fluoxetine and reported preliminary results in February 2009. The press release indicated that fluoxetine was no better than placebo in the trial of 158 subjects between the ages of five and 17 with autistic disorder. This announcement was clearly a disappointment to the company, which hoped to show that this new formulation would be helpful to repetitive behavior in children with pervasive developmental disorders. This study also used the CYBOCS-PDD as the primary outcome measure.

Citalopram

The Studies to Advance Autism Research and Treatment (STAART) consortium recently completed a placebo control trial of citalopram in 149 children with pervasive developmental disorders, ages five to 17 (King et al. 2009). This trial, funded by the National Institute of Health and the National Institute of Child Health and Development, focused on repetitive behavior. The primary outcome measures were the improvement item on the Clinical Global Impression (CGI-I) scale and the CYBOCS-PDD. The CGI-I is a measure of overall improvement (Guy 1976).

The medication was started at a low dose of approximately 2.5 mg per day and gradually moved up to a maximum allowable dose of 20 mg per day. The average dose over the 12-week period was 16 mg. After 12 weeks of treatment, there was no difference in either the CGI-I or the CYBOCS-PDD. Both groups began the study with a CYBOCS-PDD score of approximately 15 and both groups showed approximately one-point improvement over the 12-week period. On the CGI-I, 34% in the placebo group and 33% in the citalopram group were rated as much improved or very much improved.

Citalopram was generally well tolerated, but children in the citalopram group had a higher percentage of increased energy, impulsiveness, hyperactivity and insomnia. Over a third of the children were rated as having increased energy, nearly 20% with increased impulsiveness, 12% with hyperactivity, and 38% with insomnia. Not surprisingly, some children showed several of these behaviors.

Summary of SSRI Treatments

Collectively, these studies suggest that SSRIs are not effective for the treatment of repetitive behavior in children with PDDs. The failure to show improvement on a measure of repetitive behavior in the citalopram study or in the Neuropharm-sponsored trial of fluoxetine suggests that the repetitive behaviors in children with PDD may be qualitatively and etiologically separate from the compulsions in children with OCD. Children with OCD usually report that they would rather not continue with their compulsive behavior. In contrast, children with pervasive developmental disorders often appear to enjoy their repetitive behaviors. This fundamental difference may help to explain the difference in response to this class of medication.

It has been suggested that there might be other benefits of SSRIs, such as decreased rigidity, improved capacity of managed transitions, and improvements in

anxiety. This was not specifically tested in the citalopram trial. However, the lack of separation on the CGI-I disputes this view. Had these additional benefits emerged in several cases, they would have been picked up by the CGI-I.

Although, SSRIs are well tolerated with few medical side effects of concern, SSRI-induced activation appears common in children with pervasive developmental disorders. Furthermore, it appears dose-related. The decision to place a child with a PDD on an SSRI should be considered carefully and the target of the medication should be clear to the clinician and made clear to parents. Failure to be clear about the target of treatment hinders assessment of benefit. Based on available data, the dose should start low and move up slowly to avoid activation effects.

SERIOUS MALADAPTIVE BEHAVIOR

Serious maladaptive behavior may include tantrums, aggression toward others, and self-injury. Maladaptive behavior is likely to be multi-determined, reflecting inadequate functional communication, low frustration tolerance in the face of environmental demands or when interrupted from a preferred activity, or inability to regulate emotion. The most common class of medications used to treat these serious maladaptive behaviors are the atypical antipsychotics. There are now several atypical antipsychotics on the market including clozapine, risperidone, quetiapine, ziprasidone, olanzapine, and aripiprazole. To date, the only drug in this class of medications that has been examined in large-scale randomized clinical trials is risperidone, which has now been evaluated in three separate trials. There are open-label studies of the other medications in this class, which have somewhat mixed results. Aripiprazole has been evaluated in two industry-sponsored trials and the results are pending.

The first large-scale study of risperidone was conducted by the Research Units on Pediatric Psychopharmacology (RUPP) Autism Network (RUPP 2002). The target for risperidone in this trial was serious maladaptive behavior, such as tantrums, aggression, and self-injury. The rationale for selecting risperidone for these serious behavioral problems was based on a body of work, conducted in the 1970s and 1980s by Magda Campbell and her colleagues in New York City, which showed that haloperidol was superior to placebo in young children with autism for aggressive behavior (Campbell et al. 1982). However, the drawbacks of haloperidol are well established and therefore, in practice, it was reserved for only the most severe cases. Risperidone, which was released in 1994 to the US market, was presumed to have a better adverse effect profile than haloperidol. In addition, the initial trials in adults with schizophrenia suggested that risperidone might also help the so-called "negative" symptoms of schizophrenia. These symptoms, which include low motivation, lack of social interest, and poverty of speech, are somewhat reminiscent of the social disability in children with autism. Therefore, RUPP Autism Network investigators reasoned that if risperidone could reduce serious behavioral problems in children with autism, it could help the child be more available for other interventions. Risperidone might also have secondary benefits in the social domain.

The trial included 101 children (82 males and 19 females) who met criteria for autistic disorder; the mean age was 8.8 years (range 5–17 years). To be eligible for the trial, the children had to rate high on the Aberrant Behavior Checklist (ABC) irritability subscale. This subscale, which contains behaviors reflecting tantrums, aggression, and self-injury, includes 15 items rated from zero to three. Therefore,

the scores range from 0 to 45, with higher scores reflecting greater symptom severity. At the start of the study, both groups scored approximately 26 on the ABC irritability subscale. This is roughly two standard deviations above the norm for tantrums, aggression, and self-injury in children with developmental disabilities. After 8 weeks of treatment, the risperidone group improved approximately 57% to a mean score of 11.3. By contrast, the placebo group improved about 14%. This difference reflects a large effect size of $d = 1.3$, which is statistically significant. These findings were replicated in a trial of risperidone conducted by the Janssen company in a sample of 79 subjects (Shea et al. 2004).

The mean dose of risperidone at week 8 was 1.8 mg per day. The medication dose schedule was determined by the subject's weight. For children over 45 kg, the medication started at 0.5 mg with gradual increases thereafter. In children between 20 and 45 kg, the medication also started at 0.5 mg at bedtime, but moved up more slowly. Children less than 20 kg began with 0.25 mg and moved up gradually. For all weight groups, the dose escalation was completed by week 4. This is noteworthy because the graphical display of results in the published paper shows that there was continued improvement even after there were no additional increases in medication from study week 4 to week 8.

During the 8-week, double-blind phase, investigators monitored adverse affects. Of particular interest were the neurological adverse effects, such as dyskinesia, tremor, parkinsonism and dystonia, so commonly reported in children treated with haloperidol. In addition, early studies with risperidone in children suggested that weight gain also warranted close monitoring. During the 8-week trial, half of the parents reported that children on risperidone had some increase in appetite. This compares to approximately a quarter of the children in the placebo group. However, when parents were queried further about the increased appetite, nearly 25% (12 out of 49) of the children in the risperidone group were described as having increased appetite that was a problem. This compares to only 4% in the placebo group. Risperidone treatment was associated with a 2.7 kg increase in weight compared to 0.8 kg in the placebo group. In addition to these adverse effects on appetite and weight gain, other adverse effects included tiredness and drowsiness, which occurred in approximately half of the subjects in the risperidone group. Drooling occurred in approximately 25% of the risperidone group. Parents reported tremor in 14% of the children in the risperidone group, compared to 2% in the placebo group, however the tremor was not reproduced by any of the children during follow-up visits. In addition, on examination, there was no evidence of dyskinesia or dystonia. Drooling reported in children in the risperidone group is an adverse affect that is somewhat puzzling. The atypical antipsychotic medication clozapine has been shown to cause an actual increase in salivation. In contrast, the older antipsychotic medications are sometimes associated with drooling due to a lowered frequency of swallowing and hypotonia. Therefore, it is unclear whether it is appropriate to consider this a neurological adverse affect on swallowing or an actual increase in the production of saliva.

This study also evaluated the longer-term benefits of risperidone in a 4-month, open-label trial for subjects who were classified as positive responders in the double-blind phase. Children could also enter the 4-month, open-label extension, if they were originally randomized to placebo and did not show any benefits. These "placebo non-responders" were first evaluated in an 8-week, open-label trial that used the dosing and visit schedule for subjects in the double-blind phase. At the end of this 8-week, open-label period, children who showed a positive response to risperidone,

were invited into the 4-month extension phase. Primary questions to be answered during this 4-month extension was whether the gains observed during the first 8 weeks were enduring over a total 6 months of treatment and whether it would be necessary to increase the dose of the medication to maintain these gains. The results showed that gains were stable over 6 months and it was not necessary to increase the dose to maintain these gains. The ABC irritability score remained unchanged during the extension phase and the dose of risperidone increased slightly from 1.8 mg/day at the end of the first 8 weeks of treatment to 1.96 mg/day at the end of 6 months of treatment (RUPP 2005b).

Sixty three subjects remained in the study for six months. After 6 months of treatment, the average weight gain was 5.6 ± 3.9 kgs. Recalling that subjects randomized to placebo in the eight-week, double-blind phase gained 0.8 kg on average, the expected weight gain for a six-month period could be estimated at 2.4 kg. The observed weight gain of 5.6 kg is clearly more than twice the "expected" weight gain.

The final phase of the trial evaluated whether it would be possible to discontinue the medication after 6 months of beneficial treatment. To accomplish this aim, children who continued to show benefit after 6 months of treatment were randomly assigned to gradual substitution with placebo or continued treatment with risperidone under double-blind conditions. The withdrawal took place over 3 weeks. The outcome of interest was a re-emergence of the target problems (tantrums, aggression, self-injury). The return of these symptoms constituted relapse and the blind was broken for that child. A child on placebo who showed relapse was restarted on risperidone. In a planned interim analysis, with a sample size of 32, relapse showed in ten of 16 children who withdrew from active treatment compared to two of 16 that remained on risperidone. This difference in the rate of relapse was statistically significant and the discontinuation phase of the trial was halted as per the design in the protocol.

In conclusion, the results of this multiphase RUPP Autism Network Study suggest that risperidone is effective for reducing tantrums, aggression, and self-injurious behavior in children with autism. Indeed approximately 70% of children with autism accompanied by these target problems are likely to show benefit and the expected magnitude of improvement is about 50% compared to baseline. These gains are stable over time and relapse is likely if the medication is withdrawn at 6 months. The medication is generally well tolerated but weight gain is emerging as an important concern. The weight gain appears to be directly related to increased appetite, therefore, selection of food is particularly important. Weight gain and diet should be monitored during treatment. Recent guidelines also suggest that prior to beginning treatment with an atypical antipsychotic, fasting samples of blood lipids and glucose should be measured. These indices should be monitored periodically during treatment.

Based on the results of the RUPP Autism Network studies (RUPP 2002, 2005b; McDougle et al. 2005) and the study by Shea et al. (2004), risperidone was approved by the US Food and Drug Administration (FDA) for the treatment of children between the ages of five and 17 with autism accompanied by tantrums, aggression, and self injury. The official labeling of risperidone for the treatment of serious behavioral problems in children with autism is explained in the package insert and included in the Physicians' Desk Reference (http://www.pdr.net). As with all newly approved drugs, the language in the package insert reflects the negotiation between the FDA and the pharmaceutical company. Examination of the package insert reveals a more conservative dosing strategy than what was described in the RUPP Autism Network

trial. The more conservative dosing strategy described in the package insert may reduce the risk of some adverse effects and perhaps result in a lower maintenance dose. However, the more conservative approach may prolong the time to benefit. Prescribing clinicians have to balance the risk of adverse effects and the acuity of the child's clinical picture.

The approval of risperidone for the treatment of children with autism accompanied by tantrums, aggressions, and self-injury led to a second RUPP Autism Network Study in which the additive benefits of parent training were evaluated compared to risperidone only (Scahill, Aman et al. 2009; Aman et al. 2009). As a prerequisite to conducting this study, the investigators developed a treatment manual for parent training and conducted a pilot trial to examine the feasibility of the treatment manual (Johnson et al. 2007; RUPP 2007). Once the RUPP Autism Network demonstrated that the parent training intervention would be acceptable to parents (as evidenced by their active participation in the program) and that the parent training program could be delivered uniformly across sites, the investigators proceeded with the large-scale, double-blind trial.

They randomly assigned 124 children aged 4 to 13 with PDDs (autism, Asperger disorder or PDD-NOS) to 6 months of treatment with risperidone plus parent training ($N=75$) or risperidone only ($N=49$) (for a detailed description of the design, see the work of Scahill, Aman et al. (2009)). The model for this study was that the medication would reliably decrease the tantrums, aggression, and self-injurious behavior. The decrease in these challenging maladaptive behaviors could set the stage for parent training to improve compliance and everyday living skills. This conceptual framework suggests that the two treatments are directed and related but do not give the same outcomes. To be eligible for the trial, children had to show at least a moderate score on the ABC irritability subscale, be physically healthy, medication-free and have a PDD diagnosis. The mean age of the sample was 7.5 years old; 85% (N = 105) were boys and 43% (N = 53) of the subjects had intellectual disabilities. The mean ABC irritability subscale score at baseline was 29, which was higher than the mean score on entry in the prior study. These children were also rated as non-compliant as evidenced by relatively high scores on the Home Situations Questionnaire (HSQ). This 25-item, parent-rated questionnaire provides information on the child's response to everyday demands.

The design is described in detail in a paper by Scahill et al. (2009). Briefly, therapists and families were not blinded to their random assignment (risperidone only or risperidone plus parent training), but subjects were assessed by independent evaluators who were not aware of the treatment condition. To minimize attrition, children who did not show a positive response to risperidone would be allowed to stay in the study through a switch to aripiprazole. Although aripiprazole has pharmacological properties that are similar to risperidone, it is somewhat different. Therefore, this medication might in fact be successful when risperidone was not. (Note: only 12 subjects switched to aripiprazole, see the work of Aman et al. (2009)).

On the CGI-I at week 24, 77% of the children in the medication-only group were rated as much improved or very much improved by a rater who was blind to treatment assignment. This compared to 87% of children in the combined treatment group. This difference of 10% was not statistically significant. However, on parent ratings of noncompliance on the HSQ and serious behavioral problems on the ABC irritability subscale, children in the combined treatment group showed significant improvement compared to children in the medication-only group (Aman et al. 2009). A graphic display of the results suggest that both groups showed benefit within weeks of starting the trial but, over time, there was a slight loss of benefit in the medication-only group and continued improvement in the combined treatment group resulting in the significant difference. At baseline, both groups were given a score of 29 on the ABC irritability subscale. After 24 weeks of treatment, both groups showed substantial improvement on this subscale (63% decline for the combined treatment group and 51% decline for the medication-only group). On the HSQ, the medication-only group showed a 60% drop from baseline to week 24 compared to 71% improvement in the combined treatment group.

In one of the few trials of young children, Luby et al. (2006) examined the safety and effectiveness of risperidone in a 6-month trial in children (n = 23) with autism or PDD. The subjects ranged from 2.5 to 6.0 years of age. Outcome measures included the Childhood Autism Rating Scale (CARS) and the Gilliam Autism Rating Scale. Risperidone was administered in low doses and adjusted by an unblinded child psychiatrist, due to the young age of the children (the total daily dose ranged from 0.5 to 1.5 mg). The mean final daily dose of risperidone was 1.14 ± 0.32 mg, generally given twice a day. There were no serious adverse events during the 6-month trial, although the adverse effects included increased appetite, weight gain (mean gain 2.96 kg from baseline against 0.61 kg in the control group), drooling, increased serum prolactin levels and sedation. Result of the CARS over two time points (baseline and 6-month endpoint) showed significant differences between the study groups, with greater improvement in the risperidone group compared to the placebo. In addition to the small sample size, there were differences between the two groups at baseline despite randomization. Given these design limitations, the findings should be viewed with caution and may not serve as a guide to clinical practice.

In conclusion, risperidone appears to be an effective medication for the treatment of tantrums, aggression and self-injury in children with PDDs. All three studies in school-aged children suggest that a high percentage of children with PDD complicated by the presence of these behaviors will show significant improvement with risperidone. This improvement will be evident early in treatment and tends to endure at least over 6 months. Discontinuation of the medication after 6 months of treatment is likely to result in relapse. Current results do not provide clear guidance on the duration of treatment after 6 months, but periodic attempts to lower the dose warrant consideration. When using this medication in school-aged children, the dose schedule shown in the package insert is an appropriate starting place. However, if using this conservative dose scheme is not effective, a slightly more aggressive dose should be considered before discontinuing the medication.

The apparent improvement with the addition of parent training raises several issues. First, it appears that indeed the medication can be relied upon to decrease the challenging maladaptive behaviors in these children. However, there were clear benefits from the addition of a systematic parent training program in these children with PDD and serious behavioral problems. Parent training may also remediate the functional deficits in this population.

REFERENCES

Aman, M. G., Lam, K., & Collier-Crespin, A. (2003). Prevalence and patterns of use of psychoactive medicines among individuals with autism in the autism society of Ohio. *Journal of Autism and Developmental Disorders, 33*(5), 527–534.

Aman, M. G., McDougle, C. J., Scahill, L., Handen, B., Arnold, L. E., et al. (2009). Medication and parent training in children with pervasive developmental disorders and serious behavioral problems: Results from a random-

ized clinical trial. *Journal of the American Academy of Child and Adolescent Psychiatry, 48*(12), 1143–1154.

APA. (2000). *Diagnostic and Statistical Manual of Mental Disorders* (4th ed. – text revision). Washington, DC: American Psychiatric Association.

Biederman, J., Melmed, R. D., Patel, A., et al. (2008). A randomized, double-blind, placebo-controlled study of guanfacine extended release in children and adolescents with attention-deficit/hyperactivity disorder. *Pediatrics, 121*(1), e73–e84.

Brown, E., Aman, M., & Havercamp, S. (2002). Factor analysis and norms for parent ratings on the Aberrant Behavior Checklist-Community for young people in special education. *Research in Developmental Disabilities, 23*, 45–60.

Bussing, R., Fernandez, M., Harwood, M., Hou, W., Garvan, C., & Eyberg, S. (2008). Parent and teacher SNAP-IV ratings of attention deficit hyperactivity disorder symptoms: Psychometric properties and normative ratings from a school district sample. *Assessment, 15*(3), 317–328.

Campbell, M., Anderson, L., & Cohen, I. (1982). Haloperidol in autistic children: Effects on learning, behavior, and abnormal involuntary movements. *Psychopharmacology Bulletin, 18*(1), 110–111.

Fombonne, E. (2005). Epidemiology of autistic disorder and other pervasive developmental disorders. *Journal of Clinical Psychiatry, 66*(Suppl. 10), 3–8.

Guy, W. (1976). *ECDEU Assessment Manual for Psychopharmacology, revised*. Rockville, MD: National Institute of Mental Health. on p. 243

Handen, B. L., Sahl, R., & Hardan, A. Y. (2008). Guanfacine in children with autism and/ or intellectual disabilities. *Journal of Developmental and Behavioral Pediatrics, 29*(4), 303–308.

Hollander, E., Phillips, A., Chaplin, W., Zagursky, K., Novotny, S., & Wasserman, S. (2005). A placebo controlled crossover trial of liquid fluoxetine on repetitive behaviors in childhood and adolescent autism. *Neuropsychopharmacology, 30*(3), 582–589.

Horrigan, J. P., & Barnhill, L. J. (1995). Guanfacine for treatment of attention-deficit hyperactivity disorder in boys. *Journal of Child and Adolescent Psychopharmacology, 5*(3), 215–223.

Jaselskis, C., Cook, E., Fletcher, K., & Leventhal, B. L. (1992). Clonidine treatment of hyperactive and impulsive children with autistic disorder. *Journal of Clinical Psychopharmacology, 12*, 322–327.

Johnson, C. R., Handen, B. L., Butter, E., Wagner, A., Mulick, J., & Sukhodolsky, D. G. (2007).

Development of a parent management training program for children with pervasive developmental disorders. *Behavioral Interventions, 22*, 1–21.

King, B. H., Hollander, E., Sikich, L., McCracken, J. T., Scahill, L., et al. (2009). Lack of efficacy of citalopram in children with autism spectrum disorders and high levels of repetitive behavior: Citalopram ineffective in children with autism. *Archives of General Psychiatry, 66*(6), 583–590.

Kolevzon, A., Mathewson, K., & Hollander, E. (2006). Selective serotonin reuptake inhibitors in autism: A review of efficacy and tolerability. *Journal of Clinical Psychiatry, 67*, 407–414.

Levy, S., & Hyman, S. (2005). Novel treatments for autistic spectrum disorders. *Mental Retardation and Developmental Disabilities Research Reviews, 11*, 131–142.

Luby, J., Mrakotsky, C., Salets, M., Belden, A., Heffelfinger, A., & Williams, M. (2006). Risperidone in preschool children with autistic disorders: An investigation of safety and efficacy. *Journal of Child and Adolescent Psychopharmacology, 16*(5), 575–587.

Mandell, D. S., Morales, K. H., Marcus, S. C., Stahmer, A. C., Doshi, J., & Polsky, D. E. (2008). Psychotropic medication use among Medicaid-enrolled children with autism spectrum disorders. *Pediatrics, 121*(3), e441–448.

McDougle, C. J., Scahill, L., Aman, M. G., McCracken, J. T., Tierney, E., et al. (2005). Risperidone for the core symptom domains of autism: Results from the RUPP Autism Network study. *American Journal of Psychiatry, 162*, 1142–1148.

MTA Cooperative Group. (1999). A 14-month randomized clinical trial of treatment strategies for attention-deficit/hyperactivity disorder. *Archives of General Psychiatry, 56*, 1073–1086.

Neuropharm Group. (2009). *Phase III SOFIA study of NPL-2008 in Autistic Disorder.* Retrieved August, 2009 from http://www.neuropharm.co.uk/media_centre/news_release/?page=2&id=3542

Oswald, D. P., & Sonenklar, N. A. (2007). Medication use among children with autism spectrum disorders. *Journal of Child and Adolescent Psychopharmacology, 17*(3), 348–355.

Posey, D., Aman, M., McCracken, J., Scahill, L., Tierney, E., et al. (2007). Positive effects of methylphenidate on inattention and hyperactivity in pervasive developmental disorders: An analysis of secondary measures. *Biological Psychiatry, 61*(4), 538–544.

RUPP. (2002). Risperidone in children with autism and serious behavioral problems. Research Units on Pediatric Psychopharmacology (RUPP) Autism Network. *New England Journal of Medicine, 347*(5), 314–321.

RUPP. (2005a). Randomized, controlled, cross-over trial of methylphenidate in pervasive developmental disorders with hyperactivity. Research Units on Pediatric Psychopharmacology (RUPP) Autism Network. *Archives of General Psychiatry, 62*(11), 1266–1274.

RUPP. (2005b). Risperidone treatment of autistic disorder: longer term benefits and blinded discontinuation after six months. Research Units on Pediatric Psychopharmacology (RUPP) Autism Network. *American Journal of Psychiatry, 162*, 1361–1369.

RUPP. (2007). A pilot study of parent management training in children with pervasive developmental disorder. Research Units on Pediatric Psychopharmacology (RUPP) Autism Network. *Behavioral Interventions, 22*, 179–199.

Scahill, L., & Martin, A. (2005). Psychopharmacology. In F. R. Volkmar, R. Paul, A. Klin, & D. J. Cohen (Eds.), *Handbook of Autism and Pervasive Developmental Disorders* (3rd ed., pp. 1102–1117). Hoboken, NJ: Wiley.

Scahill, L., Aman, M. G., McDougle, C. J., McCracken, J. T., Tierney, E., et al. (2006). A prospective open trial of guanfacine in children with pervasive developmental disorders. *Journal of Child and Adolescent Psychopharmacology, 16*(5), 589–598.

Scahill, L., Aman, M., McDougle, C., Arnold, L., McCracken, J., & Handen, B. (2009). Trial design challenges when combining medication and parent training in children with pervasive developmental disorders. *Journal of Autism and Developmental Disorders, 39*(5), 720–729.

Scahill, L., Chappell, P. B., Kim, Y. S., Schultz, R. T., Katsovich, L., et al. (2001). A placebo-controlled study of guanfacine in the treatment of children with tic disorders and attention deficit hyperactivity disorder. *American Journal of Psychiatry, 158*(7), 1067–1074.

Scahill, L., McDougle, C. J., Williams, S. K., Dimitropoulos, A., Aman, M. G., et al. (2006). Children's Yale-Brown obsessive compulsive scale modified for pervasive developmental disorders. *Journal of the American Academy of Child and Adolescent Psychiatry, 45*(9), 1114–1123.

Scahill, L., Riddle, M. A., McSwiggin-Hardin, M., Ort, S. I., King, R. A., et al. (1997). Children's Yale-Brown Obsessive Compulsive Scale: reliability and validity. *Journal of the American Academy of Child and Adolescent Psychiatry, 36*(6), 844–852.

Shea, S., Turgay, A., Carroll, A., Schulz, M., Orlik, H., et al. (2004). Risperidone in the treatment of disruptive behavioral symptoms in children with autistic and other pervasive developmental disorders. *Pediatrics, 114*(5), e634–e641.

CHAPTER 9

Interventions That Address Sensory Dysfunction for Individuals with Autism Spectrum Disorders: Preliminary Evidence for the Superiority of Sensory Integration Compared to Other Sensory Approaches

Roseann C. Schaaf

ABBREVIATIONS

ADOS	Autism Diagnostic Observation Schedule
ANOVA	Analysis of variance
ASDs	Autism spectrum disorders
DBC	Developmental behavior checklist
DSM-IV-TR	Diagnostic and Statistical Manual of Mental Disorders, 4th edition
GSR	Galvanic skin response
ICD-10	International Classification of Diseases and Related Health Problems, 10th edition
MANOVA	Multivariate analysis of variance
PDD	Pervasive developmental disorder
PPVT	Peabody picture vocabulary test
SD	Sensory dysfunction
SSED	Single subject experimental design
SSQ	Sound sensitivity questionnaire

INTRODUCTION

It is estimated that 80–90% of individuals with autism spectrum disorders (ASD) demonstrate sensory-related problem

B. Reichow et al. (eds.), *Evidence-Based Practices and Treatments for Children with Autism*,
DOI 10.1007/978-1-4419-6975-0_9, © Springer Science+Business Media, LLC 2011

behaviors such as self-stimulating behaviors (finger flicking or excessive rocking), avoiding behaviors (such as placing hands over ears in response to typical levels of auditory input), sensory seeking behaviors (twirling, chewing, etc.), "tuning out" behaviors such as not responding to their name or other environmental cues, and difficulty enacting purposeful plans of action (Baranek et al. 2006; Huebner 2001; Kientz and Dunn 1997; O'Neill and Jones 1997; Ornitz 1974, 1989; Rogers et al. 2003; Tomchek and Dunn 2007). These behaviors, which may have a sensory basis, are termed sensory dysfunction (SD) and findings show that they limit participation in play, social, self-care and learning activities (Adrien et al. 1987; Baranek 1999, 2002; Edelson et al. 1999; Grandin 1995; Leekam et al. 2007; McClure and Holtz-Yotz 1991; Leekam et al. 2007, 1997; O'Riordan and Passetti 2006; Ornitz 1974, 1989; Rapin and Katzman 1998; Rogers and Ozonoff 2005; Schaaf et al. 2010; Williams 1992, 1994). Although interventions for SD are among the most requested services for children with ASD (Mandell et al. 2005; Green et al. 2006), there is limited evidence about their efficacy (Baranek et al. 2006; Dawson and Watling 2000; Rogers and Ozonoff 2005). The National Research Council (2001, p. 131) reports that there is a "pressing need for more basic and applied research to address the sensory aspects of behavior problems (in children with ASD)." Baranek (2002) also stressed that "best practice" for children with ASD should include interventions to address SD, but that more research is needed to guide parents, teachers, and other professionals to make informed decisions about intervention. Most studies to date fail to link basic science findings to behavioral or functional changes, and thus, it is not possible to determine the specific processes underlying behavioral gains reported in intervention studies. The purpose of this chapter is to define and describe SD in ASD, evaluate the evidence for current interventions that

address SD in ASD, and discuss practice recommendations in light of these data.

What Is Sensory Dysfunction in ASD?

Courtney is a six-year-old child diagnosed with ASD who attends a public school in a semi-inclusive classroom for children with special needs. Today, like most other days, Courtney is having difficulty participating in the class activities. The teacher already reprimanded Courtney several times this morning for "fidgeting" in her seat during circle time, disrupting the other children by making silly noises with her mouth and constantly getting up to wander about the room. During snack time, at 10 am, Courtney has an outburst and refuses to eat the graham crackers and milk provided by the school. The ticklish sensation of the milk on her lips is bothersome and the graham crackers are "too rough" for her liking. Instead of participating in snack time, Courtney sits by herself. During morning recess at 11 am, Courtney keeps to herself and is afraid to play on the slide with the other children. Finally, she runs to the swings and uses them to spin in circles. At 11:30 am, when the lunch bell rings, Courtney places her hands over her ears and runs into the closet, bothered by the noise. A classmate tries to comfort her but Courtney shoves the girl away and hurts her. In the cafeteria, Courtney becomes increasingly agitated. She sits alone with her hands over her ears until she feels able to negotiate the lunch line. After the crowd subsides, with the help of the classroom aide, Courtney manages to select a few items from the menu and place them on her tray. On the way back to her seat, Courtney trips over a backpack lying in the aisle and spills her tray. The other children begin to laugh. Courtney runs from the cafeteria with her hands covering her ears.

The teacher finds her in the gym wedged under several gym mats that she has piled on top of herself. Her hands are over her ears and she is rocking.

Courtney is a child with ASD and a SD that contributes to her disability. Families indicate that SD is one of the most significant factors limiting their ability to participate in home and community activities (Mandell et al. 2005). For example, one parent of a child with ASD and SD stated, "(After) our last commercial flying experience, we both swore off of it. Never again. His sensory sensitivity made it unbearable. He was just inconsolable." (Benevides et al. 2010). Others indicate that they must orchestrate their family routines and outings to accommodate the child's SD. They are unable to participate as a family in mealtimes (they must feed the child with ASD earlier than the others due to food sensitivities), family outings such as going to the movies are impossible (the child is unable to tolerate typical levels of noise and stimulation of crowds), or socialization with friends ("our child's self-stimulating behaviors make it impossible to be comfortable visiting with friends or meeting other children for a play date") (Larson 2006; Schaaf et al. (in press); Schaaf and Nightlinger 2007). Self-reports from individuals with ASD confirm these findings and are particularly potent in their descriptions of the impact of SD on participation in daily life activities (Grandin 1995; O'Neill and Jones 1997; Williams 1992, 1994). These self-reported data portray how SD limits the ability of individuals with ASD to participate fully in society. For example, Temple Grandin, a high functioning woman with ASD, articulates how her unusual processing of auditory, visual, and tactile information impedes social conversation because she is over-stimulated and distracted by the non-essential stimuli (Grandin 1995). As a result, she does not enjoy or participate in many of the daily activities of her peers.

INTERVENTIONS TO ADDRESS SENSORY DYSFUNCTION

It is widely accepted that a comprehensive educational program for children with ASD is the most effective in achieving optimal outcomes (National Research Council 2001). In addition to educational, speech and language, and behavioral services, a comprehensive program for individuals with ASD often includes occupational therapy services to address SD and other sensory-motor delays. In fact, Mandell et al. (2005) and Green et al. (2006) found that occupational therapy to address SD is among the top three services requested by families of children with ASD. Schwenk and Schaaf (2003) found that 99% of the therapists surveyed who work in public school settings with children with ASD used strategies to address SD as part of their therapeutic approach.

Occupational therapists follow a professional clinical reasoning framework to evaluate and design interventions for children with SD. Treatment follows a well-documented theoretical framework (Ayres 1979, 1989; Schaaf et al. 2010) directed by a set of principles that guide the therapists' clinical reasoning and interactions with the child (Schaaf and Miller 2005). The therapist chooses individually tailored sensory-motor activities for the child based on areas of need identified by systematic assessment. For example, for a child who is constantly rocking in his seat, systematic assessment might suggest a greater need for vestibular input. To address this issue the therapist generally takes a three-pronged approach:

- Work directly with the child using specialized equipment in a clinic that allows the child to experience vestibular input such as swings, bolsters, or scooter boards

- Provide environmental adaptations such as a small inflated cushion for the child to sit on in the classroom (thereby providing needed vestibular input and decreasing disruptive rocking behaviors)
- Provide consultation to the parent or teacher, for example, to suggest that the school team provide greater opportunities for the child to access playground equipment, such as swings, to provide regular intervals of the needed input and thus decrease the rocking behaviors (environmental adaptation)

It is worth noting that the prescribed activities are meaningful to the child (i.e., developmentally appropriate and contextualized in play) and embedded within the daily routine when possible. The therapist maintains data on whether these strategies are effective in reducing the disruptive behaviors and improving the child's attention and participation in class or home and community activities. Thus, by engaging the child in individually tailored sensory-motor activities, it is hypothesized that the child's nervous system is better able to modulate, organize, integrate and utilize information from the environment, and thus, is not driven to seek or avoid sensation in maladaptive ways. Adequate processing of sensory information, in turn, provides a foundation for further adaptive responses and participation in activities through adaptive neuroplastic mechanisms (Baranek 2002). Parent education and environmental adaptations are provided in tandem with direct intervention to support the child's sensory-motor needs.

This approach is child-centered and provides a just-right challenge (scaffolding) to facilitate progressively more sophisticated adaptive sensory-motor responses while engaging the child in affectively meaningful and developmentally appropriate play interactions. The child's focus is intended to be placed on play (intrinsically motivated) and not on cognitive-behavioral strategies or repetitive drills; thus, gains made during treatment are expected to be generalized to everyday life situations. Treatment goals focus on improving the ability to process and utilize sensory information, so that the child can develop better sensory modulation for attention and behavioral control, or the ability to form perceptual schemas and practical abilities as a foundation for greater participation in school, social, and daily living activities (Baranek 2002; Mailloux 2006). Thus, the sensory-integrative approach is utilized within a professional domain of practice, such as occupational therapy, and is focused on improving the child's participation in activities through the use of individually prescribed sensory motor activities.

Although this approach is based on solid theoretical principles that are contextualized within the professional framework of occupational therapy (Baranek 2002;), there is no manualized protocol and, thus, its utility and efficacy has not been systematically tested. Therefore, the evidence to support this approach is sparse and the studies that do exist have methodological flaws including that they do not explicitly describe the intervention and do not have a measure of fidelity, making it difficult to determine if the intervention provided was in keeping with the theoretical principles of the sensory-integrative approach. Evaluation of the evidence that does exist is further complicated by the fact that there are several techniques that utilize sensory stimulation but are not in keeping with the sensory-integrative approach and which are confused with it (Cox et al. 2009). These techniques usually provide passive stimulation to one sensory system rather than the holistic, child-directed, playful approach to intervention that is contextualized within a professional framework that is the hallmark of the sensory-integrative approach. The sensory-integrative approach is guided by the set of principles outlined in Table 9.1 (Parham et al. in press). The reader is referred to the work of Schaaf et al. (2010) for a full description of the sensory-integrative approach and the principles that guide the intervention.

EVIDENCE FOR THE SENSORY-INTEGRATIVE APPROACH

Like many other therapeutic interventions utilized with children with ASD, solid evidence for interventions to address SD in ASD is just beginning to surface and data

TABLE 9.1 Principles of Ayres sensory integration (Adapted from Parham et al. in press)

Item	Description
Ensures physical safety	The therapist anticipates physical hazards and attempts to ensure that the child is physically safe through manipulation of protective and therapeutic equipment or the therapist's physical proximity and actions. An existing safe room is important as is the therapist's attention to the child's abilities and potential dangers.
Presents sensory opportunities	The therapist presents the child with at least two of the following types of sensory opportunity, tactile, vestibular, or proprioceptive, in order to support the development of self regulation, sensory awareness, or movement in space.
Helps attain appropriate levels of alertness	The therapist helps the child to attain and maintain appropriate levels of alertness, as well as an affective state that supports engagement in activities.
Challenges postural, ocular, oral and bilateral motor control	The therapist supports and challenges postural control, ocular control, or bilateral development. At least one of the following types of challenge are intentionally offered: postural, resistive whole body, ocular-motor, bilateral, oral, or projected action sequences.
Challenges praxis and organization of behavior	The therapist supports and presents challenges to the child's ability to conceptualize and plan novel motor tasks, and to organize his or her own behavior in time and space.
Collaborates in activity choice	The therapist negotiates activity choices with the child, allowing the child to choose equipment, materials, or specific aspects of an activity. Activity choices and sequences are not determined solely by the therapist.
Tailors activity to present a just-right challenge	The therapist suggests or supports an increase in complexity of challenge when the child responds successfully. These challenges are primarily tailored to the child's postural, ocular, or oral control; sensory modulation and discrimination; or praxis developmental level.
Ensures that activities are successful	The therapist presents or facilitates challenges that focus on sensory modulation or discrimination; postural, ocular, or oral control; or praxis, in which the child can be successful in making an adaptive response to challenge.
Supports intrinsic motivation to play	The therapist creates a setting that supports play as a way to fully engage the child in the intervention.
Establishes a therapeutic alliance	The therapist promotes and establishes a connection with the child that conveys a sense of working together towards one or more goals in a mutually enjoyable partnership. The therapist and child relationship goes beyond pleasantries and feedback on performance such as praise or instruction.

are mainly from case reports, studies using single subject experimental designs (SSED), or small group design studies. To access available studies, we utilized Ovid Medline, PsychInfo, and OTSearch from 1995 forward using the search terms of "sensory integration," "sensory therapy," "sensory occupational therapy," "occupational therapy sensory integration," "auditory integration training," "vestibular therapy," "brushing," "visual therapy," "tactile therapy," "tactile treatment," "deep pressure," "and pressure vest." We have included one classic study of the sensory-integrative approach that dates back to 1980 because it was completed by the author of the sensory integration theory and thus we felt that it was important to include (Ayres and Tickle 1980). Our search yielded studies using both the sensory-integrative approach and sensory stimulation techniques.

In the following sections, we report first on studies of intervention using a sensory-integrative approach and then on those that used a sensory stimulation technique.

Table 9.2 lists the studies that utilized the sensory-integrative frame of reference within occupational therapy, specifically investigated interventions for SD, and show emerging evidence. Collectively, they report that individuals with ASD and SD who receive occupational therapy using a sensory-integrative approach demonstrated gains in play, individualized goals, and social interaction (Ayres and Tickle 1980; Case-Smith and Bryan 1999; Linderman and Stewart 1999; Schaaf and Nightlinger 2007; Watling and Dietz 2007) and a decrease in sensory symptoms (Smith et al. 2005; Fazlioglu and Baran 2008).

Schaaf and Nightlinger (2007) case study reports on a child who received occupa-

TABLE 9.2   Studies that investigate the use of sensory integration in occupational therapy in children with ASD

Study	Participants	Outcome	Evidence-based rating	Discussion
Ayres and Tickle 1980	$N=10$ mean age 7.4 years with ASD	Subjects with average- to hyper-responsive patterns to the stimuli (e.g., touch, movement, gravity, and air puff) showed better outcomes than those with a hypo-responsive pattern.	Weak	Descriptions of participants, intervention and outcome measures are not clearly provided.
Case-Smith and Bryan 1999	$N=5$ males aged 4–5;3 with autism	Independent coding of videotaped observations of free play indicated that three of the five boys demonstrated significant improvements in mastery play and four demonstrated less "non-engaged" play.	Adequate	• Clear descriptions of the participants, the outcome measures and the intervention are provided. The data analysis is linked to the research questions. Use of visual inspection is relevant and appropriate. • However, detailed information on the intervention is not provided and generalizations of the findings are limited by the (single subject) design.

(Continued)

TABLE 9.2 (Continued)

Study	Participants	Outcome	Evidence-based rating	Discussion
Linderman and Stewart 1999	*N* = 2 aged 3;3 and 3;9 with mild and severe ASD, respectively	Participant 1 (who was noted to have tactile hypersensitivity) demonstrated gains in all intended outcomes (social interactions, approach to new activities, and response to holding). Participant 2 (who had both hypo-responsiveness to vestibular and hyper-responsiveness to tactile sensations) made gains in activity level and social interaction, but not in functional communication.	Adequate	• Participant characteristics are described. The dependent measure is described and can be replicated. The baseline measurement is adequate. The analysis uses visual inspection. The inter-rater reliability has Kappa of .63. There is good social validity as it measures functional behaviors during daily activities. • However, there is no specific information about the diagnoses or the treatment; no consideration is given to the effect of other interventions; the sample size is small and homogenous; there is no fidelity measure; and raters are not blind to condition.
Smith et al. 2005	*N* = 7 (four males, three females) aged 8–19 years diagnosed with PDD	Videotape analysis of 15 min and 1 h after intervention showed a decrease in the frequency of self-stimulating behaviors. Teachers reported fewer self-stimulating behaviors and self-injurious behaviors during the treatment phase.	Adequate	• Intervention is described and is in keeping with the principles of sensory integration. • However, the sample was small and homogenous; there was no fidelity measure and no mention of whether the raters were blinded as to the treatment and control weeks.
Schaaf and Nightlinger 2007	*N* = 1 (male) 4 years of age with ASD	Measurable improvements were observed in individual goals and in post-treatment testing of sensory processing. Qualitative data (parent interview) also reported striking improvements in child and family's participation in activities and outings.	Adequate	• Intervention is detailed in a replicable way and follows the theoretical principles of the sensory integrative approach. Outcomes have social validity (child gains had an impact on his everyday life and the mother was extremely satisfied with the results). • However, findings cannot be generalized, there is no measure of fidelity and the rater is not blind to intervention.

(Continued)

TABLE 9.2   (Continued)

Study	Participants	Outcome	Evidence-based rating	Discussion
Watling and Dietz 2007	$N = 4$ males aged 3 and 4; 4 with ASD	There were improvements in ability to handle transitions, socialization, compliance and behavioral regulation. No decrease in undesirable behavior or increase in engagement was found.	Adequate	• Participant characteristics are described in detail. Dependent and independent variables are identified. There is a reliable measurement of fidelity. The comparable condition (a play scenario) is well described, activity choices are individualized and • presented in a random order and dependent variables are described in detail and are individually determined. There is good procedural reliability and social validity. • However, specific diagnostic information is missing; there is a limited use of standardized test scores; detailed information on the intervention is not provided; and generalizations of the findings are limited by the (single subject) design.
Fazlioglu and Baran 2008	$N = 30$ children aged 7–11 years old diagnosed with autism according to the DSM-IV criteria	Statistically significant differences were recorded in the Sensory Evaluation Form for Children with Autism, with the treatment group $p < .05$.	Adequate	• Subject randomization is valid; the protocol for intervention is described in a manner that can be replicated (the principles and philosophy are described); data analysis is linked to the research questions and there is good social validity. • However, there is no fidelity measure or mention of whether the raters were blind to the group assignment.

tional therapy using a sensory-integrative approach and showed improvements in the hypothesized direction in several behaviors. The child in this study demonstrated improved motor skills, social skills, and adaptive behaviors (e.g., improved ability to tolerate foods and thus improved participation in mealtime with the family, as measured by individual Goal Attainment scales, and decreased SD, as measured by the sensory profile scores and individual Goal Attainment scales). The results obtained were consistent with anecdotal reports from parents and other sources describing how quality of life for the family improved because the child's sensory over-responsive behaviors decreased and his ability to tolerate and participate in family activities improved (e.g., he was able to maintain self-regulation during grooming activities and to interact with other children during community playgroup activities). This study is promising in terms of its evidence for a sensory-integrative approach for ASD as it details the intervention in a replicable way and demonstrates how the intervention follows the theoretical principles of the sensory-integrative approach. In addition, the outcomes have social validity in that the child made gains that had an impact on his everyday life and the mother was extremely satisfied with the results. However, the study is limited in that it is a case study report, there is no measure of fidelity, and the rater was not blind to intervention.

Fazlioglu and Baran (2008) using a randomized two-group design, this study found statistically significant ($p < 0.05$) improvements between the groups in sensory-related behaviors pre- and post-intervention as measured by the Sensory Evaluation Form for Children with Autism. The study used a combination of sensory integration strategies (individually designed vestibular, somatosensory, and other sensory activities where the child was an active participant) and a "sensory diet" (systematically applied sensory stimuli) with 30 children diagnosed with low-functioning autism according to the criteria of the *Diagnostic and Statistical Manual of Mental Disorders*, 4th edition (DSM-IV-TR; APA 2000). This study is promising in terms of its evidence for a sensory-integrative approach for ASD as the subject randomization is valid, the protocol for intervention is described

in a manner that can be replicated (the principles and philosophy are described), the data analysis is linked to the research questions, and there is good social validity. However, there is no fidelity measure or mention of whether the raters were blind to the group assignment.

Smith et al. (2005) study considered seven subjects with ASD, aged 8–19 years. The study utilized a single subject withdrawal design (A–B–A–B) where weeks 1 and 3 represented the control sessions (30 min/day of table-top activities) and weeks 2 and 4 were the treatment sessions consisting of 30 min per day for 5 days per week. They video recorded the participants and performed frequency counts for presence and number of self-stimulating behaviors. They found that the overall frequency of self-stimulating behaviors decreased over the 4 weeks. Teachers also reported fewer self-stimulating and self-injurious behaviors during the treatment. This study was promising in that it describes the intervention and it is clear that it was in keeping with the principles of sensory integration (Smith et al. 2005, p. 421):

> Subjects engaged in sensory based treatment that included a variety of tactile, proprioceptive and vestibular input, based on their unique sensory needs. This is distinguished from sensory stimulation programs in that treatment was individualized based on assessment results, and the type or types of sensation and specific activities used.... Vestibular, tactile and proprioceptive based activities were primarily used, which is consistent with the accepted characteristics of intervention.

However, the study was limited by the small, homogenous sample and lack of a fidelity measure. In addition, there was no mention as to whether the raters were blinded to the treatment versus control weeks.

Linderman and Stewart (1999) study used a single subject A–B design to explore the effects of occupational therapy using a sensory-integrative approach on the functional behaviors of two young children (aged 3 years 3 months and 3 years 9 months) with pervasive developmental disabilities (PDD). They used the revised Functional Behavioral Assessment for Children with Sensory Integrative Dysfunction (Cook 1991) to evaluate the duration, quality and frequency of targeted sensory behaviors. Participant 1 demonstrated major improvements in social interactions, approach to new activities and responses to hugging and holding. Participant 2 displayed improvements in social interaction and response to movement. Although the authors state that treatment was in keeping with the sensory-integrative principles (i.e., child-directed treatment and active participation of the child) there is no specific information about the treatment, no consideration was given to the effect of other interventions (e.g., one subject enrolled in a preschool and another started a vitamin regimen), and the sample size was small and homogenous.

Case-Smith and Bryan (1999) conducted a study with a single subject A–B design of five subjects with autism, at 4 and 5 years of age. Baseline measures of play, non-engaged behaviors, child–adult interactions, and peer interactions were obtained via video-coding for a 3-week period. Data were analyzed by plotting behaviors on line graphs, computing means for each phase, and then calculating regressions for each phase. Data from each phase were compared using the Wilcoxon signed rank test to assess differences in the means for each phase. Results were mixed as there were improvements in some areas but not in others. For example, following intervention, three of the five children showed significant improvements in mastery play, four of the children demonstrated significantly decreased non-engaged behaviors, and only one participant demonstrated a significant increase in adult interactions.

None of the participants demonstrated significant increases in peer interactions. Despite the mixed findings, this study is promising in that it clearly describes the participants and the outcome measures and the intervention is described in detail. The data analysis is linked to the research questions and use of visual inspection is relevant and appropriate.

Watling and Dietz (2007) study used a withdrawal SSED (A–B–A–B) with four boys between the ages of 3 and 4.4 years of age who were diagnosed with ASD (criteria for diagnosis not known) to examine the immediate effects of occupational therapy using a sensory-integrative approach (Ayres Sensory Integration[1]) on undesirable behaviors and engagement. Target behaviors were operationalized and coded. The target behaviors included: changes in individually defined undesirable behaviors that interfere with task engagement and participation in daily activities; and engagement defined as intentional, persistent, active, and focused interaction with the environment, people and objects. The study consisted of familiarization, baseline phase 1 and treatment phase 1, followed by baseline phase 2 and treatment phase 2. Baseline consisted of developmentally appropriate toys selected individually for each child. Intervention consisted of three, 40-min sessions of Ayres Sensory Integration per week followed by a 10-min table-top activity segment during which outcome data was collected. Data for each subject were plotted on a line graph and interpreted through visual inspection. In addition, data in a study log from researchers and weekly reports of the participant's behavior in the home environment were reviewed. Visual inspection of the data for undesirable behaviors and engagement indicates considerable overlap in the number of intervals in which the behavior was observed in all phases; thus, Ayres Sensory Integration did not have a significantly different effect from the play scenarios on target behaviors. Data from study logs suggested that the intervention had a positive effect on transitions, socialization, compliance, and general behavior regulation, however, given the anecdotal nature of this data, the findings from this study cannot be interpreted to provide evidence for Ayres Sensory Integration. This study was promising in that participant characteristics were described in detail and dependent and independent variables were identified, however specific diagnostic information was missing and there was limited use of standardized test scores other than the Sensory Profile score that was used as an inclusion criterion. The information on the intervention was not provided except to mention that it followed the Ayres Sensory Integration approach. There was reliable measurement of fidelity. The comparable condition (a play scenario) was well described, the activity choices were individualized and presented in a random order, and the dependent variables were described in detail and also individually determined. There was good procedural reliability (above 99% for all phases). The social validity of this study was good in that dependent variable behaviors were identified based on parent interview and the data from study logs indicates an impact on daily life, however, the generality of the findings are limited by the design (single subject).

Ayres and Tickle (1980) study investigated whether the type of sensory processing disturbance predicted the response to sensory-integrative therapy. The subjects were ten children with autism aged between 3.5 and 13 years (mean age was 7.4). Subjects' responses to sensory input were evaluated through the use of a test constructed by the researchers solely for this purpose. The test consisted of 14 specific sensory stimuli (e.g., response to light touch, response to pain, and response to sound of white noise) and rating was on a scale of 1–5 (no reaction to definite over-reaction). The test was administered by the investigator at least twice to enhance accuracy. Intervention was 1 year of occupational therapy using a sensory-integration approach "that focused on carefully providing somatosensory and vestibular sensory experiences and on eliciting an adaptive response to these stimuli" (Ayres and Tickle 1980, p. 378). Results were reported by individual subject changes on the test of responses to specific sensory stimuli and, in some cases, post-test scores on motor performance and vocabulary tests. A stepwise discriminant analysis was conducted to determine the parameters that best discriminated between subjects who were good responders to therapy versus those who were not. The good versus the poor responders had statistically significant ($p < 0.05$) differences on the presence of tactile defensiveness. There were no significant differences in the proposed direction for reactions to touch pressure, vibration, and movement. The best discriminators between the good and the poor responders were tactile defensiveness, reaction to movement, gravitational insecurity, and reaction to an air puff. Subjects who had normal or over-reactions to stimuli were better responders to therapy than non-responders. This study is interesting in that it is one of the first studies conducted to evaluate the effects of the sensory-integrative approach for children with autism and provides some preliminary data suggesting that children who are over responsive to stimuli will respond better than those who are under responsive. However, the study was weak in that it failed to adequately describe the participants' characteristics and the independent variable (treatment) was not described. The dependent variables (measures) did not have reliability or validity, there was no comparison condition, and there was no calculation of power. The study has high social validity in that it is an area of high interest for clinicians and serves to provide preliminary guidelines for future studies in this area.

Conclusion

Although these studies provide promising evidence, it is not possible to draw strong practice implications because of small sample sizes, failure to adequately characterize the sample, lack of a detailed, replicable intervention protocol with a fidelity measure, and other methodological and design flaws. Future studies must address these issues and, fortunately, several efforts are underway to do so. For example, a Fidelity to Treatment Measure has been developed to evaluate whether intervention follows the sensory-integrative principles established in the literature (Parham et al. 2007). This fidelity scale evaluates constructs related to sensory-integration interventions, details the training of the people administering the intervention, and specifies the environment in which the treatment is conducted. It will ensure that future studies evaluating the sensory-integrative approach attain rigorous standards that include fidelity. A pilot version of this fidelity scale was used in the Watling and Dietz (2007) study. A manualized protocol has also been developed and is being tested for its utility and effectiveness for SD in ASD (Schaaf et al. in preparation). This manual is in keeping with the recommendations in the literature for intervention with the ASD population as outlined by Lord et al. (2005): it outlines key theoretical principles; it describes the objectives for each principle; it describes the clinical reasoning for each principle; and it is flexible in its application to allow for individualization of the treatment – an important aspect of interventions for ASD. An earlier version of the manual was used in a randomized pilot study for a non-ASD group (Miller et al. 2007; Miller et al. 2007). The findings show that, following a 10-week, 30-session intervention, children

in the treatment group ($n=7$) made gains that were significantly greater than the children in the other two groups (no treatment ($n=10$) and active control ($n=7$)) on Goal Attainment scales ($p<0.01$). They also increased more than the other groups on attention, measured by Leiter-R (Roid and Miller 1997), with $p=0.03$ compared to $p=0.07$ for no treatment. Data showed trends in the predicted direction for the treatment group on sensory behaviors and the cognitive/social composite score on the Leiter-R. The treatment group showed a trend toward greater reduction in electrodermal activity (a measure of sensory responsivity) than the other groups.

Finally, to address the need for sensitive, meaningful outcome measures that are function-oriented and in keeping with the principles of the sensory-integrative approach, Goal Attainment Scaling (Kiresuk et al. 1994) has been adapted and applied for use with the sensory-integrative approach (Mailloux et al. 2007). Goal Attainment Scaling provides a means to monitor intervention goals that are specifically relevant to individuals and their families and thus holds promise as an effective, replicable outcome measure to evaluate the efficacy of the sensory-integrative approach for individuals with autism. The Goal Attainment scale provides a mechanism for assuring that outcomes have high social validity.

EVIDENCE FOR SPECIFIC SENSORY TECHNIQUES

A number of studies examine the effects of specific sensory strategies on reducing self-stimulating behaviors, improving attention and engagement in tasks, and decreasing sensory aversions for individuals with ASD. To reiterate, these interventions should be distinguished from the sensory-integrative approach in that they utilize stimulation of one specific sensory system rather than the holistic, integrated approach that is consistent with sensory integration. Broadly, these studies can be grouped into four categories: interventions that utilize touch (i.e., massage or touch therapy); interventions that utilize weighted vests; auditory interventions; and other interventions (the Wilbarger Protocol, therapy balls, and sensory diet). Again, the majority of the studies utilized case study, SSED, or group design protocols and are limited by small sample sizes and other methodological flaws. Thus, it is difficult to draw practice implications.

Touch-Based Treatments

The four studies summarized in Table 9.3 utilize massage, touch therapy, or deep pressure stimulation.

Escalona et al. (2001) examined whether nightly massage improved the sleeping habits and behaviors of children with autism. Twenty subjects with autism between the ages of 3 and 6 years of age were randomly assigned to either a control group or a massage therapy group. Parents were trained in the massage therapy and provided it every night for 15 min prior to bedtime for 1 month. Control subjects were read a story for 15 min by parents. Outcome measures were the Revised Conners Scales (Conners 1997) and observation of classroom behaviors (pre- and post-intervention). Parents also kept sleep diaries. The treatment group showed improvements on the Conners Scale ($p<0.05$) and in observation measures of play behaviors including a greater decrease in stereotypical behaviors ($t=2.01$, $p<0.05$) and a greater increase in on-task behavior ($t=2.13$, $p<0.05$), and better sleeping patterns as evidenced by more time spent in deep sleep and less night wakening. The latter results do not report statistical significance.

Field et al. (1997) examined the effects of touch therapy on inattention, touch aversion, and withdrawal in 22 children

with autism who had an average age of 4.5 years. Subjects were randomly assigned to either touch therapy or control. Touch therapy consisted of 15 min of touch in the form of moderate pressure and smooth strokes along the entire body. Children were assessed on the first and last day of intervention using the Autism Behavior Checklist (Krug et al. 1993) and the Early Social Communication Scales (Seibert et al. 1982). Touch aversion, off-task behavior, and orientating to irrelevant stimuli decreased in both groups although significantly ($p<0.05$) more in the treatment group. Only children in the touch-therapy group showed decreased scores on the sensory scale and the Autism Behavior Checklist. Children in the treatment group also showed significant ($p<0.05$) changes on the Early Social Communication Scales in the area of joint attention ($p<0.05$), behavioral regulation ($p<0.01$), social behavior ($p<0.05$), and initiating behavior ($p<0.01$).

Silva et al. (2009) completed a multisite, randomized control trial of massage, using a specific type of massage, Qigong Massage. They conducted a randomized controlled study of 46 children diagnosed with ASD and measured the effects of the treatment (Qigong massage) on adaptive behavior, sensory symptoms, digestion and sleep (all evaluated by parent and teacher report). Teacher report (blinded) showed that treated children had significant improvements in the language and social skills domains of the Vineland ($p<0.01$) and reduction in autistic behaviors ($p<0.03$) compared to controls. Parent data confirmed the findings and showed stability of results at 10 months. This study is strong methodologically as subjects were randomly assigned, interventionists were trained, and data were collected pre-treatment, post-treatment, and at 5 months following intervention; it thus provides emerging evidence for the use of Qigong Massage on the stated outcomes.

TABLE 9.3   Studies of touch-based treatments

Study	Participants	Outcome	Evidence-based rating	Quality indicators present
Escalona et al. 2001	$N=20$ children aged 3–6 years with ASD	Dependent Variables: off-task behavior and sleep problems via the Conner's Scale and teachers' observations. *Results*: children who received massage therapy showed increases in on-task behavior, attentiveness and better sleeping patterns	Adequate	• Primary: independent variable, comparison condition exists but does not specifically indicate what it was, dependent variable, use of statistical tests • Secondary: random assignment
Field et al. 1997	$N=22$ children (12 male, 10 female) average age of 4.5 years with ASD	Touch aversion, off-task behavior, orienting to irrelevant sounds, and stereotypic behaviors decreased in both groups (orienting to irrelevant sounds and stereotypic behaviors decreased significantly more in the touch therapy group). Only children in the touch therapy group showed decreased scores on the sensory scale, relating scale, and the total scores of the ABC. Children in the touch therapy group showed significant changes in joint attention, behavior regulation, social behavior, and initiating behavior.	Strong	• Primary: participant information, independent variable, comparison condition, dependent variable, use of statistical tests, link better research question and data analysis • Secondary: random assignment
Silva et al. 2009	$N=26$ children aged 3–6 years with an educational diagnosis of autism but no additional medical diagnoses	Pre-test to post-test differences on standardized measures (adaptive behavior, sensory impairment and autistic behavior) were all found to be statistically significant at .003 level or better. Trainers and parents were able to administer intervention in a reliable manner.	Strong	• Primary: participant information, independent variable, dependent variable, use of statistical tests (pre–post test differences on objective, standardized measures), link research question, and data analysis • Secondary: fidelity rating, social validity • Weakness: No comparison group, pre–post design
Edelson et al. 1999	$N=12$ children (nine male, three female) aged 4–13 years with a physician diagnosis of autism	Experimental group showed non-significant decreases in anxiety and tension after treatment; control group did not. Greater arousal (measured by galvanic skin response) may predict greater efficacy of deep pressure.	Weak	• Primary: participant characteristics, independent variable, comparison condition, dependent variable, use of statistical tests • Secondary: random assignment.

Edelson et al. (1999) reported a study of the effects of deep pressure on arousal and anxiety. The study used the Grandin hug machine (Grandin 1992), a device that allows for self-administration of lateral body pressure. Twelve subjects (nine males and three females ranging from 4 to 13 years of age) with a physician diagnosis of autism participated but there was no detail of the methods used for diagnosis. Five subjects were in the experimental condition and subjects were matched on age and gender. Prior to administration of treatment, both groups showed statistically similar levels of arousal and anxiety. Outcome measures were galvanic skin response (GSR) measured before and immediately after each session, the Conners' parent rating scale (Goyette et al. 1978), and a side effects questionnaire to measure any side effects of the deep pressure. Data from the Conners' scale was assessed using a 2×3 (group × time) MANOVA (pre-, mid-, and post-session time points) and showed that the tension and anxiety decreased in the experimental group ($p < 0.05$ and $p < 0.10$ respectively). Results of GSR are difficult to evaluate as they rely on demonstrating that physiological and behavioral measures converged prior to treatment and remain highly correlated with each other throughout the study. Further, in evaluating changes in GSR between the groups, there were non-significant differences but the authors did note that variability in GSR increased in the treatment group and decreased in the control group. They felt that this observation suggested that individuals within the treatment group responded differently to the intervention and thus, divided them into responders or non-responders based on their initial levels of anxiety or arousal. They found a marginally significant difference between those who benefited and those who did not – those who benefited were more likely to have higher GSR – but the sample sizes for this analysis are very small. They

suggest that greater arousal may predict greater efficacy of deep pressure. This study is weak in that many of the study characteristics were not described (participant characteristics, inter-rater reliability) and random assignment was not detailed. The study did identify the independent and dependent variables, describe the comparison condition, and statistical tests, but findings were weak and liberties were taken in the interpretation of the findings.

Collectively, the studies using touch as the intervention show encouraging evidence in that improvements in target behaviors are noted. In general, the studies describe an intervention that can be replicated, describe the subject characteristics in detail, and utilize accepted statistical procedures in the data analysis and interpretation. Drawing strong conclusions from this data is limited, however, by the variability in intervention (touch pressure vs. massage) and the lack of an active control group or fidelity measure.

Interventions That Utilize Weighted Vests

Six studies, shown in Table 9.4, examined the effect of using weighted vests in children with ASD on attention, self-stimulatory behaviors, or on-task behaviors. One confounding factor in interpretation of these studies is that the weighted vest, although it provides mainly proprioception (the weight of the vest requires that increased muscle activity be utilized and thus increases the proprioceptive signals from the muscles, joints and tendons) may also provide some amount of pressure touch (due to the vest being placed on the torso) and thus, it is difficult to determine the nature of the stimuli that is being studied.

Fertel-Daly et al. (2001) examined the effects of weighted vests on five subjects with PDD (aged 2–4 years old) using an

TABLE 9.4 Studies of weighted vest treatments

Study	Participants	Outcome	Evidence-based rating	Quality indicators present
Ferrel-Daly et al. 2001	$N = 5$ children aged 2–4 diagnosed with PDD; one also with autism	During intervention, focused attention to task increased; during intervention withdrawal, it decreased but stayed above the baseline level. During intervention, the number of distractions decreased; during intervention withdrawal, it increased but stayed below the baseline level. During intervention, four participants showed a decrease in the duration of self-stimulatory behaviors and one showed an increase. During intervention withdrawal, self-stimulatory behaviors increased. Parent and teacher behavioral reports were all positive for children who received intervention with weighted vests and reported gains in areas not directly tested by this study.	Adequate	• Primary: participant characteristics, independent variable, dependent variable, link between research question and data analysis • Secondary: inter-observer agreement, social validity
Kane et al. 2004–05	$N = 4$; three subjects with autism and one participant with PDD A–B–C design: no vest, vest with no weight, weighted vest	No significant improvements in attention or decreases in stereotypic behaviors with the use of a weighted vest.	Adequate	• Primary: participant characteristics, independent variable, dependent variable, link between research question and data analysis • Secondary quality indicator: social validity • Weakness: no interobserver agreement assessed
Olson and Moulton 2004	$N = 514$ pediatric occupational therapists	The majority of weighted vests used support therapeutic and occupational goals. Protocols for using weighted vests varied and were difficult to follow, although the majority of respondents (73%) recommended wearing the vest for less than 1 h each time.	Not applicable	Evidence-based rating is not applicable as this is a survey of occupational therapists' perspectives on the use of weighted vests.

Study	Subjects	Findings	Rating	Notes
Stephenson and Carter 2009	Subjects described in the individual studies	Four articles claimed the weighted vests proved ineffective in reducing problem behaviors. One article produced mixed results. Two articles claimed the weighted vests proved effective in reducing problem behaviors.	Not applicable	Evidence-based rating is not applicable as this is a review of current research.
Cox et al. 2009	$N=3$ subjects of elementary school age, with a diagnosis of autism and intellectual disability and sensory processing abnormalities (as measured by the Short Sensory Profile)	The weighted vest did not have an effect on in-seat behavior. The behavioral intervention (noncontingent reinforcement) improved in-seat behavior.	Adequate	• Primary: participant characteristics, independent variable, dependent variable, link between research question and data analysis • Secondary: social validity strong, interobserver agreement assessed • Weakness: single subject case study, autism diagnosis was made using different assessments at varied locations, assessment of sensory processing inadequate
Reichow et al. in press	$N=3$ subjects, ages 2–6 years, with an educational or medical diagnosis of autism or developmental delay	For one subject, there was an increase in problematic behaviors when wearing the vest and a decrease in stereotypic behaviors. There were no differences for the other two subjects in any of the observed behaviors among the three conditions.	Strong	• Primary: participant characteristics, independent variable, comparison condition, dependent variable, link between research question and data analysis, use of statistical tests • Secondary: random assignment, inter-rater agreement, social validity

A–B–A withdrawal single subject study. Observations of focused attention to task, number of distractions, and duration and type of self-stimulatory behaviors during a 5-min fine motor activity were collected and plotted for visual analysis. Data for the intervention began in the third week of the study. The intervention consisted of wearing the weighted vest (four quarter-pound weights) three times per week for 2 weeks. Vests were worn for 2 h as soon as the child arrived at school and data were collected after 1.5 h of wearing the vest. Intervention was discontinued in the fifth week of the study and data were collected for two additional weeks. Results compared mean duration of focused attention, number of distractions, and duration of self-stimulatory behavior during each phase of the study. The authors concluded through visual analysis that all subjects' data "supports the clinical observation that a weighted vest had a positive effect on at least two measures of attention for all five participants" (Fertel-Daly et al. 2001, page 638). An additional finding was that the increase in focused attention that occurred during the intervention was not sustained when the vest was removed and four participants had an abrupt drop in the duration of focused attention to task. The article concluded that a weighted vest "appeared to be beneficial... for five children with PDD who had difficulty attending to tasks and who exhibited self-stimulatory behaviors."

Kane et al. (2004–05) conducted a single subject study with an A–B–C (no vest, vest with no weight, weighted vest) counterbalanced design with three subjects with autism and one participant with PDD using a vest specifically made for the study that was 5% of the child's weight. The findings indicated no significant improvements in attention or decreases in stereotypic behaviors with the use of a weighted vest and the authors conclude that their study does not support the use of a weighted vest to decrease stereotypic behaviors or improve attention. The study design was single subject and thus the generality of these findings is limited. In addition, the study is flawed in that inter-observer agreement was not assessed. It is difficult to assess if findings are specifically related to the weight of the vest or to other qualities of the study (the vest was noted to be distracting to some subjects, activities provided to evaluate attention were not counterbalanced), nonetheless, this study is methodologically strong in its adherence and use of the single subject A–B–C design.

Reichow et al. (in press) completed a study of three subjects (aged 2–6 years), with an educational or medical diagnosis of autism or developmental delay, to determine if wearing a weighted vest increased engagement during a table-top activity. The vest was 5% of the child's weight. This study was methodologically strong in that it utilized an alternating treatments design with three conditions (vest with weight, vest with no weight, and no vest), controlled for the vest-with-no-weight condition to ensure that there were no visually perceived differences between this and the weighted-vest conditions and thus the observers were blind to the study condition, and the conditions were randomly assigned based on a 5-day schedule (for example, one child might have 2 days with no vest, then 2 days with a vest and 1 day without the vest whereas another subject might have a different schedule). Videotape recordings of behavior during table-top activities were utilized and raters coded for engagement, non-engagement, stereotypic behaviors, and problem behaviors. Each behavior was defined. Interobserver agreement was excellent (0.93–0.96). Findings are reported by subject. For one subject there was an increase in problematic behaviors when wearing the vest and a decrease in stereotypic behaviors. There were no differences for the other two subjects in any of the observed behaviors among the three conditions. Findings do not provide any evidence of positive gain from the vest and suggested the possibility of negative outcomes (i.e., decreased engagement). This study provides emerging evidence that weighted vests are not effective for improving engagement during table-top activities. The quality of the study is high given the attention to methodological issues stated above, however, the ability to generalize is limited by the SSED methodology and would be strengthened by including a greater number of sessions. The observers were graduate students and it is not clear if they were blind to the opinions of the other members of the research team. The social validity of the study is high in that it is an area of high interest for teacher, clinicians, and families.

Cox et al. (2009) examined the effects of a weighted vest, a vest with no weights and no vest on in-seat behavior during a group activity on three elementary-age students with autism, intellectual disabilities, and sensory processing difficulties. This study was methodologically strong as it used an alternating treatments design to compare the effects of the three conditions – the three conditions are randomly and rapidly alternated and counterbalanced across participants to control for sequence effects – and then utilized a generalization condition to determine if effects would generalize to a different group activity. In-seat behavior was defined and evaluated by viewing videotapes of observed behaviors in 10-s intervals. Interobserver agreement on occurrence (94.7% average agreement) and nonoccurrence ratings of behaviors (88.2% average agreement) was good. The percentage of intervals for appropriate in-seat behavior was visually displayed for baseline and each condition and the percentage overlap between conditions was calculated by counting the number of data points in the second condition that fall within the range of the first condition and then multiplying by 100. High percentages of overlap were found and, thus,

the authors concluded that the weighted vest did not have an effect on appropriate in-seat behavior for the participants. A second experiment was conducted to evaluate whether a behaviorally based intervention (noncontingent reinforcement, where subjects were given the choice of two highly preferred objects that they were allowed to access during the group activity) had an effect on in-seat behavior. Findings indicated that this strategy did improve in-seat behavior in the subjects. The authors concluded that, for these participants, the behavioral intervention had a stronger effect on in-seat behavior than the sensory intervention even though participants were identified as having sensory processing abnormalities.

This study is limited by the use of single subject methodology and thus the findings cannot be generalized. Another limitation is that the subjects were diagnosed with autism using different assessments and at different institutions. In addition, in-seat behavior was scored based on the subjects remaining in their seat for a full 10 s, which may limit the ability to detect changes that occur in smaller time increments. Finally, the study suggests that they were evaluating the effects of "sensory integration" whereas they are studying the effects of one sensory modality; they suggest that the study evaluates "deep pressure" on in-seat behavior, although it is difficult to determine if deep pressure (from the tightness of the vest) was provided at all or if the major sensory system stimulated was proprioception (as is generally the case with a weighted vest). This is important because it points to confusion about the use of sensory integration as opposed to sensory-based (single sensory system) strategies and the need to tailor treatment strategies to the individual needs of the child. For example, based on the information provided, it is impossible to evaluate whether the choice of the weighted vest was made based on the subjects scoring deficient in proprioceptive processing or some other criteria. Of note, only one subject scored in the "definite difference" range on tactile sensitivity and there is no information about proprioceptive processing. This issue speaks to the importance of individually tailoring sensory-based interventions to the child's specific needs rather than utilizing a strategy for all subjects universally. Further, this issue speaks to the importance of a comprehensive assessment of the child's ability to process and integrate sensory information that includes not only a measure of sensory modulation (as in the Short Sensory Profile) but a more comprehensive assessment of processing and integration of sensation and its effects on praxis and behavior.

Of the remaining two reports on weighted vests used with an ASD population, one article was a review of existing studies (Stephenson and Carter 2009) and another was a survey of therapists (members of the School-Based Special Interest Section or the Sensory Integration Special Interest Section of the American Occupational Therapy Association, AOTA) to determine their protocols and clinical reasoning for using weighted vests (Olson and Moulton 2004). These two reviews are shown in Table 9.4 but not elaborated on here.

Overall, the use of weighted vests to improve attention and self-stimulating behaviors is difficult to evaluate as few studies were found for children with ASD and they were conducted using SSED.

Auditory Interventions

Four studies, shown in Table 9.5, report on auditory interventions with children with ASD. Conclusions from this group of studies are difficult because they utilize different types of auditory intervention with varying levels of rigor, however, there is a trend that auditory interventions do not demonstrate any notable improvements in behaviors over either no treatment or a control condition of auditory input.

Mudford et al. (2000) reported a crossover experimental design study of 16 children with autism using an auditory integration training developed by Berard (1993). The intervention program involved playing modified music through headphones for 30-min sessions twice a day for 10 days whereas the control condition played music in the room but not through the training device or headphones. The study is promising in that participants were adequately described (ages 5.7–13.9 years with an average age of 9.42); the diagnosis of autism was confirmed based on the *International Classification of Diseases and Related Health Problems*, 10th edition (ICD-10; World Health Organization 1992) and DSM-IV (APA 1994) classifications; and measures of cognitive abilities and adaptive behavior were used. Dependent variables were the Aberrant Behavior Checklist (Aman et al. 1996) and direct observational recordings of behavior for an average of 3.82 h across the 14 months of the study. They reported seven statistically significant effects from 32 dependent variables, but none of the effects favored the auditory intervention. For example, they found that parent-rated behaviors on the Aberrant behavior checklist decreased more following the control condition compared to the auditory training intervention (Wilcoxon $z = 1.91$, $p = 0.06$, two-tailed) and that ear occlusion increased after the auditory intervention ($p = 0.03$). Overall IQ scores on the Leiter did not increase significantly (decreased from 68 to 66) and Vineland Adaptive Behavior Composite scores decreased but not significantly. The authors concluded that the control condition was more beneficial than the auditory integration training.

Corbett et al. (2008) reported a study designed to test the effects of the Tomatis Method on language skills. Eleven subjects

TABLE 9.5 Studies of auditory interventions

Study	Participants	Outcome	Evidence-based rating	Quality indicators present
Bettison 1996	$N = 80$ children (66 male and 14 female) Aged 3.9–17.1 years, with a primary diagnosis from an independent agency of autism, significant autism symptoms, or Asperger syndrome	There were marked improvements in the behavioral measures for both groups at 1 month but there was a general lack of differences between the groups.	Strong	*Primary*: participant characteristics, independent variable, comparison condition, dependent variable, power analysis, and use of statistical tests *Secondary*: random assignment, inter-rater agreement, social validity
Mudford et al. 2000	$N = 16$ children (17 male, 4 female) Aged 5.75–13.92 years, with a diagnosis of autism	ABC scores were lower following control treatment than AIT. Much of the change in behavior was not statistically significant. Overall, researchers state no behavioral benefits from AIT therapy.	Adequate	*Primary*: Participant characteristics, independent variable, comparison condition, dependent variable, use of statistical tests *Secondary*: random assignment, blind raters
Sinha et al. 2006	Subjects described in the individual studies	Two studies did not find consistent improvement in behavior. Three trials found small improvements when groups were compared to control. Measures of cognitive ability and hearing sensitivity did not differ when compared between groups.	Not applicable	Evidence-based rating is not applicable as this is a review of current research
Corbett et al. 2008	$N = 11$ children (9 male and 2 female) Aged between 3.5 and 7.2 years, with autism	No significant difference found between treatment and placebo groups on language tests. All subjects showed progression in verbal reception over the course of the study; however, this progression did not correlate with the administration of Tomatis Sound Therapy.	Strong	

with autism (based on DSM-IV criteria (APA 1994)), which was corroborated by the Autism Diagnostic Observation Schedule (ADOS; Lord et al. 2002) and clinical judgment. Subjects were aged 3.5–7.2 years; nine subjects were male and two were female. Outcomes were measured using the ADOS, the Stanford-Binet intelligence scale (Thorndike et al. 1986), the Peabody Picture Vocabulary Test (PPVT; Dunn and Dunn 1997), and the expressive one-word picture vocabulary test (Brownell 2000). They use a randomized, double-blind, placebo-controlled crossover design. Tomatis training was administered by trained assistants and researchers and parents were blind to condition. In keeping with the Tomatis Method, the combination of filtered music listened to through an "electronic ear" headphones and auditory feedback should result in enhanced auditory perception. However, no significant difference was found between treatment and control groups on the PPVT or the Expressive one-word picture vocabulary test and, thus, the authors concluded that their results do not provide evidence for the treatment.

Bettison (1996) reported a study of the long-term effects of auditory training on 80 children (66 males and 14 female), aged 3.9–17.1 years. All children had a primary diagnosis of autism, significant autism symptoms, or Asperger syndrome from an independent agency (no further information on autism diagnosis was provided). There were no differences between the groups on age, sex, or educational program attended. Auditory training followed the Berard (1993) method, which involved listening to filtered music on 16 CDs (up to 14 frequencies). The control group received structured listening to unmodified music under the same conditions as the treatment group (two half-hour sessions at least 4 h apart each day for 10 consecutive days). Measures included the Autism Behavior Checklist (ABC) (Krug et al. 1993), the Developmental behavior checklist (DBC),

parent and teacher (Brereton et al. 2002), subtests from the PPVT (Dunn and Dunn 1981), and the Leiter international performance scale (Roid and Miller 1997). Sensory behaviors were assessed using the sensory problems checklist and the sound sensitivity questionnaire (SSQ; Rimland and Edelson 1994). Scores on each child's audiogram were also assessed pre- and post-intervention. Inter-rater reliability was established for each measure and ranged from 0.90 to 0.99. T-tests to compare pre- and post-test scores were conducted at 1, 3, 6, and 12 months after intervention. Overall, there were marked improvements in the behavioral measures for both groups at 1 month, but there was a general lack of statistically significant differences between the groups. The authors suggested that the lack of difference between the groups suggests that, "some aspect of both conditions was operating to cause these changes" (Bettison 1996, p. 370). Of interest, the IQ scores as measured by the Leiter improved in both groups, however, the magnitude of improvement was greater for the intervention group. The authors felt that this may suggest an intervention effect on IQ score although they also noted that practice obtained during intervention cannot be ruled out as a factor influencing this finding. For example, for the ABC, statistically significant improvements were found at 1 month and these were maintained through 6 months but reverted to levels at 1 month when tested at 12 months. The main finding from this study is that both the auditory training and the structured listening may lead to reductions in auditory sensitivities but that further research is needed to confirm this finding. This study is strong in that it contains several primary quality indicators: participant characteristics are described, independent variable, intervention and comparison condition, and dependent variable are described, and the link between research question and data analysis is clear. The use of statistical tests is appropriate and several secondary quality indicators are present including random assignment and inter-rater agreement. The social validity is high in that the research addresses a question that is of high interest in the field.

Other Sensory Techniques

In this section, we consider three studies that each examined one specific other intervention (the Wilbarger Protocol, therapy balls, and sensory diet). They are summarized in Table 9.6.

Kimball et al. (2007) conducted a study to evaluate the Wilbarger protocol, which provides "very deep pressure input to the skin with a specially manufactured non-scratching brush followed by compression of the major joints" (Wilbarger and Wilbarger 2001, p. 406). They evaluated changes in salivary cortisol after 4 weeks of treatment. The protocol is designed to be administered every 1.5–2 h but it was administered only once per week in the morning so as to keep with the routine of the subjects. The study used a single subject A–B design with a convenience sample of four boys (aged 3–5 years) showing signs of sensory defensiveness as indicated by their primary occupational therapist. Sensory defensiveness was confirmed using the short sensory profile but no cut-off scores were mentioned. They also administered the Conners' Rating Scale (Conners 1997) to examine correlates of behavioral issues pre- and post-intervention. Although all children's salivary cortisol levels moved in the direction expected after application of the Wilbarger-based protocol, no statistical significance is reported. This study is very weak in that it lacked adequate subject descriptions, failed to report statistical significance, the protocol was not carried out in the way intended, the link between research question and data analysis was not clear and there was no mention of inter-rater agreement. The social validity is high

in that the research addresses a question that is of high interest in the field.

Schilling and Schwartz (2004) conducted a study to evaluate the use of therapy balls used as a seating alternative for young children with ASD on engagement and in-seat behavior. Four male subjects (aged from 3 years 11 months to 4 years 2 months) participated in a withdrawal SSED. Each subject had a physician diagnosis of ASD but no further detail about the diagnostic criteria was mentioned. Each participant's characteristics were described in detail and participants were selected for the study based on teacher reports of difficulty with engagement and in-seat behavior and the intervention was individualized based on each participant's situation (e.g., participant 1 received intervention during art activities in his extended day program and, since the length of time for each art activity varied, the data collection varied from 5 to 10 min). Data on dependent variables (sitting and engagement) were collected via real time sampling and interobserver agreement ranged from 82% to 100%. Intervention (use of therapy ball for classroom sitting during an individually chosen activity) was implemented for a minimum of 2 weeks. Three of the four participants showed immediate and substantial improvements for in-seat behavior with the implementation of therapy balls. These three individuals also showed a marked return to baseline levels upon withdrawal. This study is strong in that primary quality indicators such as independent variable, dependent variable, description of participants, and adherence to study design are evident as is the link between research question and data analysis. Social validity is directly addressed in the design of the study and data on social validity is collected via staff questionnaire.

Ingersoll et al. (2003) studied the effects of sensory feedback on immediate object imitation for children with ASD. Sensory feedback was achieved through the use of toys with flashing lights and sound. The

TABLE 9.6 Studies of other sensory techniques

Technique	Study	Participants	Outcome	Evidence-based rating	Quality indicators present
Wilbarger protocol	Kimball et al. 2007	N = 4 boys (receiving services at the Community Occupational Therapy Clinic, University of New England) aged 3–5 years, two with PDD or autism; all showed signs of sensory defensiveness, according to their primary occupational therapist	Although all children's salivary cortisol levels moved in the direction expected after application of the Wilbarger-based protocol, there is no statistical significance reported.	Weak	*Primary*: dependent variable *Secondary*: social validity
Therapy balls	Schilling and Schwartz 2004	N = 4 male children aged 3;11–4;2, with a physician diagnosis of ASD and reported by teachers as having trouble with in-seat behavior and difficulty with task engagement.	Three of the participants showed immediate and substantial improvements in in-seat behavior with the implementation of therapy balls. These individuals also showed a marked return to baseline levels upon withdrawal.	Strong	*Primary*: participant characteristics, independent variable, dependent variable, link between research question and data analysis *Secondary*: inter-observer agreement, social validity
Sensory feedback	Ingersoll et al. 2003	N = 15 children (nine boys, six girls) with autism and 14 children (five boys, nine girls) developing typically ages ranged from 23 to 53 months	Although overall imitation performance did not differ significantly between the two groups, the imitation performance of the participants with autism was significantly higher with sensory toys than with no sensory toys. Both groups played significantly more with the sensory toys during free play, suggesting that sensory toys were more reinforcing for both groups. It is argued that children with autism may be less motivated to imitate by social interaction but may be motivated to imitate to receive a nonsocial reward (sensory feedback).	Weak	*Primary*: participant characteristics, independent variable, dependent variable *Secondary*: social validity

subjects were 15 children (nine boys and six girls) with ASD and 14 typically developing children (five boys and nine girls). Subjects with ASD were previously diagnosed and confirmed by the study author. Participants ranged in age from 23 to 53 months and there were no differences between the groups on mental age. The experiment compared imitation using toys that had sensory feedback versus the same toy with no sensory feedback using the motor imitation scale (Stone et al. 1997). Analysis used mixed-model repeated measures ANOVA and although overall imitation performance did not differ significantly between the two groups, the imitation performance of the participants with autism was significantly higher with sensory toys than with non-sensory toys ($p < 0.02$). The imitation performance of typically developing participants did not differ between the two sets of toys and both groups played significantly more with the sensory toys during free play, indicating that the sensory toys were more reinforcing for both groups. Additional results demonstrated that typical children used significantly more social behaviors during imitation than children with autism, but they did not differ in object-oriented behaviors, replicating previous findings. It is argued that children with autism may be less motivated to imitate by social interaction, but may be motivated to imitate to receive a nonsocial reward (sensory feedback). Although inter-rater reliability was calculated (it ranged from 0.71 to 0.95) and the experimental conditions were clearly described, the diagnosis of autism was not confirmed, and the study did not report on a number of other primary and secondary quality indicators.

CONCLUSION

Overall, the data supporting the sensory-integrative approach is promising, whereas the data related to isolated sensory strategies is problematic. Several factors have limited the conduct of rigorously controlled studies of the sensory integration approach, including lack of a specific intervention protocol, the absence of a fidelity measure, and the paucity of meaningful outcome measures that are in keeping with the theoretical principles of the intervention and that describe changes at the levels of activity and participation as recommended by the World Health Organization (2001). These issues were discussed in the introductory section of this chapter, as were the efforts that are underway to fill these voids and lay the foundation for rigorous controlled studies. However, from the findings of the majority of studies that investigated the sensory-integrative approach, it is felt that there is emerging evidence to support the use of the sensory-integrative approach for individuals with ASD, in particular to impact sensory and motor outcomes and individual client-centered goals.

Overall, the studies of other sensory techniques, with the exception of Qigong Massage, do not establish the techniques as evidence-based and they should be regarded as still in the experimental stages. The strongest support comes from the group of studies using touch-based intervention; however, given that each study used different interventions, it is not possible to draw strong conclusions. Thus, touch-based interventions should also be used cautiously. In general, interventions that use isolated sensory techniques should be recommended cautiously and, when used, systematic data should be collected and analyzed frequently to assess utility. Given that many children with ASD are receiving treatment for their SD to help deal with behavioral issues and sensory sensitivities and parents and funding agencies are spending a great deal of money and time on these, the need for solid research has reached a critical level.

Acknowledgements

The author wishes to thank Amanda Pallotta for her assistance with the preparation of the manuscript.

REFERENCES

Adrien, J. L., Ornitz, E., Barthelemy, C., Sauvage, D., & Lelord, G. (1987). The presence or absence of certain behaviors associated with infantile autism in severely retarded autistic and nonautistic retarded children and very young normal children. *Journal of Autism and Developmental Disorders, 17*(3), 407–416.

Aman, M. G., Tasse, M. J., Rojahn, J., & Hammer, D. (1996). The Nisonger CBRF: A child behavior rating form for children with developmental disabilities. *Research in Developmental Disabilities, 17*(1), 41–57.

APA. (1994). *Diagnostic and statistical manual of mental disorders* (4th ed. – text revision). Washington, DC: American Psychiatric Association.

APA. (2000). *Diagnostic and statistical manual of mental disorders* (4th ed. – text revision). Washington, DC: American Psychiatric Association.

Ayres, A. J. (1979). *Sensory integration and the child.* Los Angeles, CA: Western Psychological Services.

Ayres, A. J. (1989). *The sensory integration and praxis tests.* Los Angeles, CA: Western Psychological Services.

Ayres, A. J., & Tickle, L. S. (1980). Hyperresponsivity to touch and vestibular stimuli as a predictor of positive response to sensory integration procedures by autistic children. *The American Journal of Occupational Therapy, 34*(6), 375–381.

Baranek, G. T. (1999). Autism during infancy: A retrospective video analysis of sensory-motor and social behaviors at 9–12 months of age. *Journal of Autism and Developmental Disorders, 29*(3), 213–224.

Baranek, G. T. (2002). Efficacy of sensory and motor interventions for children with autism. *Journal of Autism and Developmental Disorders, 32*(5), 397–422.

Baranek, G. T., David, F. J., Poe, M. D., Stone, W. L., & Watson, L. R. (2006). Sensory experiences questionnaire: Discriminating sensory features in young children with autism, developmental delays, and typical development. *Journal of Child Psychology and Psychiatry and Allied Disciplines, 47*(6), 591–601.

Benevides, T., Schaaf, R., Toth-Cohen, S., Johnson, S. L., & Madrid, G. (2010) The everyday routines of families of children with autism: Examining the impact of sensory processing difficulties in children with autism on the family. Presented at 9th International Meeting for Autism Research, Philadelphia, PA, May 2010.

Berard, G. (1993). *Hearing equals behaviour.* New Canaan, CT: Keats Publishing.

Bettison, S. (1996). The long-term effects of auditory training on children with autism. *Journal of Autism and Developmental Disorders, 26*(3), 361–374.

Brereton, A. V., Tonge, B. J., Mackinnon, A. J., & Einfeld, S. L. (2002). Screening young people for autism with the developmental behavior checklist. *Journal of the American Academy of Child and Adolescence Psychiatry, 41*(11), 1369–1375.

Brownell, R. (2000). *Expressive one-word picture vocabulary test.* Novato, CA: Academic Therapy Publications.

Case-Smith, J., & Bryan, T. (1999). The effects of occupational therapy with sensory integration emphasis on preschool-age children with autism. *The American Journal of Occupational Therapy: Official Publication of the American Occupational Therapy Association, 53*(5), 489–497.

Conners, K. (1997). *Conners' rating scales – revised.* North Tonawanda, NY: Multi-Health Systems.

Cook, D. G. (1991). The assessment process. In W. Dunn (Ed.), *Pediatric occupational therapy: Facilitating effective service provision* (pp. 35–72). Thorofare, NJ: Slack.

Corbett, B. A., Shickman, K., & Ferrer, E. (2008). Brief report: The effects of Tomatis sound therapy on language in children with autism. *Journal of Autism and Developmental Disorders, 38*(3), 562–566.

Cox, A. L., Gast, D. L., Luscre, D., & Ayres, K. M. (2009). The effects of weighted vests on appropriate in-seat behaviors of elementary-age students with autism and severe to profound intellectual disabilities. *Focus on Autism and Other Developmental Disabilities, 24*(1), 17–26.

Dawson, G., & Watling, R. (2000). Interventions to facilitate auditory, visual, and motor integration in autism: A review of the evidence. *Journal of Autism and Developmental Disorders, 30*(5), 415–421.

Dunn, L. M., & Dunn, L. M. (1981). *The peabody picture vocabulary test* (2nd ed.). Bloomington, MN: Pearson Assessments.

Dunn, L. M., & Dunn, L. M. (1997). *The peabody picture vocabulary test* (3rd ed.). Bloomington, MN: Pearson Assessments.

Edelson, S. M., Edelson, M. G., Kerr, D. C., & Grandin, T. (1999). Behavioral and physiological effects of deep pressure on children with autism: A pilot study evaluating the efficacy of Grandin's hug machine. *The American Journal of Occupational Therapy, 53*(2), 145–152.

Escalona, A., Field, T., Singer-Strunck, R., Cullen, C., & Hartshorn, K. (2001). Brief report: Improvements in the behavior of children with autism following massage therapy. *Journal of Autism and Developmental Disorders, 31*(5), 513–516.

Fazlioglu, Y., & Baran, G. (2008). A sensory integration therapy program on sensory problems for children with autism. *Perceptual and Motor Skills, 106*(2), 415–422.

Fertel-Daly, D., Bedell, G., & Hinojosa, J. (2001). Effects of a weighted vest on attention to task and self-stimulatory behaviors in preschoolers with pervasive developmental disorders. *The American Journal of Occupational Therapy, 55*(6), 629–640.

Field, T., Lasko, D., Mundy, P., Henteleff, T., Kabat, S., et al. (1997). Brief report: Autistic children's attentiveness and responsivity improve after touch therapy. *Journal of Autism and Developmental Disorders, 27*(3), 333–338.

Goyette, C. H., Conners, C. K., & Ulrich, R. F. (1978). Normative data on revised Conners parent and teacher rating scales. *Journal of Abnormal Child Psychology, 6*(2), 221–236.

Grandin, T. (1992). Calming effects of deep touch pressure in patients with autistic disorder, college students, and animals. *Journal of Child and Adolescent Psychopharmacology, 2*(1), 63–72.

Grandin, T. (1995). *Thinking in pictures: And other reports from my life with autism.* New York: Random House.

Green, V. A., Pituch, K. A., Itchon, J., Choi, A., O'Reilly, M., & Sigafoos, J. (2006). Internet survey of treatments used by parents of children with autism. *Research in Developmental Disabilities, 27*(1), 70–84.

Huebner, R. (2001). *Autism: A sensorimotor approach to management.* Gaithersburg, MD: Aspen.

Ingersoll, B., Schreibman, L., & Tran, Q. H. (2003). Effect of sensory feedback on immediate object imitation in children with autism. *Journal of Autism and Developmental Disorders, 33*(6), 673–683.

Kane, A., Luiselli, J. K., Dearborn, S., & Young, N. (2004–05). Wearing a weighted vest as intervention for children with autism/pervasive developmental disorder: Behavioral assessment of stereotypy and attention to task. *The Scientific Review of Mental Health Practice, 3*(2), 19–24.

Kientz, M. A., & Dunn, W. (1997). A comparison of the performance of children with and without autism on the sensory profile. *The American Journal of Occupational Therapy, 51*(7), 530–537.

Kimball, J. G., Lynch, K. M., Stewart, K. C., Williams, N. E., Thomas, M. A., & Atwood, K. D. (2007). Using salivary cortisol to measure the effects of a Wilbarger protocol-based procedure on sympathetic arousal: A pilot study. *The American Journal of Occupational Therapy, 61*(4), 406–413.

Kiresuk, T. J., Smith, A., & Cardillo, J. E. (1994). *Goal attainment scaling: Applications, theory and measurement.* Hillsdale, NJ: Lawrence Erlbaum.

Krug, D., Arick, J., & Almond, P. (1993). *Autism screening instrument for educational planning.* Austin, TX: Pro-ed.

Larson, E. (2006). Caregiving and autism: How does children's propensity for routinization influence participation in family activities? *Occupational Therapy Journal of Research: Occupation, Participation and Health, 26*(2), 69–79.

Leekam, S. R., Nieto, C., Libby, S. J., Wing, L., & Gould, J. (2007). Describing the sensory abnormalities of children and adults with autism. *Journal of Autism and Developmental Disorders, 37*(5), 894–910.

Linderman, T. M., & Stewart, K. B. (1999). Sensory integrative-based occupational therapy and functional outcomes in young children with pervasive developmental disorders: A single subject study. *The American Journal of Occupational Therapy, 53*(2), 207–213.

Lord, C., Rutter, M., DiLlavore, P. C., & Risi, S. (2002). *Autism diagnostic observation schedule.* Los Angeles, CA: Western Psychological Services.

Lord, C., Wagner, A., Rogers, S., Szatmari, P., Aman, M., et al. (2005). Challenges in evaluating psychosocial interventions for autistic spectrum disorders. *Journal of Autism and Developmental Disorders, 35*(6), 695–711.

Mailloux, Z. (2006). Setting goals and objectives around sensory integration concerns. In R. C. Schaaf & S. Smith Roley (Eds.), *Sensory integration: Applying clinical reasoning to practice with diverse populations* (pp. 63–70). Austin, TX: PsychCorp.

Mailloux, Z., May-Benson, T. A., Summers, C. A., Miller, L. J., Brett-Green, B., et al. (2007). Goal attainment scaling as a measure of meaningful outcomes for children with sensory integration disorders. *The American Journal of Occupational Therapy, 61*(2), 254–259.

Mandell, D. S., Novak, M. M., & Levey, S. (2005). Frequency and correlates of treatment use among a community sample of children with autism. Paper presented at the International Meeting for Autism Research, Boston, MA.

McClure, M. K., & Holtz-Yotz, M. (1991). The effects of sensory stimulatory treatment on an autistic child. *The American Journal of Occupational Therapy, 45*(12), 1138–1142.

Miller, L. J., Coll, J. R., & Schoen, S. A. (2007). A randomized controlled pilot study of the effectiveness of occupational therapy for children with sensory modulation disorder. *The American Journal of Occupational Therapy, 61*, 228–238.

Miller, L. J., Schoen, S. A., James, K., & Schaaf, R. C. (2007). Lessons learned: A pilot study on occupational therapy effectiveness for children with sensory modulation disorder. *The American Journal of Occupational Therapy, 61*(2), 161–169.

Mudford, O. C., Cross, B. A., Breen, S., Cullen, C., Reeves, D., et al. (2000). Auditory integration training for children with autism: No behavioral benefits detected. *American Journal of Mental Retardation, 105*(2), 118–129.

National Research Council. (2001). *Educating young children with autism*. Washington, DC: National Academy Press.

O'Neill, M., & Jones, R. S. (1997). Sensory-perceptual abnormalities in autism: A case for more research? *Journal of Autism and Developmental Disorders, 27*(3), 283–293.

O'Riordan, M., & Passetti, F. (2006). Discrimination in autism within different sensory modalities. *Journal of Autism and Developmental Disorders, 36*(5), 665–675.

Olson, L. J., & Moulton, H. J. (2004). Use of weighted vests in pediatric occupational therapy practice. *Physical & Occupational Therapy in Pediatrics, 24*(3), 45–60.

Ornitz, E. M. (1974). The modulation of sensory input and motor output in autistic children. *Journal of Autism and Childhood Schizophrenia, 4*(3), 197–215.

Ornitz, E. M. (1989). *Autism: Nature, diagnosis, and treatment*. New York: Guilford.

Parham, D., & Mailloux, Z. (1995). Sensory integrative principles in intervention with children with autistic disorder. In J. Case-Smith, A. S. Allen, & P. N. Pratt (Eds.), *Occupational therapy for children* (3rd ed., pp. 329–382). St. Louis, MO: Mosby.

Parham, L. D., Cohn, E. S., Spitzer, S., Koomar, J. A., Miller, L. J., et al. (2007). Fidelity in sensory integration intervention research. *The American Journal of Occupational Therapy, 61*(2), 216–227.

Parham, L. D., Smith Roley, S., May Benson, T., Koomar, J., et al. (in press) Development of a fidelity measure for research on effectiveness of Ayres Sensory Integration intervention. *The American Journal of Occupational Therapy*.

Rapin, I., & Katzman, R. (1998). Neurobiology of autism. *Annals of Neurology, 43*(1), 7–14.

Reichow, B., Barton, E. E., Neeley, J., Good, L., & Wolery, M. (in press). Effects of wearing a weighted vest on engagement in young children with developmental disabilities. *Focus on Autism and Other Developmental Disabilities*.

Reichow, B., Barton, E. E., Neeley, J., Good, L., & Wolery, M. (2010). Effects of wearing a weighted vest on engagement in young children with developmental disabilities. *Focus on Autism and Other Developmental Disabilities, XX*(X) 1–9. http://www.sagepub.com/journalsPermissions.navDOI: 10.1177/1088357609353751

Rimland, B., & Edelson, S. M. (1994). The effects of auditory integration training on autism. *American Journal of Speech-Language Pathology, 3*, 16–24.

Rogers, S. J., & Ozonoff, S. (2005). Annotation: What do we know about sensory dysfunction in autism? A critical review of the empirical evidence. *Journal of Child Psychology and Psychiatry and Allied Disciplines, 46*(12), 1255–1268.

Rogers, S. J., Hepburn, S., & Wehner, E. (2003). Parent reports of sensory symptoms in toddlers with autism and those with other developmental disorders. *Journal of Autism and Developmental Disorders, 33*(6), 631–642.

Roid, G. H., & Miller, L. J. (1997). *Leiter international performance scale-revised*. Wood Dale, IL: Stoelting.

Schaaf, R. C., & Miller, L. J. (2005). Occupational therapy using a sensory integrative approach for children with developmental disabilities. *Mental Retardation and Developmental Disabilities Research Reviews, 11*(2), 143–148.

Schaaf, R. C., & Nightlinger, K. M. (2007). Occupational therapy using a sensory integrative approach: A case study of effectiveness. *The American Journal of Occupational Therapy, 61*(2), 239–246.

Schaaf, R.C, Benevides, T., Johnson S., Madrid, G., Toth-Cohen, S. (2010). The everyday routines of families of children with autism: Examining the impact of sensory processing difficulties on the family. Presented at 9th International Meeting for Autism Research, Philadelphia, PA, May 2010.

Schaaf, R.C, Benevides, T., Johnson S., Madrid, G.; Toth-Cohen, S. (in press – accepted for publication). The everyday routines of families of children with autism: examining the impact of sensory processing difficulties on the family. *Autism Research*

Schaaf, R. C., Schoen, S. A., Smith Roley, S., Lane, S. J., Koomar, J. A., & May-Benson, T. A. (2010). A frame of reference for sensory integration. In P. Kramer & J. Hinojosa (Eds.), *Frames of reference for pediatric occupational therapy* (3rd ed.). Philadelphia, PA: Lippincott Williams & Wilkins.

Schaaf, R. C., Blanche, E. I., Mailloux, Z., Benevides, T., Burke, J. P., et al. (in preparation). The sensory integration intervention manual.

Schilling, D. L., & Schwartz, I. S. (2004). Alternative seating for young children with autism spectrum disorder: Effects on classroom behavior. *Journal of Autism and Developmental Disorders, 34*(4), 423–432.

Schwenk, H.A. & Schaaf, R.C. (2003). Assessments used by occupational therapists working with children with autism. Pennsylvania Occupational Therapy Association Annual Conference, Pittsburg, PA.

Seibert, A., Hogan, E., & Mundy, P. C. (1982). Assessing interactional competencies: The early social-communication scales. *Infant Mental Health Journal, 3*(4), 244–258.

Silva, L. M., Ayres, R., & Schalock, M. (2009). Outcomes of a pilot training program in a qigong massage intervention for young children with autism. *The American Journal of Occupational Therapy, 62*(5), 538–546.

Sinha, Y., Silove, N., Wheeler, D., & Williams, K. (2006). Auditory integration training and other sound therapies for autism spectrum disorders: A systematic review. *Archives of Disease in Childhood, 91*(12), 1018–1022.

Smith Roley, S., & Mailloux, Z. (2007). Understanding Ayres sensory integration. *Occupational Therapy Practice, 12*(17), CE1–CE7.

Smith, S. A., Press, B., Koenig, K. P., & Kinnealey, M. (2005). Effects of sensory integration intervention on self-stimulating and self-injurious behaviors. *The American Journal of Occupational Therapy, 59*(4), 418–425.

Stephenson, J., & Carter, M. (2009). The use of weighted vests with children with autism spectrum disorders and other disabilities. *Journal of Autism and Developmental Disorders, 39*(1), 105–114.

Stone, W. L., Ousley, O. Y., & Littleford, C. D. (1997). Motor imitation in young children with autism: What's the object? *Journal of Abnormal Child Psychology, 25*(6), 475–485.

Thorndike, R. L., Hagen, E. P., & Sattler, J. M. (1986). *Stanford-Binet intelligence scale* (4th ed.). Itasca, IL: Riverside Publishing.

Tomchek, S. D., & Dunn, W. (2007). Sensory processing in children with and without autism: A comparative study using the short sensory profile. *The American Journal of Occupational Therapy, 61*(2), 190–200.

Watling, R. L., & Dietz, J. (2007). Immediate effect of Ayres's sensory integration-based occupational therapy intervention on children with autism spectrum disorders. *The American Journal of Occupational Therapy, 61*(5), 574–583.

Wilbarger, P. L., & Wilbarger, J. L. (2001). *Sensory defensiveness: A comprehensive treatment approach.* Panorama City, CA: Avanti Educational Programs.

Williams, D. (1992). *Nobody nowhere: The extraordinary autobiography of an autistic.* New York: Crown.

Williams, D. (1994). *Somebody somewhere: Breaking free from the world of autism.* New York: Crown.

World Health Organization. (1992). *International classification of diseases and related health problems* (10th ed.). Geneva, Switzerland: WHO.

World Health Organization. (2001). *International classification of functioning, disability and health.* Geneva, Switzerland: WHO.1Ayres Sensory Integration was trademarked in an effort to clarify the concepts that reflect Ayres's sensory integration framework and to distinguish it from other sensory approaches that do not use Ayres work in the way it was intended (Smith Roley and Mailloux 2007)

CHAPTER 10

Dietary, Complementary and Alternative Therapies

Susan L. Hyman and Susan E. Levy

ABBREVIATIONS

ADHD	Attention deficit hyperactivity disorder
ASDs	Autism spectrum disorders
CAM	Complementary and alternative medical treatments
CGI	Clinical global improvement
DAN	Defeat Autism Now
GFCF	Gluten-free casein-free
HBOT	Hyperbaric oxygen therapy
NCCAM	National Center for Complementary and Alternative Medicine
NIH	National Institutes of Health
RCT	Randomized control trial

INTRODUCTION

Few treatments for autism generate as much controversy and consternation among families and caregivers than the group of treatments considered as complementary and alternative medical (CAM) treatments. Evidence-based practice should guide all treatments used for symptoms of autism, including behavioral, educational, medical biologic or complementary therapies. All interventions should be held to the same standards of evidence. This chapter discusses commonly used CAM therapies, reports the prevalence for use in children, reviews the factors promoting its use, and discusses the evidence-based evaluation of efficacy of treatments.

In an effort to advance the scientific rigor of the study of complementary and alternative medical practices, the National Center for Complementary and Alternative Medicine (NCCAM) of the National Institutes of Health (NIH) was established in 1998. Their mission is to "explore practices in the context of rigorous science, train CAM researchers, and disseminate authoritative information to public and professionals" (http://nccam.nih.gov). NCCAM defines complementary medicine as "practices that are outside traditional western medical practice that are used with

B. Reichow et al. (eds.), *Evidence-Based Practices and Treatments for Children with Autism*, DOI 10.1007/978-1-4419-6975-0_10, © Springer Science+Business Media, LLC 2011

conventional medicine" and alternative medicine as "practices used in place of conventional medicine." CAM therapies fall into five categories: alternative medical systems, biologically based practices, energy medicine, manipulative and body-based practices, and mind–body medicine. As interest in the use of CAM therapies has increased, the scientific evaluations in the literature have also increased.

EPIDEMIOLOGY OF CAM

It is difficult to determine the true prevalence of CAM use in the general population. Survey studies suffer from a lack of uniform definitions of CAM, differing types of treatments included in the categories of CAM, and differences in the populations under study (e.g., the general population or children with special health care needs) (Ernst 1999). Population-based estimates of the use of CAM among adults vary from 1.8% (Davis and Darden 2003) to 62% (Barnes et al. 2004). When prayer used specifically for health reasons is excluded, the rate of CAM usage dropped to 36% (Barnes et al. 2004), with biologically based therapies the most commonly reported. A recent online, self-administered survey of adolescents revealed lifetime rates of CAM use of 79% and current use of 48.5% (Wilson et al. 2006). Population-based data for the prevalence of use of CAM in younger children is not available. Surveys of pediatric-clinic-based populations report rates in 1994 of 11% (Spigelblatt et al. 1994) increasing to 41–51% in 2001 (Cincotta et al. 2006) and 58% in 2006 (Zuzak et al. 2008) Children with chronic illnesses report high rates in disorders such as cancer (20–90%) (Kelly 2007), juvenile rheumatoid arthritis (70–92%) (Rouster-Stevens et al. 2008) and diabetes mellitus (18%) (Dannemann et al. 2008) Children with developmental disabilities have among the highest reported rates

for use of CAM. Disorder-specific rates reported include: ADHD (12–64%) (Weber and Newmark 2007), cerebral palsy (56%) (Liptak 2005), Down syndrome (87%) (Roizen 2005), and ASD (30–90%) (Hanson et al. 2007; Weber and Newmark 2007; Wong and Smith 2006).

DECISION TO USE CAM FOR SYMPTOMS OF ASD

Many families choose to use CAM therapies for their children with ASD based on their perception of its safety, the belief that there are fewer side effects and the feeling that it is "natural" (Hanson et al. 2007; Rhee et al. 2004). Some families reported that they elected for CAM interventions because of a desire for more control over treatment selection, based on information obtained on the internet or from friends or families of other children with ASD, or the promise of a cure (Cincotta et al. 2006). Other motivating factors for the choice of CAM therapies may be the promise of treatment of significant comorbid symptoms, such as gastrointestinal difficulties, that are not acknowledged by their primary health care provider (Levy and Hyman 2005). Predictive factors for the use of CAM include use of CAM by a parent (often the mother), higher educational levels of the parents (Barnes et al. 2004), and greater severity of diagnosis reported by parents (Hanson et al. 2007).

EVALUATION OF CAM THERAPIES

The principles used for review of the evidence supporting other interventions for ASD can, and should, be applied to CAM therapies. While the hierarchy of evidence used for assessment of interventions for ASD has been examined in Chaps. 1–3, there are particular caveats that are unique to the evaluation of CAM therapies. Many practitioners who support CAM therapies come from outside traditional medical and scientific backgrounds and believe that scientific methodology used to assess other types of interventions cannot be used for CAM therapy because of the number of modifying variables and the complex interactions between components of therapy (Patel and Curtis 2007). Some proponents of CAM therapies argue that the randomized control trial is less appropriate than a randomized comparison trial, quasi-experimental designs, or non-experimental designs to assess and evaluate therapeutic practices (Hyland 2003). Special considerations in reviewing the evidence regarding CAM therapies include:

Characterization of the Population Under Study

As age, phenotypic variation within ASD, and other medical comorbidities may affect response to therapy, it is important that consistent diagnosis and careful description of the recruited population are used to define the population studied. This may not be the case in reports of community ascertained populations or studies led by researchers with limited clinical science expertise in ASD diagnosis (Gupta et al. 1996; Sandler et al. 2000).

Standard Dosage

Biologic treatments including vitamins and herbs are not regulated for quality as medications are. Unless concentration of active substance, bioavailability, and activity is measured, it is not known if the intervention is providing consistent dosing. Unknown dosing makes interpretation of studies of supplements obtained commercially difficult to interpret (Adams and Holloway 2004). Similarly, when therapies

are based on an interaction with a therapist, manualization is important to understand the components of that intervention and allow for replication. Most studies of CAM interventions have not addressed this aspect of design, as in the example of Qigong massage therapy (Silva and Cignolini 2005).

Hierarchy of Study Design

While conventional pharmacologic interventions hold the randomized controlled trial (RCT) as the most rigorous test of a therapy, CAM practices are often prescribed in an interdependent fashion making it difficult to tease out the effect of a component therapy. Careful and stepwise assessment of each therapy and the interaction between them would both be costly and extend the time for well-designed studies to be completed. An example of this barrier to appropriate use of conventional study design is the DAN! Protocol (http://www.defeatautismnow.com).

Placebo Control

Sandler and Bodfish (2000) discussed the importance of placebo in the assessment of CAM therapies. The relationship with the provider, the time that families spend with their children in implementing CAM and the effects of other concomitant therapies make it even more important for placebo control conditions to be used in studies of CAM therapies. A single blind trial, such as that conducted by Knivsberg et al. (2002), is difficult to interpret because the family and school staff knew which participants were randomized to dietary treatments. Placebo conditions have been effectively used to study CAM therapies as diverse as hyperbaric oxygen therapy (Granpeesheh et al. 2009; Rossignol, Rossignol et al. 2009) and auditory integration training (Sinha et al. 2004,2006).

Use of Valid Outcome Measures

Investigators trained in other areas of science who enter clinical autism research may compromise the potential importance of their observations by use of inappropriate or nonstandard outcome measures. The children treated with B12 injections by James et al. (2004) in a metabolic evaluation of methylation demonstrated altered biochemical parameters which might be indicative of differences in metabolic pathways in at least a subgroup of children with ASD. However, absence of standard and valid outcome measures preclude their data from serving as support for this therapy clinically. Many CAM practitioners maintain that appropriate outcome measures that assess more holistic parameters of response to therapy are not yet available (Verhoef et al. 2006).

Appropriate Statistical Analysis

As discussed in prior chapters, confounding interventions, phenotypic variation, and the use of appropriate statistical analyses and sample size need to be considered in reviewing reports of interventions for ASD. This is especially true in examining the literature related to CAM therapies. For example, an inadequate sample size impacts the support that Amminger et al. (2007) can provide for treatment with omega-3 fatty acids. Rossignol, Rossignol et al. (2009) reported statistical improvement in behaviors in children with ASD treated with hyperbaric oxygen therapy based on improvement in clinician ratings of clinical global improvement (CGI) compared to controls. However more conservative statistical interpretation might be argued given the multiple comparisons, effect perceived by the parents during the placebo condition, and the absence of statistical difference in other measures such as the Aberrant Behavioral Checklist and the Autism Treatment Evaluation Checklist (ATEC) between groups. The ATEC is as yet not validated but it is used primarily in studies examining CAM for autism to assess change with treatment (Autism Research 2005). The importance of appropriate statistical methodology and relating statistical change to clinical effect in clinical trials needs to be emphasized for both CAM and traditional interventions (Kazdin 2004). It is difficult to disprove the null hypothesis, that there is no difference between the outcome of two treatments or conditions. Given the influence of study design issues (e.g., sample size, representativeness of the larger population, use of appropriate statistical measures or comparisons, and others), it is much harder to prove something will not happen than to demonstrate it has happened in a few instances.

Challenges to Recruitment for Studies Evaluating CAM Therapies

There are unique challenges to the evidence-based evaluation of CAM therapies. While recruiting study participants is challenging for all clinical trials, there may be additional hesitancy on the part of families suspicious of conventional medicine. Advocates of CAM are increasingly promoting evidence-based examination of interventions (Kemper et al. 2008; Rossignol, Rossignol et al. 2009) but individual CAM practitioners may discourage their clients from participating in trials that they may perceive as attempting to prove the null hypothesis. Families who are considering CAM therapies have often read positive anecdotal reports in the media and may be unwilling to consider a trial where their child might get a placebo or delayed access to a "cure." Studies that examine how families use evidence, personal interactions, and media to decide on therapeutic choices will be important both in recruitment for future clinical trials and in knowing how to effectively disseminate scientific information that may impact family choices related to therapies. As with other areas of intervention, the literature contains studies and reports regarding CAM interventions of varying quality.

Evidence for Common CAM Treatments

For the purposes of this review, we discuss CAM therapies from the five categorical areas of NCCAM convention. We do not discuss alternative medical systems, which include Ayurveda (traditional Indian medicine), traditional Chinese medicine, homeopathic treatment and naturopathy. The rationales for these systems of belief are different from those used to support conventional medical practice. There is little data in the peer-reviewed, scientific literature to allow for comment on the validity of these systems or their role in the care of people with autism. This review does not include every CAM therapy used for symptoms of ASD but selects CAM therapies from each of the NCCAM categories for representative discussion.

Biologically Based Therapies

The most frequently reported CAM therapies for people with ASD are biologically based (vitamin supplementation and diet) and nonstandard use of medical therapies (Brown and Patel 2005). Prescription medications which have been the subject of off-label use include secretin (Williams et al. 2005), vancomycin (Sandler et al. 2000), and antifungal agents.

Elimination of grain products containing the peptide gluten (wheat, barley, rye) and dairy products which contain casein is a common intervention for ASD. Almost one third of children with ASD are treated with diet (Levy et al. 2003). While the initial hypothesis was that opiate peptides were absorbed across a leaky intestinal lining, this has not been substantiated (Cass et al. 2008). Many families empirically report clinical improvement with dietary elimination of gluten and casein (Christison and Ivany 2006). It is plausible that some children with ASD may have common pediatric problems, such as lactose intolerance or milk allergy, for example, and sleep, stool quality, or mood may be improved with less discomfort. It is plausible that other aspects of dietary change that accompany the elimination of gluten and casein may alter stool consistency or, perhaps, behavior (McCann et al. 2007)

Two small studies have examined the effect of a gluten-free, casein-free (GFCF) diet. A single-blind study of 20 children with ASD, randomized to a GFCF or a regular diet, suggested improvement in features of ASD after 1 year (Knivsberg et al. 2002). This study is compromised by the single-blind design, the lack of control for other therapies, and an absence of medical data regarding the participants, other than the presence of urinary peptides. Elder et al. (2006) published data on 15 children who completed a double-blind, placebo-controlled, crossover study. Limited information regarding medical factors was reported and outcome measures were limited in the capacity to detect change. While the dietary removal of dairy products places children at risk for decreased calcium and vitamin D intake and subsequent bone growth, it is possible to ingest adequate nutrition on this diet.

Table 10.1 briefly lists the trials that have taken place. Additional research is necessary to determine if behavioral effects of dietary elimination are detectable in subgroups of children with ASD and what those effects are.

Vitamins and Other Supplements

Almost half of families of children with ASD report giving their child vitamins or supplements (Green et al 2006). Given the

TABLE 10.1   Biological treatments or diets

	Rating	Study	Participants	Design, Outcome and Comment
GFCF diet				
Randomized Controlled Trials	× Rv	Millward et al. (2008)	*N* = 35	*Design:* Two RCT studies Outcome: Improvement in autistic traits, social isolation, ability to communicate and interact *Comment:* Evidence for efficacy is poor
	O	Knivsberg et al. (2002)	*N* = 10 diet, *N* = 10 control; all ASD; 5–12 years old	*Design:* Single-blind randomized trial *Outcome:* Improvement in language and symptoms of ASD *Comment:* Methodological problems—no controls for interventions or nutritional status; no assurance that controls did not use diet
	O	Elder et al. (2006)	*N* = 15; ASD; 2–16 years old	*Design:* RDB/PC crossover diet trial, 12 weeks *Outcome:* No difference in group data for autistic symptoms or urinary peptide levels; some subjective improvement
	×	Whiteley et al. (1999)	*N* = 22 on GF diet; autism, ASP, ASD; *N* = 6 no-diet control; autism, ASD	*Design:* OL diet trial *Outcome:* subjective improvement in some, from questionnaires and observation measures; no decrease in urinary peptides *Comment:* Methodological problems—blinding, subject definition, many others
GI meds, digestive enzymes				
Treatment Trial	×	Brudnak et al. (2002)	*N* = 46; ASD; 5–31 years old	*Design:* OL trial of "Enzymaid" supplement for 12 weeks *Outcome:* Subjective improvement, mostly to socialization and hyperactivity *Comment:* Methodological problems—37% dropouts, 40% on GFCF diet, 6 of 29 had adverse effects
Secretin				
Treatment Trials	● Rv	Williams et al. (2005)	14 studies; MA	RCTs have not shown improvements for core features of autism
	● Rv	Esch and Carr (2004)	*N* = 600; 17 studies; MA	Twelve of the 13 PC studies failed to demonstrate differential efficacy of secretin

KEY: ● = Strong, O = moderate, × = unacceptable
DB = double blind, *RDB* = randomized double blind, *PC* = placebo-controlled, *RCT* = randomized controlled trial, *Rv* = systematic review, *NDD* = neurodevelopmental disability, *MA* = meta-analysis, *OL* = open label

popularity of nutritional supplements as a treatment for symptoms of ASD, however, there are relatively few well-designed trials to support this practice. Vitamins and nutritional supplements are perceived as improving specific symptoms such as gastrointestinal and sleep behaviors (Adams and Holloway 2004). The societal pressure towards acceptance of "natural" interventions and the increasing education of conventional practitioners regarding CAM is leading to more acceptance and recommendation of nutritional approaches to management of symptoms. Almost half of pediatricians responding to a survey reported that they encourage their patients with ASD to take multivitamins, 25% report encouraging omega-3 fatty acids or melatonin, and 19% encourage use of probiotics (Golnik and Ireland 2009). Nutritional interventions may have biologic effects that affect behavioral and medical symptoms. Studies examining nutritional interventions need to include potential explanations for effects that reflect what is known about metabolism and biochemistry in addition to carefully looking at the role of comorbid disease states and subgroups with true metabolic abnormalities (James et al. 2009). The potential for side effects (e.g. loose stool with magnesium and other supplements) needs to be addressed in future studies. Table 10.2 briefly lists the trials that have taken place.

Immune-Mediated Treatment

The potential role of immune events during brain development that may impact the development of autism has led to both CAM therapies and nonstandard use of conventional therapies that are purported to enhance immune function. Family members have been reported to have increased rates of autoimmune disorders on self-reported inventories (Sweeten et al. 2003). No increased rate of clinically significant immune dysfunction or allergy has been documented in children with ASD (Bakkaloglu et al. 2008; Jyonouchi 2009) although there are reports of decreased immunoglobins and other parameters measured in the laboratory that have been examined relative to behaviors (Heuer et al. 2008). While there is an active research agenda investigating whether prenatal or atypical immunologic events are related to the neurobiology of ASD (Wills et al. 2007) neither biologic interventions marketed to enhance immune function nor general immune enhancement with products such as intravenous immunoglobulin (IVIg) have evidence to support their use for symptoms of ASD at this time. Table 10.3 briefly lists the trials that have taken place.

Chelation Therapy and Hyperbaric Oxygen Therapy

Table 10.4 briefly lists the trials of chelation and hyperbaric oxygen therapy that have taken place.

While there is no evidence in the peer-reviewed literature to support chelation therapy for symptoms of ASD, it remains a popular and very controversial complementary intervention. The lack of evidence to support an association of autism with administration of vaccines containing the preservative thimerosal is beyond the scope of this chapter (Fombonne 2008; Schechter and Grether 2008). Because of the concern held by many families that the ethylmercury preservative commonly used in pediatric vaccines in the United States prior to 2001 resulted in mercury toxicity and caused autism, chelation regimens became part of CAM practice. Although blood levels of mercury are not elevated in people with ASD, proponents of this theory believe that excretion of mercury compounds maybe faulty and there may be increased tissue stores (Adams et al. 2007). A clinical trial to assess safety and efficacy

TABLE 10.2 Vitamins and other supplements

	Rating	Study	Participants	Design, Outcome and Comment
B6/magnesium (Mg++)				
Treatment Trials	× Rv	Nye and Brice (2005)	N=41; 3 studies; MA	*Findling et al. (1997):* DB/PC, questionnaires; no group differences. *Kuriyama et al. (2002):* PC; significant difference in IQ score. *Review:* few studies, methodological problems with no recommendation for use of B6-Mg
	×	Mousain-Bosc et al. (2006)	N=33 treatment; PDD or autism; 1–10 years; N=36 control; typical	*Design:* Treatment B6/Mg++, no treatment in control. *Outcome:* Improved lab (increased intra-erthrocyte Mg++) and behavioral symptoms; when treatment stopped, symptoms reappeared. *Comment:* Methodological problems — change based on non-standardized measure, inappropriate controls
	O	Martineau et al. (1985)	N=60; autism; 3–14 years	*Design:* Crossed-sequential DB treatment trials (B6 and/or Mg++). *Outcome:* Improved rating scales, urinary excreted HVA, evoked potentials. *Comment:* Methodological problems — no placebo control
Dimethylglycine (DMG)				
Treatment Trials	O	Kern et al. (2001)	N=37; autism or PDD; 3–11 years; matched controls	*Design:* DB/PC trial, 4 weeks. *Outcome:* no group differences; both showed improvement on Vineland maladaptive behavior domain and ABC
	O	Bolman and Richmond (1999)	N=8; autism; males; 4–30 years	*Design:* DB/PC crossover, low dose DMG. *Outcome:* No group differences in rating scale. *Comment:* Methodological problems — low dose, small N
Vitamin C				
Treatment Trials	×	Adams and Holloway (2004)	N=11 treatment; ASD; 3–8 years; N=9 control	*Design:* RDB/PC trial, 3 months. *Outcome:* Improved sleep, GI by parent questionnaire. *Comment:* Methodological problems — dropout, small N
	O	Dolske et al. (1993)	N=18; autism; 6–19 years; residential school	*Design:* DB/PC, 30 weeks, Ritvo-Freeman scale. *Outcome:* Decrease in sensory motor symptoms. *Comment:* Methodological problems — sample, confounding variables, dependent measures

Category / Type	Rating	Study	Sample	Details
Carnosine Treatment Trial	○	Chez et al. (2002)	N=31; autism, PDD; 3–12 years	*Design:* DB/PC oral carnosine. *Outcome:* significant changes in observation and questionnaires. *Comment:* Methodological problems — confounds (some with epilepsy)
Omega-3 fatty acids Treatment Trial	○ ●	Amminger et al. (2007)	N=13; autism, severe behavior problems; 5–17 years	*Design:* RDB/PC, Omega-3 FA, EPA,DHA, 6 weeks. *Outcome:* Less hyperactivity, stereotypy; no adverse effects. *Comment:* Methodological problems — small N; short treatment. Risk–benefit ratio appears tolerable
Melatonin Treatment Trials	●	Wasdell et al. (2008)	N=51; NDD (with ASD); 2–18 years	*Design:* RDB/PC, crossover, followed by OL 3 months. *Outcome:* Improvement in somnologs, actigraphs, clinician and parent ratings
	●	Garstang and Wallis (2006)	N=7; ASD; 4–16 years	*Design:* RDB/PC crossover trial. *Outcome:* Reduced sleep latency and awakenings and increased total sleep time
	○	Andersen et al. (2008)	N=107; ASD; 2–18 years	*Design:* Retrospective case series and OL treatment. *Outcome:* Improvement 87%, continued problems 13%, worse 1%; safe, well-tolerated
	×	Giannotti et al. (2006)	N=25; autism; 2.5–9.5 years	*Design:* OL treatment. *Outcome:* Improved sleep patterns in all; maintained gains at 12 and 24 months; well tolerated
Oxidative stress Treatment Trial	×	James et al. (2009)	N=40; autism	*Design:* OL treatment with methylcobalamin. *Outcome:* Improvement metabolites and glutathione redox status; subjective behavior improvement (not quantified). *Comment:* Methodological problems — no correlation to clinical outcome
Folate Treatment Trial	×	Moretti et al. (2005)	N=1; autism; 6 years	*Design:* OL folinic acid, case study. *Outcome:* Pre-treatment low folate (CSF and blood); post-treatment corrected CSF abnormalities, improved motor skills

KEY: ● = Strong, ○ = moderate, × = unacceptable

DB=double blind, RDB=randomized double blind, PC=placebo controlled, RCT=randomized controlled trial, Rv=systematic review, NDD=neurodevelopmental disability, MA=meta-analysis, OL=open label

TABLE 10.3   Immune-mediated treatments

	Rating	Study	Participants	Design, Outcome and Comment
Anti-infectives (e.g., antibiotics, antifungal, anti-virals)				
Treatment trial	×	Sandler et al. (2000)	N = 11; autism regressive onset; 3.5–7 years	*Design*: OL short term oral vancomycin. *Outcome*: Short-term improvement; not suggested as useful therapy (potential resistance)
Case series	×	Niehus and Lord (2006)	N = 75 ASD; N = 29 ASD with regression; N = 24 typical controls	*Design*: Record review. *Outcome*: For ASD more otitis, antibiotic use, fewer fevers; no group difference in age of vaccination
Immunoglobulins				
Treatment trial	×	Plioplys (1998)	N = 10 autism (8 regressives); 4–17 years	*Design*: Open treatment trial, IVIg infusion every 6 weeks (4 infusions). *Outcome*: 5 subjects — no change; 4 subjects — mild improvement in attention span; no parents wanted to continue infusions post study. *Comment*: Methodological problems — small sample; not recommended as treatment
	○	DelGiudice-Asch et al. (1999)	N = 7; autism; 3.5–6 years	*Design*: OL trial, IVIg infusion, 6 months. *Outcome*: severity scales, questionnaires; no benefit identified
	×	Schneider et al. (2006)	N = 12; autism; 2–8 years	*Design*: OL trial, 8 weeks, fixed dose. *Outcome*: 50% response or remission; 25% dropout. Methodological issues
	●	Handen et al. (2009)	N = 125; autism and GI symptoms; 2–17 years	*Design*: RDB/PC, parallel groups, dose-ranging oral immunoglobulin. *Outcome*: no significant group differences

KEY: ● = Strong, ○ = moderate, × = unacceptable
DB = double blind, RDB = randomized double blind, PC = placebo controlled, RCT = randomized controlled trial, Rv = systematic review, NDD = neurodevelopmental disability, MA = meta-analysis, OL = open label

TABLE 10.4 Chelation and hyperbaric oxygen therapy

	Rating	Study	Participants	Design, Outcome and Comment
Chelation				
Case series	×	Geier and Geier (2007a)	N = 9	*Outcome:* observational, hypothetical mercury exposure
Treatment Trial	×	Geier and Geier (2007b)	N = 71	*Design:* OL treatment trial *Outcome:* Lab studies urinary porphyrins, with reductions noted post-chelation *Comment:* Methodological problems—no clinical correlation
	×	Geier and Geier (2006)	N = 11; autism; 6–11 years	*Design:* OL treatment trial with Lupron and DMSA (heavy metal chelator) *Outcome:* lab measurements, behavioral symptoms improved *Comment:* Methodological problems—subject diagnosis, small N, potential untoward side-effects
	O	Soden et al. (2007)	N = 15, autism; N = 4, typical control; 3–7 years	*Design:* OL DMSA provoked excretion test *Outcome:* Urinary levels—12 autism no elevation, 2 minor other heavy metal, 1 with mercury (after 1 month without fish ingestion, level normal) *Comment:* No evidence for excess body burden of mercury
Hyperbaric Oxygen Therapy (HBOT)				
Treatment trial	O	Rossignol, Rossignol, et al. (2007)	N = 18; autism; 3–16 years	*Design:* OL treatment, 40 hyperbaric sessions *Outcome:* no changes in lab measures oxidative stress; improvement c-reactive protein (CRP); parental report of improvements
	O	Rossignol, Rossignol, et al. (2009)	N = 62; ASD; 2–7 years	*Design:* RDB/PC, HBOT or slightly pressurized air for 40 sessions *Outcome:* improvement in multiple questionnaires for HBOT compared to control *Comment:* Methodological problems — including financial interest, confounds of other therapies and multiple comparisons, parent and clinician CGI inconsistent
	●	Granpeesheh et al. (2009)	N = 34; ASD; 2–11 years	*Design:* RDB/PC, HBOT or air in chamber, controlled for other interventions *Outcome:* questionnaires, observation, no difference in groups

KEY: ● = Strong, O = moderate, × = unacceptable
DB = double blind, RDB = randomized double blind, PC = placebo controlled, RCT = randomized controlled trial; Rv = systematic review, NDD = neurodevelopmental disability, MA = meta-analysis, OL = open label

of chelation in children with ASD was terminated because of concerns regarding safety of the participants (Mitka 2008). Conventional chelating agents bind to heavy metals and allow for excretion in the urine or stool. In medical practice, chelating agents are used for documented heavy metal toxicity such as lead poisoning. If clinical mercury toxicity is suspected on the basis of exposure, conventional blood measurement and not hair or urine studies are necessary for diagnosis (Ng et al. 2007).

Hyperbaric oxygen therapy (HBOT) is used by complementary practitioners to increase oxygen delivery to the brain of children by means of increased oxygen concentration delivered at increased pressure in specialized sealed chambers. Additional hypotheses have been generated regarding correction of oxidative stress response. Two recent randomized clinical trials have been completed that attempt to provide evidence for this intervention but come to opposite conclusions. Rossignol (Rossignol et al. 2009) randomized 62 children with ASD to HBOT or sham sessions. They report improvement in behavior and symptoms of autism in the study population compared to the controls on the clinician completed Clinical Global Index. This difference does not reach statistical significance for the other measures used or in the parent CGI although improvement in scores is noted over the course of the study. Granpeesheh et al. (2009) also randomized 34 children with ASD to HBOT or sham sessions. Like Rossignol (Rossignol et al. 2009) this group used the Clinical Global Index and Aberrant Behavior Checklist to monitor response but they also collected objective data on behavioral change. No difference between treatment and control groups was reported. The risks of HBOT include ear pain from the increased pressure and anxiety from the enclosed space as well as the substantial cost of the therapy. Repeat exposure to increased pressure and oxygen

for the adult who enters the chamber to comfort the child for each of 40 or more sessions has unknown health risks. A recent incident of explosion and fire involved a child with cerebral palsy receiving HBOT with a caregiver. Additional study is necessary to determine if HBOT results in benefit to children with ASD.

Manipulative and Body-Based Therapies

Chiropractic care by licensed chiropractors is covered by most insurers and can be accessed by families for their children with ASD. While there are anecdotal reports of benefit, there have been no trials to assess efficacy.

Craniosacral manipulation purports to alter the spinal fluid movement and pressure by external manipulation. This phenomenon has not been demonstrated (Downey et al. 2006). No data permits comment on the safety or effectiveness of this approach for children with autism. There are anecdotal supporters.

People with ASD are often described as craving pressure or finding touch aversive. Strategies that attempt to use sensory preferences may have some theoretical basis as part of an intervention plan, as discussed in Chap. 9. Evidence-based studies have not been performed to support the use of massage as an intervention for ASD. However, families report anecdotal benefits of touch and massage that allow them to enhance emotional bonding with their children (Cullen et al. 2005). Qigong, a Chinese therapy that teaches an integration of position in space and calming strategies, may have promise if pilot studies of small sample size are expanded (Silva et al. 2007). Further studies of interventions in this modality are clearly indicated.

Programmatic provision of sound through earphones with certain frequencies altered has been advocated as a means of improving symptoms of people with ASD.

While initial trials demonstrated improvement, these findings are not uniformly replicated in studies with control conditions (Sinha et al. 2004, 2006). It is not yet known whether there may be subgroups within ASD, such as children with hyperacusis, who might demonstrate specific areas of benefit from auditory integration training.

Vagal nerve stimulation has become an important therapy for control of recalcitrant seizures in neurologic practice. Increased alertness has been observed in some individuals with ASD whose seizures respond to this intervention (Park 2003). This has not been uniformly observed (Danielsson et al. 2008). Further studies with careful outcome criteria would be indicated given the potential physiologic relationship of vagal activity with reactivity and potential impact on development of behaviors important to social interaction (Field and Diego 2008).

Table 10.5 briefly lists the trials of manipulative and body-based therapies that have taken place.

Mind- and Body-Based Therapies

There are no studies in the current scientific literature that specifically address the impact of meditation or yoga on the symptoms of ASD. Yoga did not demonstrate an effect on attention or behavior in a pilot study of boys with ADHD (Jensen and Kenny 2004). The use of other self-regulation techniques, such as hypnosis, has widespread clinical utility in behavioral health practice, for example management of headaches (Daniel and Robert 2007). Research regarding implementation and effectiveness of self-regulation approaches may be especially useful in children and youth with anxiety especially when pharmacologic interventions are not successful.

Music therapy may have a role in the educational and behavioral program provided to students with ASD to enhance behavioral control and communication development. Neurobiologic research is examining how music is processed in the brains of people with and without ASD. An educational approach has been developed based on clinical observation that music can reinforce behaviors and provide auditory structure for learning other tasks (Gold et al. 2006). The evidence supporting music therapy is encouraging. Future studies will benefit from larger sample sizes, use of valid outcome measures, and study designs that allow for addressing confounding interventions and the endurance of the observed benefits. Table 10.6 briefly lists the music therapy trials that have taken place.

Energy Healing Therapy

Reiki is a form of spiritual healing in which the practitioner channels "universal life energy" to the recipient through light touch. It is thought to balance the biofield and enhance both wellness and self healing. It is often categorized with healing touch and therapeutic touch. While data supports the possibility of benefit from these modalities in the management of pain in adults (So et al. 2008) there is no data at this time regarding general use for anxiety or mood.

CONCLUSION

In the age of translational medicine, we need to integrate the empirical observations made by patients, families and clinicians regarding apparent response to novel therapies with what science has demonstrated regarding the causality and pathophysiology of the underlying disorder. Some empiric observations related to response to CAM therapies *may* be substantiated by careful study: the observation that limes prevented scurvy predated the understanding of the pathophysiology of

TABLE 10.5 Manipulative and body-based therapies

	Rating	Study	Participants	Design, Outcome and Comment
Massage/Qigong				
Treatment trials	O	Escalona et al. (2001)	N=20; autism; 3–6 years	*Design:* Random assignment to massage and reading attention groups; parents trained *Outcome:* Less stereotypic behavior, more social relatedness, fewer sleep problems *Comment:* Methodological problems—potential bias
	×	Cullen and Barlow (2002)	N=14 parents, N=13 children	*Design:* Training and Support Program (TSP) for touch therapy *Outcome:* Sleep benefits, improved comfort with their child *Comment:* Methodological problems—uncontrolled
	O	Cullen et al. (2005)	N=12; ASD (and comorbidity); 2–13 years	*Design:* Convenience sample; parents administered touch program; 8 weeks *Outcome:* Parent report less touch aversive, activities of daily living easier *Comment:* Methodological problems—multiple confounders, uncontrolled
	×	Silva and Cignolini (2005)	N=8; autism; under 6 years old	*Design:* Qigong massage from physician practitioner and trained parents *Outcome:* Decreased behaviors, increased language, improved motor and sensory function and general health *Comment:* Methodological problems—uncontrolled
	×	Silva et al. (2007)	N=8; autism; N=7 control; 3–6 years	*Design:* Open treatment trial, daily Qigong massage, 5 months *Outcome:* Improved sensory impairment; both groups improved social skills and language *Comment:* Methodological problems—controls, questionnaires
	×	Williams (2006)	N=12; autism; 12–15 years; residential school	*Design:* Open treatment trial, aromatherapy massage *Outcome:* No beneficial effect on sleep *Comment:* Methodological problems—no controls
Auditory Integration Training (AIT)				
Treatment trial	O Rv	Sinha et al. (2004, 2006)	N=171; 3–39 years	*Design:* MA not possible due to heterogeneous or unusable data *Outcome:* No benefit over control in 3 studies; improvement by ABC total mean score in 3 studies *Comment:* Methodological problems
Vagus nerve stimulation				
Treatment trial	×	Danielsson et al. (2008)	N=8; autism and epilepsy; 5–18 years	*Design:* OL trial vagus stimulation *Outcome:* No change in seizure frequency, no positive cognitive effects; 3 with minor behavioral improvement; 1 increased seizures, worse behavior *Comment:* Prospective studies needed

KEY: ● =Strong, O =moderate, × = unacceptable
DB =double blind, *RDB* =randomized double blind, *PC* =placebo controlled, *RCT* =randomized controlled trial, *Rv* =systematic review, *NDD* =neurodevelopmental disability; *MA* =meta-analysis, *OL* =open label

TABLE 10.6   Music therapy

	Rating	Study	Participants	Design, Outcome and Comment
Treatment trials	● Rv	Whipple (2004)	N=76; ASD; 4–21 years; MA, 9 studies	*Design*: Open treatment trials, with control (no music) condition *Outcome*: Improved social, communication, repetitive behaviors
	○ Rv	Gold et al. (2006)	3 studies, ASD, N=24, 2–9 years	*Design*: RCT, music therapy vs. placebo *Outcome*: Improved verbal and gestural skills improved

KEY: ● = Strong, ○ = moderate, × = unacceptable

DB = double blind, *RDB* = randomized double blind, *PC* = placebo controlled, *RCT* = randomized controlled trial, *Rv* = systematic review, *NDD* = neurodevelopmental disability, *MA* = meta-analysis, *OL* = open label

the disorder and understanding of vitamin C metabolism (Baron 2009). We must respect clinical observation as a means for hypothesis generation and use careful study design to test CAM therapies used for symptoms of ASD for both safety and efficacy. Clinicians and scientists must also respect the data from appropriately designed clinical trials examining CAM therapy even when it counters conventional medical belief.

While promoting evidence-based treatment is the goal of this volume, it is acknowledged that there is no uniform agreement as to what constitutes evidence among families and CAM providers. The American Academy of Pediatrics promoted guidelines (AAP Committee on Children with Disabilities 2001) for practitioners to set up a dialog with families seeking CAM therapies, even when there is disagreement, so that the interests of the child can remain in focus.

CAM use continues to increase. More research regarding CAM therapies is needed. This research must include appropriately designed clinical trials, examination of potential scientific explanations, as well as understanding of how to present evidence from scientific studies in a way that will impact the practice behaviors of complementary and allopathic practitioners as well as therapy choice by potential consumers of CAM therapies.

REFERENCES

AAP Committee on Children with Disabilities. (2001). Counseling families who choose complementary and alternative medicine for their child with chronic illness or disability. American Academy of Pediatrics. *Pediatrics, 107*(3), 598–601.

Adams, J. B., & Holloway, C. (2004). Pilot study of a moderate dose multivitamin/mineral supplement for children with autistic spectrum disorder. *Journal of Alternative and Complementary Medicine, 10*(6), 1033–1039.

Adams, J. B., Romdalvik, J., Ramanujam, V. M., & Legator, M. S. (2007). Mercury, lead, and zinc in baby teeth of children with autism versus controls. *Journal of Toxicology and Environmental Health, Part A: Current Issues, 70*(12), 1046–1051.

Amminger, G. P., Berger, G. E., Schafer, M. R., Klier, C., Friedrich, M. H., & Feucht, M. (2007). Omega-3 fatty acids supplementation in children with autism: A double-blind randomized, placebo-controlled pilot study. *Biological Psychiatry, 61*(4), 551–553.

Andersen, I. M., Kaczmarska, J., McGrew, S. G., & Malow, B. A. (2008). Melatonin for insomnia in children with autism spectrum disorders. *Journal of Child Neurology, 23*(5), 482–485.

Autism Research Institute (2005) *Autism Treatment Evaluation Checklist (ATEC) Report*. Retrieved from http://www.autism.com/ind_atec_report.asp.

Bakkaloglu, B., Anlar, B., Anlar, F. Y., Oktem, F., Pehlivanturk, B., et al. (2008). Atopic features in early childhood autism. *European Journal of Paediatric Neurology, 12*, 476–479.

Barnes, P. M., Powell-Griner, E., McFann, K., and Nahin, R. L. (2004) *Complementary and alternative medicine use among adults: United States, 2002: Advance data from vital and health statistics.* Retrieved from http://www.nccam.nih.gov.

Baron, J. H. (2009). Sailors' scurvy before and after James Lind: a reassessment. *Nutrition Reviews, 67*(6), 315–332.

Bolman, W. M., & Richmond, J. A. (1999). A double-blind, placebo-controlled, crossover pilot trial of low dose dimethylglycine in patients with autistic disorder. *Journal of Autism and Developmental Disorders, 29*(3), 191–194.

Brown, K. A., & Patel, D. R. (2005). Complementary and alternative medicine in developmental disabilities. *Indian Journal of Pediatrics, 72*(11), 949–952.

Brudnak, M. A., Rimland, B., Kerry, R. E., Dailey, M., Taylor, R., et al. (2002). Enzyme-based therapy for autism spectrum disorders: Is it worth another look? *Medical Hypotheses, 58*(5), 422–428.

Cass, H., Gringras, P., March, J., McKendrick, I., OHare, A. E., et al. (2008). Absence of urinary opioid peptides in children with autism. *Archives of Disease in Childhood, 93*, 745–750.

Chez, M. G., Buchanan, C. P., Aimonovitch, M. C., Becker, M., Schaefer, K., et al. (2002). Double-blind, placebo-controlled study of L-carnosine supplementation in children with autistic spectrum disorders. *Journal of Child Neurology, 17*(11), 833–837.

Christison, G. W., & Ivany, K. (2006). Elimination diets in autism spectrum disorders: Any wheat amidst the chaff? *Journal of Developmental and Behavioral Pediatrics, 27*(2 Suppl), S162–171.

Cincotta, D. R., Crawford, N. W., Lim, A., Cranswick, N. E., Skull, S., et al. (2006). Comparison of complementary and alternative medicine use: Reasons and motivations between two tertiary children's hospitals. *Archives of Disease in Childhood, 91*(2), 153–158.

Cullen, L., & Barlow, J. (2002). 'Kiss, cuddle, squeeze': The experiences and meaning of touch among parents of children with autism attending a touch therapy programme. *Journal of Child Health Care, 6*(3), 171–181.

Cullen, L. A., Barlow, J. H., & Cushway, D. (2005). Positive touch, the implications for parents and their children with autism: An exploratory study. *Complementary Therapies in Clinical Practice, 11*(3), 182–189.

Daniel, P. K., & Robert, Z. (2007). Self-hypnosis training for headaches in children and adolescents. *Journal of Pediatrics, 150*(6), 635–639.

Danielsson, S., Viggedal, G., Gillberg, C., & Olsson, I. (2008). Lack of effects of vagus nerve stimulation on drug-resistant epilepsy in eight pediatric patients with autism spectrum disorders: A prospective 2-year follow-up study. *Epilepsy and Behavior, 12*(2), 298–304.

Dannemann, K., Hecker, W., Haberland, H., Herbst, A., Galler, A., et al. (2008). Use of complementary and alternative medicine in children with type 1 diabetes mellitus: Prevalence, patterns of use, and costs. *Pediatric Diabetes, 9*(3 Pt 1), 228–235.

Davis, M. P., & Darden, P. M. (2003). Use of complementary and alternative medicine by children in the United States. *Archives of Pediatric and Adolescent Medicine, 157*(4), 393–396.

DelGiudice-Asch, G., Simon, L., Schmeidler, J., Cunningham-Rundles, C., & Hollander, E. (1999). Brief report: A pilot open clinical trial of intravenous immunoglobulin in childhood autism. *Journal of Autism and Developmental Disorders, 29*(2), 157–160.

Dolske, M. C., Spollen, J., McKay, S., Lancashire, E., & Tolbert, L. (1993). A preliminary trial of ascorbic acid as supplemental therapy for autism. *Progress in Neuro-Psychopharmacology and Biological Psychiatry, 17*, 765–774.

Downey, P. A., Barbano, T., Kapur-Wadhwa, R., Sciote, J. J., Siegel, M. I., & Mooney, M. P. (2006). Craniosacral therapy: The effects of cranial manipulation on intracranial pressure and cranial bone movement. *Journal of Orthopaedic and Sports Physical Therapy, 36*(11), 845–853.

Elder, J. H., Shankar, M., Shuster, J., Theriaque, D., Burns, S., & Sherrill, L. (2006). The gluten-free, casein-free diet in autism: Results of a preliminary double blind clinical trial. *Journal of Autism and Developmental Disorders, 36*(3), 413–420.

Ernst, E. (1999). Prevalence of complementary/alternative medicine for children: A systematic review. *European Journal of Pediatrics, 158*(1), 7–11.

Escalona, A., Field, T., Singer-Strunck, R., Cullen, C., & Hartshorn, K. (2001). Brief report: Improvements in the behavior of children with autism following massage therapy. *Journal of Autism and Developmental Disorders, 31*(5), 513–516.

Esch, B. E., & Carr, J. E. (2004). Secretin as a treatment for autism: A review of the evidence. *Journal of Autism and Developmental Disorders, 34*(5), 543–556.

Field, T., & Diego, M. (2008). Vagal activity, early growth and emotional development. *Infant Behavior and Development, 31*, 361–373.

Findling, R. L., Maxwell, K., Scotese-Wojtila, L., Huang, J., Yamashita, T., & Wiznitzer, M.

(1997). High-dose pyridoxine and magnesium administration in children with autistic disorder: An absence of salutary effects in a double-blind, placebo-controlled study. *Journal of Autism and Developmental Disorders, 27*(4), 467–478.

Fombonne, E. (2008). Thimerosal disappears but autism remains. *Archives of General Psychiatry, 65*(1), 15–16.

Garstang, J., & Wallis, M. (2006). Randomized controlled trial of melatonin for children with autistic spectrum disorders and sleep problems. *Child: Care, Health and Development, 32*(5), 585–589.

Geier, D. A., & Geier, M. R. (2006). A clinical trial of combined anti-androgen and anti-heavy metal therapy in autistic disorders. *Neuroendocrinology Letters, 27*(6), 833–838.

Geier, D. A., & Geier, M. R. (2007a). A case series of children with apparent mercury toxic encephalopathies manifesting with clinical symptoms of regressive autistic disorders. *Journal of Toxicology and Environmental Health, Part A: Current Issues, 70*(10), 837–851.

Geier, D. A., & Geier, M. R. (2007b). A prospective study of mercury toxicity biomarkers in autistic spectrum disorders. *Journal of Toxicology and Environmental Health, Part A: Current Issues, 70*(20), 1723–1730.

Giannotti, F., Cortesi, F., Cerquiglini, A., & Bernabei, P. (2006). An open-label study of controlled-release melatonin in treatment of sleep disorders in children with autism. *Journal of Autism and Developmental Disorders, 36*(6), 741–752.

Gold, C., Wigram, T., and Elefant, C. (2006) Music therapy for autistic spectrum disorder. *Cochrane Database of Systematic Reviews,* 2:CD004381.

Golnik, A. E., & Ireland, M. (2009). Complementary alternative medicine for children with autism: A physician survey. *Journal of Autism and Developmental Disorders, 39*(7), 996–1005.

Granpeesheh, D., Bradstreet, J. J., Tarbox, J., Dixon, D. R., Allen, S., & Wilke, A. E. (2009) *Randomized placebo-controlled trial of hyperbaric oxygen therapy.* Paper presented at the IMFAR, Chicago, IL.

Green, V. A., Pituch, K. A., Itchon, J., Choi, A. O., Reilly, M., Sigafoos, J., (2006). Internet survey of treatments used by parents of children with autism. *Res Dev Disabil.* 27(1):70-84

Gupta, S., Aggarwal, S., & Heads, C. (1996). Dysregulated immune system in children with autism: Beneficial effects of intravenous immune globulin on autistic characteristics. *Journal of Autism and Developmental Disorders, 26*(4), 439–452.

Handen, B. L., Melmed, R. D., Hansen, R. L., Aman, M. G., Burnham, D. L., et al. (2009). A double-blind, placebo-controlled trial of oral human immunoglobulin for gastrointestinal dysfunction in children with autistic disorder. *Journal of Autism and Developmental Disorders, 39*(5), 796–805.

Hanson, E., Kalish, L. A., Bunce, E., Curtis, C., McDaniel, S., et al. (2007). Use of complementary and alternative medicine among children diagnosed with autism spectrum disorder. *Journal of Autism and Developmental Disorders, 37*(4), 628–636.

Heuer, L., Ashwood, P., Schauer, J., Krakowiak, P., Hertz-Picciotto, I., et al. (2008). Reduced levels of immunoglobulin in children with autism correlates with behavioral symptoms. *Autism Research, 1*(5), 275–183.

Hyland, M. E. (2003). Methodology for the scientific evaluation of complementary and alternative medicine. *Complementary Therapies in Medicine, 11*(3), 146–153.

James, S. J., Cutler, P., Melnyk, S., Jernigan, S., Janak, L., et al. (2004). Metabolic biomarkers of increased oxidative stress and impaired methylation capacity in children with autism. *American Journal of Clinical Nutrition, 80*(6), 1611–1617.

James, S. J., Melnyk, S., Fuchs, G., Reid, T., Jernigan, S., et al. (2009). Efficacy of methylcobalamin and folinic acid treatment on glutathione redox status in children with autism. *American Journal of Clinical Nutrition, 89*(1), 425–430.

Jensen, P. S., & Kenny, D. T. (2004). The effects of yoga on the attention and behavior of boys with attention-deficit/hyperactivity disorder (ADHD). *Journal of Attention Disorders, 7*(4), 205–216.

Jyonouchi, H. (2009). Food allergy and autism spectrum disorders: Is there a link? *Current Allergy and Asthma Reports, 9*(3), 194–201.

Kazdin, A. E. (2004). Evidence-based treatments: Challenges and priorities for practice and research. *Child and Adolescent Psychiatric Clinics of North America, 13*(4), 923–940.

Kelly, K. M. (2007). Complementary and alternative medicines for use in supportive care in pediatric cancer. *Support Care Cancer, 15*(4), 457–460.

Kemper, K. J., Vohra, S., Walls, R., & the Task Force on Complementary and Alternative Medicine, and the Provisional Section on Complementary, Holistic, and Integrative Medicine. (2008). The use of complementary and alternative medicine in pediatrics. *Pediatrics, 122*(6), 1374–1386.

Kern, J. K., Miller, V. S., Cauller, L., Kendall, R., Mehta, J., & Dodd, M. (2001). Effectiveness of N, N-Dimethylglycine in autism and pervasive developmental disorder. *Journal of Child Neurology, 16*(3), 169–173.

Knivsberg, A. M., Reichelt, K. L., Hoien, T., & Nodland, M. (2002). A randomised, controlled study of dietary intervention in autistic syndromes. *Nutritional Neuroscience, 5*(4), 251–261.

Kuriyama, S., Kamiyama, M., Watanabe, M., Tamabashi, S., Muraguchi, I., et al. (2002). Pyridoxine treatment in a subgroup of children with pervasive developmental disorders. *Developmental Medicine and Child Neurology, 44*(4), 283–286.

Levy, S., & Hyman, S. (2005). Novel treatments for autistic spectrum disorders. *Mental Retardation and Developmental Disabilities Research Reviews, 11*, 131–142.

Levy, S. E., Mandell, D. S., Merhar, S., Ittenbach, R. F., & Pinto-Martin, J. A. (2003). Use of complementary and alternative medicine among children recently diagnosed with autistic spectrum disorder. *Journal of Developmental and Behavioral Pediatrics, 24*(6), 418–423.

Liptak, G. S. (2005). Complementary and alternative therapies for cerebral palsy. *Mental Retardation and Developmental Disabilities Research Reviews, 11*(2), 156–163.

Martineau, J., Barthelemy, C., Garreau, B., & Lelord, G. (1985). Vitamin B6:magnesium and combined B6-Mg: Therapeutic effects in childhood autism. *Biological Psychiatry, 20*(5), 467–478.

McCann, D., Barrett, A., Cooper, A., Crumpler, D., Dalen, L., et al. (2007). Food additives and hyperactive behaviour in 3-year-old and 8/9-year-old children in the community: A randomised, double-blinded, placebo-controlled trial. *Lancet, 370*(9598), 1560–1567.

Millward, C., Ferriter, M., Calver, S., & Connell-Jones, G. (2008) Gluten- and casein-free diets for autistic spectrum disorder. *Cochrane Database of Systematic Reviews, 2*:CD003498.

Mitka, M. (2008). Chelation therapy trials halted. *Journal of the American Medical Association, 300*(19), 2236.

Moretti, P., Sahoo, T., Hyland, K., Bottiglieri, T., Peters, S., et al. (2005). Cerebral folate deficiency with developmental delay, autism, and response to folinic acid. *Neurology, 64*(6), 1088–1090.

Mousain-Bosc, M., Roche, M., Polge, A., Pradal-Prat, D., Rapin, J., & Bali, J. P. (2006). Improvement of neurobehavioral disorders in children supplemented with magnesium-vitamin B6: II. Pervasive developmental disorder – autism. *Magnesium Research, 19*(1), 53–62.

Ng, D. K., Chan, C. H., Soo, M. T., & Lee, R. S. (2007). Low-level chronic mercury exposure in children and adolescents: Meta-analysis. *Pediatrics International, 49*(1), 80–87.

Niehus, R., & Lord, C. (2006). Early medical history of children with autism spectrum disorders. *Journal of Developmental and Behavioral Pediatrics, 27*(2 Suppl), S120–127.

Nye, C., & Brice, A. (2005) Combined vitamin B6-magnesium treatment in autism spectrum disorder. *Cochrane Database of Systematic Reviews, 4*:CD003497.

Park, Y. D. (2003). The effects of vagus nerve stimulation therapy on patients with intractable seizures and either Landau-Kleffner syndrome or autism. *Epilepsy and Behavior, 4*(3), 286–290.

Patel, K., & Curtis, L. T. (2007). A comprehensive approach to treating autism and attention-deficit hyperactivity disorder: A prepilot study. *Journal of Alternative and Complementary Medicine, 13*(10), 1091–1097.

Plioplys, A. V. (1998). Intravenous immunoglobulin treatment of children with autism. *Journal of Child Neurology, 13*(2), 79–82.

Rhee, S. M., Garg, V. K., & Hershey, C. O. (2004). Use of complementary and alternative medicines by ambulatory patients. *Archives of Internal Medicine, 164*(9), 1004–1009.

Roizen, N. J. (2005). Complementary and alternative therapies for Down syndrome. *Mental Retardation and Developmental Disabilities Research Reviews, 11*(2), 149–155.

Rossignol, D. A., Rossignol, L. W., James, S. J., Melnyk, S., & Mumper, E. (2007). The effects of hyperbaric oxygen therapy on oxidative stress, inflammation, and symptoms in children with autism: An open-label pilot study. *BMC Pediatrics, 7*(1), 36.

Rossignol, D. A., Rossignol, L. W., Smith, S., Schneider, C., Logerquist, S., et al. (2009). Hyperbaric treatment for children with autism: A multicenter, randomized, double-blind, controlled trial. *BMC Pediatrics, 9*, 21.

Rouster-Stevens, K., Nageswaran, S., Arcury, T. A., & Kemper, K. J. (2008). How do parents of children with juvenile idiopathic arthritis (JIA) perceive their therapies? *BMC Complementary and Alternative Medicine, 8*, 25.

Sandler, A. D., & Bodfish, J. W. (2000). Placebo effects in autism: Lessons from secretin. *Journal of Developmental and Behavioral Pediatrics, 21*(5), 347–350.

Sandler, R. H., Finegold, S. M., Bolte, E. R., Buchanan, C. P., Maxwell, A. P., et al. (2000). Short-term benefit from oral vancomycin treatment of regressive-onset autism. *Journal of Child Neurology, 15*(7), 429–435.

Schechter, R., & Grether, J. K. (2008). Continuing increases in autism reported to California's developmental services system: Mercury in retrograde. *Archives of General Psychiatry, 65*(1), 19–24.

Schneider, C. K., Melmed, R. D., Barstow, L. E., Enriquez, F. J., Ranger-Moore, J., & Ostrem, J. A. (2006). Oral human immunoglobulin for children with autism and gastrointestinal dysfunction: A prospective, open-label study. *Journal of Autism and Developmental Disorders, 36*(8), 1053–1064.

Silva, L. M., & Cignolini, A. (2005). A medical Qigong methodology for early intervention in autism spectrum disorder: A case series. *American Journal of Chinese Medicine, 33*(2), 315–327.

Silva, L. M., Cignolini, A., Warren, R., Budden, S., & Skowron-Gooch, A. (2007). Improvement in sensory impairment and social interaction in young children with autism following treatment with an original Qigong massage methodology. *American Journal of Chinese Medicine, 35*(3), 393–406.

Sinha, Y., Silove, N., Wheeler, D., & Williams, K. (2004) Auditory integration training and other sound therapies for autism spectrum disorders. *Cochrane Database of Systematic Reviews,* 1:CD003681.

Sinha, Y., Silove, N., Wheeler, D., & Williams, K. (2006). Auditory integration training and other sound therapies for autism spectrum disorders: A systematic review. *Archives of Disease in Childhood, 91*(12), 1018–1022.

So, P. S., Jiang, Y., & Qin, Y. (2008) Touch therapies for pain relief in adults. *Cochrane Database of Systematic Reviews,* 4:CD006535.

Soden, S. E., Lowry, J. A., Garrison, C. B., & Wasserman, G. S. (2007). 24-hour provoked urine excretion test for heavy metals in children with autism and typically developing controls: A pilot study. *Clinical Toxicology, 45*(5), 476–481.

Spigelblatt, L., Laine-Ammara, G., Pless, I. B., & Guyver, A. (1994). The use of alternative medicine by children. *Pediatrics, 94*(6 Pt 1), 811–814.

Sweeten, T. L., Bowyer, S. L., Posey, D. J., Halberstadt, G. M., & McDougle, C. J. (2003). Increased prevalence of familial autoimmunity in probands with pervasive developmental disorders. *Pediatrics, 112*(5), e420.

Tolbert, L., Haigler, T., Waits, M. M., Dennis, T. (1993) Brief REport: Lack of Response in an autistic population to a low dose clinical trial of pyridoxine and magnesium. *Journal of Autism and Developmental Disorders, 23*(1): 193-9

Verhoef, M. J., Vanderheyden, L. C., Dryden, T., Mallory, D., & Ware, M. A. (2006). Evaluating complementary and alternative medicine interventions: In search of appropriate patient-centered outcome measures. *BMC Complementary and Alternative Medicine, 6,* 6–38.

Wasdell, M. B., Jan, J. E., Bomben, M. B., Freeman, R. D., Rietveld, W. J., et al. (2008). A randomized, placebo-controlled trial of controlled release melatonin treatment of delayed sleep phase syndrome and impaired sleep maintenance in children with neurodevelopmental disabilities. *Journal of Pineal Research, 44*(1), 57–64.

Weber, W., & Newmark, S. (2007). Complementary and alternative medical therapies for attention-deficit/hyperactivity disorder and autism. *Pediatric Clinics of North America, 54*(6), 983–1006.

Whipple, J. (2004). Music in intervention for children and adolescents with autism: A meta-analysis. *Journal of Music Therapy, 41*(2), 90–106.

Whiteley, P., Rodgers, J., Savery, D., & Shattock, P. (1999). A gluten-free diet as an intervention for autism and associated spectrum disorders: Preliminary findings. *Autism, 3*(1), 45–65.

Williams, K. W., Wray, J. J., & Wheeler, D. M. (2005) Intravenous secretin for autism spectrum disorder. *Cochrane Database of Systematic Reviews,* 3:CD003495.

Williams, T. I. (2006). Evaluating effects of aromatherapy massage on sleep in children with autism: A pilot study. *Evidence-based Complementary and Alternative Medicine, 3*(3), 373–377.

Wills, S., Cabanlit, M., Bennett, J., Ashwood, P., Amaral, D., & Van de Water, J. (2007). Autoantibodies in autism spectrum disorders (ASD). *Annals of the New York Academy of Sciences, 1107,* 79–91.

Wilson, K. M., Klein, J. D., Sesselberg, T. S., Yussman, S. M., Markow, D. B., et al. (2006). Use of complementary medicine and dietary supplements among US adolescents. *Journal of Adolescent Health, 38*(4), 385–394.

Wong, H. H., & Smith, R. G. (2006). Patterns of complementary and alternative medical therapy use in children diagnosed with autism spectrum disorders. *Journal of Autism and Developmental Disorders, 36*(7), 901–909.

Zuzak, T. J., Zuzak-Siegrist, I., Simoes-Wust, A. P., Rist, L., & Staubli, G. (2008). Use of complementary and alternative medicine by patients presenting to a paediatric emergency department. *European Journal of Pediatrics, 168*(4), 431–437.

PART III

Research to Practice

Chapter 11

The Role of Adaptive Behavior in Evidence-Based Practices for ASD: Translating Intervention into Functional Success

Katherine D. Tsatsanis, Celine Saulnier, Sara S. Sparrow,
and Domenic V. Cicchetti

ABBREVIATIONS

ADHD	Attention deficit hyperactivity disorder
ADLs	Adaptive daily living skills
ADOS	Autism Diagnostic Observation Schedule
AS	Asperger Syndrome
ASDs	Autism spectrum disorders
CBT	Cognitive behavioral therapy
EIBI	Early intensive behavioral intervention
HFA	High-functioning autism
PDD-NOS	Pervasive developmental disorder not otherwise specified
SSED	Single subject experimental design
VSMS	Vineland Social Maturity Scale
VABS	Vineland Adaptive Behavior Scales

INTRODUCTION

The main diagnostic features of autism spectrum disorders (ASD) are defined in terms of qualitative impairments in social interaction, communication, and a pattern of restricted interests or repetitive behaviors. However, the particular constellation of symptoms, number, frequency, and severity differs from individual to individual. For some, an end goal in the treatment of autism spectrum disorders, whether stated explicitly or not, is to reduce autistic symptomatology and "cure" the disorder. One positive step in the discourse around treatment for ASD is a change in focus from symptom expression to measured changes in adaptive functioning. From this perspective, the intransigence of the diagnosis is not an indication of lack of success of a treatment model or educational program; rather, an emphasis is placed on functional outcomes such as helping people with

B. Reichow et al. (eds.), *Evidence-Based Practices and Treatments for Children with Autism*,
DOI 10.1007/978-1-4419-6975-0_11, © Springer Science+Business Media, LLC 2011

ASD attend school in the least restrictive environment, communicate with family and peers, enjoy leisure activities with others, attend to their daily living needs (e.g., toileting, washing, dressing, eating, and cleaning), regulate emotions and behavior, and establish and maintain relationships with others.

ADAPTIVE BEHAVIOR

Adaptive behavior can be understood as a measured construct reflecting real-life functioning. In contrast to the assessment of other abilities, such as cognitive or language functioning, measured adaptive functioning represents typical performance rather than the potential ability of the individual, i.e., what a person does on a day-to-day basis as opposed to what a person is capable of doing under optimal conditions. Adaptive behavior is defined on the basis of the everyday activities necessary to take care of oneself, communicate and get along with others. A distinction can also be made between performance-based and skill-based deficits; that is, the difference between a person who is able to perform a task but does not (e.g., because of severe depression) and a person who does not perform the task because of not having learned the necessary skills. For ASD, the latter is frequently the case: individuals either have not learned the specific skill or have not been explicitly taught how to apply that skill to their lives in a functional and meaningful way. Thus, the focus of intervention must consider both teaching skills and ensuring that the individual can independently apply those skills to daily life.

Levels of Adaptive Functioning

A typical profile of adaptive behavior in autism is marked by significant impairments in socialization, intermediate deficits in communication, and relative strengths in daily living skills (Bolte and Poustka 2002; Carter et al. 1998; Volkmar et al. 1987). The phrase "relative strengths" should be considered with caution, as daily living skills still tend to fall below age and cognitive expectations in many cases (Klin et al. 2007). This profile of deficits is well documented in the general ASD literature (Bolte and Poustka 2002; Carter et al. 1998; Freeman et al. 1999; Liss et al. 2001). Discrepant findings emerge when investigating individuals with different levels of functioning within the spectrum. For instance, significant adaptive behavior deficits have been found in samples of high-functioning individuals with ASD (such as Asperger Syndrome (AS), autism or pervasive developmental disorder, not otherwise specified (PDD-NOS)) without cognitive impairment (Klin et al. 2007; Perry et al. 2009; Saulnier and Klin 2007). In the study by Saulnier and Klin (2007), the ASD group had a mean age of 12.4 years and average verbal, performance, and full-scale IQ scores but age equivalencies for adaptive behaviors as measured using the Vineland Adaptive Behavior Scales (VABS) were, for example, 3.2 years for interpersonal skills, 5.8 years for coping skills, and 6.2 years for personal care skills. When the level of deficit in adaptive functioning is expressed in this way, the results dramatically underscore the impact of the disorder on a person's ability to function independently in the world and the need for intervention that focuses on adaptive or real-life skills.

In two more recent studies (Fenton et al. 2003; Perry et al. 2009), contrary findings have been reported in individuals who have both ASD and cognitive impairment, with adaptive behavior being on par with or above mental age in some cases. Perry et al. (2009) suggest this could be due to the group maximizing their potential better than higher-functioning individuals and/or could be the product of the specific intervention focus for these individuals. Although previous studies of lower-functioning ASD yielded the "autism profile" of adaptive deficits, with socialization skills being the lowest (Carter et al. 1998; Volkmar et al. 1987), Fenton et al. (2003) propose that the greater the gap between chronological and mental age in ASD, the less likely the "autism profile" is to manifest. More research is merited to flesh out whether or not this is truly the case, particularly in the context of earlier detection and intervention for children with ASD.

Relationship to Age

In addition to the gap between levels of cognitive and adaptive functioning, there is evidence to suggest a widening gap in meeting the increasing social demands and expectations with age (Klin et al. 2007; Szatmari et al. 2003). This pattern appears to be the case in very young children as well. In an early detection study, where children were initially evaluated at age two and followed up at age four, results suggest that despite progress in both developmental and adaptive skills, the gap between developmental skills and adaptive functioning widens with age (Saulnier et al. 2008). Furthermore, the minimal gains that were evident in functional social skills over time were independent of symptom severity. Collectively, these results reinforce the importance of a focus on adaptive behaviors as individuals with ASD get older. Additional study is needed to examine whether there are specific age transitions at which time adaptive skill instruction should be intensified, given spurts or lags in the acquisition of such skills.

Relationship Between ASD Symptomatology and Adaptive Behavior

In the study by Klin et al. (2007), Vineland Adaptive Behavior Scales (VABS) scores and age were negatively correlated, whereas scores on the Autism Diagnostic Observation Schedule (ADOS; Lord et al. 2000) did not vary over time. Thus, adaptive skills did not keep pace with chronological age, while autism symptomatology remained stable. Although social communication is assessed on both the ADOS and VABS, no relationship was found between social adaptive functioning and social or communication symptomatology on the ADOS in either of the two clinical samples studied.

While the study by Klin et al. (2007) was cross-sectional, a longitudinal study conducted by Szatmari et al. (2003) also indicated that autism-related symptoms were a weak predictor of outcome on the Vineland Adaptive Behavior Scales (VABS). When children with different levels of expression of the disorder have been compared, such as autism with PDD-NOS (Paul et al. 2004) or high-functioning autism (HFA) and AS (Saulnier and Klin 2007), few differences in adaptive function have been found despite the differences in diagnostic features. Therefore, lower levels of symptomatology do not, in and of themselves, imply higher levels of adaptive skills.

These results further underscore the importance of interventions targeting adaptive functioning for individuals with ASD regardless of subtype. They may also serve to caution against the utility of interventions that exclusively target symptom expression. Severity of symptom presentation and level of adaptive functioning do not appear to be related; it is worth considering whether a change in symptom presentation is or is not associated with gains in functional skills. The factors necessary for the acquisition of adaptive skills may be different from factors mediating the expression of ASD. Altogether, it would be desirable to distinguish those with ASD who show a successful real-life outcome from those at the same, or very similar, levels of cognitive functioning who remain quite impaired in their functional independence in order to begin to consider what variables may be at work.

EVIDENCE-BASED PRACTICES IN ADAPTIVE BEHAVIOR INTERVENTION

Existing studies that have proposed treatments for adaptive behavior tend to focus either on decreasing maladaptive or stereotypical behaviors or on teaching specific daily living skills. The former studies are addressed in other chapters of this book, including Chaps. 4 and 8. The latter studies, concerning daily living skills, typically include single subject experimental design studies (SSED) using varying techniques (e.g., prompting, self-management, stimulus control, reinforcement, punishment, conditioning, desensitization) to address a range of behaviors (e.g., toileting, dressing, feeding, on-task behavior, vocational skills). Several studies focus on teaching basic skills to individuals using self-management strategies that are explicitly and systematically taught (Mithaug and Mithaug 2003; Pierce and Schreibman 1994; Harchik et al. 1992). For instance, Pierce and Schreibman (1994) showed picture activity schedules to be effective in teaching three low-functioning children with ASD to dress themselves. Other studies utilized behavioral techniques such as graduated exposure to treat food selectivity (Paul et al. 2007), reinforcement strategies to teach toileting skills (Cicero and Pfadt 2002), and Social Stories to teach mealtime skills (Bledsoe et al. 2003). Studies using prompting methods have also been conducted to teach various adaptive skills, such as janitorial skills (Duran 1985) or self-care (Nelson et al. 1980), but too much prompting or adult assistance can also become detrimental to independent functioning (Koegel and Rincover 1976; Hume et al. 2009).

It is important to highlight that many of the studies on treatment of daily living skills involve very low-functioning individuals. For individuals with significant cognitive impairment, it is not uncommon to find that one focus of intervention is on teaching basic adaptive daily living skills (ADLs), such as dressing, eating, toileting, and self-care. As suggested by Perry et al. (2009), this could account for the less severe discrepancy between levels of adaptive and cognitive functioning observed in lower- versus higher-functioning individuals with ASD. In addition, older studies seem to have been more focused on teaching functional skills in the form of ADLs or personal care (Ando 1977; Nelson et al. 1980; Duran 1985), whereas in the past few decades the focus of autism intervention has moved toward addressing core symptomatology, such as social communication and interaction skills.

ADAPTIVE BEHAVIOR: A FUNDAMENTAL COMPONENT OF THE TREATMENT PROCESS

Adaptive skills, by their very definition, are a measure of the individual's ability to function independently in the world. From this perspective, it is not so much a matter of a "treatment method" for teaching adaptive behavior as adaptive behavior representing a fundamental step in the treatment process and adaptive functioning a fundamental measure of outcome. Adaptive behavior is addressed when an individual's repertoire of skills (explicitly taught through various treatment approaches) is applied to real-life situations in a functional and meaningful manner. Given that limited generalization is a significant feature of ASD, it cannot be assumed that building a repertoire of skills is enough. Functional application of skills across multiple contexts becomes a meaningful goal in and of itself.

According to the National Research Council (2001), one of the factors addressed in most current educational and treatment programs is the reduction of symptoms. Shifting the focus from the reduction of autistic symptomatology to an increase in adaptive functioning would mirror the difference between a disability- and ability-based definition of the disorder; between an emphasis on deviations from typical development and the processes that interfere with normative development. Given that current research indicates that autism symptomatology and level of adaptive behavior are relatively independent constructs, reducing symptoms may not in and of itself lead to changes in independent functioning; thus, leaving a major gap in the field of intervention.

Even when skill acquisition is the focus of therapies, it is usually in the form of teaching skills that are delayed or absent (e.g., speech). Less attention is given to the functional application of those skills to real life (e.g., how to speak in a job interview). In fact, in a review of 600 autism studies reported in the literature between 2000 and 2006, the authors coded outcome studies into two groups, skill acquisition and behavior reduction, and found that 60–70% of studies focused on the former (Abel et al. 2008). The authors point out that of the intervention studies that focused on the reduction of problem behaviors, many also addressed skill acquisition, which may indicate recognition of the effectiveness of teaching more functional skills to prevent or replace the maladaptive behavior. Nonetheless, the dearth of explicit adaptive skills instruction as a major component of intervention is notable.

In order to maximize potential and ensure a positive outcome, intervention must include a focus on the translation point of independently applying one's skill to real-life situations. Beyond acquiring a particular skill, it is important that interventions include the use of a skill across a variety of natural contexts (and not just in a research setting or highly supportive educational setting) and build in procedures

for the reduction of dependence on prompts from caregivers or other appropriate adults. In a recent review of factors that impede independent functioning, Hume et al. (2009) highlight vulnerabilities in executive functioning that need to be addressed. These include planning difficulties, impaired processing speed, attention to relevant stimuli, limited intrinsic motivation to learn, inability to cope with ambiguity, and cognitive inflexibility. They also highlight the pitfalls of prompt dependency. Thus, in order for an intervention to be successful, there needs to be a fading of adult management and an increase in self management and independent problem solving (e.g., through the use of self-monitoring strategies).

The previous chapters in this book underscore that when existing evidence-based interventions are put into practice effectively, functional skills can be taught and maintained with success. In Chap. 4, Powers et al. demonstrate that by identifying problematic behaviors and assessing their underlying function, more adaptive behaviors can be taught in their place that serve the same purpose. By conceptualizing each behavior as a means of communication, we can better understand the unwanted behavior's function and replace it with effective communicative strategies. Consequently, the problematic behaviors decrease and can even disappear altogether. For aberrant behaviors that interfere with an individual's ability to learn (e.g., severe aggression, self-injurious behaviors, inattention, impulsivity, hyperactivity, and dysregulation), systematically addressing these behaviors is also merited. Powers et al. discuss several evidence-based behavior modification techniques, such as noncontingent reinforcement, behavioral momentum, high-probability request sequence, and graduated extinction. In addition, in Chap. 8, Scahill and Griebell Boorin provide information on empirically tested medications that have proven to reduce challenging behaviors. In particular, risperidone has been found to significantly reduce severe aggression, self-injurious behaviors, and tantrums, while the addition of systematic parent training has been shown to simultaneously improve functional skill acquisition. In Chap. 9, Schaaf demonstrates that broad-based sensory integration therapies used effectively to address sensory processing impairments or dysregulation can result in better coping strategies, enhanced attention, and learning readiness skills.

Chapters 5 and 6 demonstrate how functional social communication and interaction skills can be taught at all stages of development, regardless of level of functioning. At the prelinguistic level of functioning, children need to be taught that communicative acts are social and functional. Behaviors such as requesting, sharing affect, and interacting through gesture, joint attention, and imitation involve another person; thus, they are social. This is why methodologies such as More than Words and Milieu Communication Training show promise. In the early language stage, in addition to functional communication training (which speaks for itself), Prelock, Paul, and Allen highlight the importance of providing augmentative and alternative communication systems (e.g., voice output devices, Picture Exchange Communication System (PECS), and sign language) to the more severely verbally impaired individuals, defying the misconception that these methods might impede their ability to eventually develop speech. On the contrary, these systems provide individuals with an alternative to the aberrant behaviors that communicate their needs, often to the detriment of their own safety or the safety of others (eventually requiring the treatments set forth by Powers et al. to undo the maladaptive behavior).

Finally, for individuals with more advanced language, Prelock, Paul, and Allen and Ferraioli and Harris sift through the expansive literature of social communication and social skills interventions utilized across development to outline the most promising methods that not only teach these skills, but more importantly, foster the utility and application of these skills to real-life contexts. This involves both teaching social cognition and metalinguistic skills to the individual with ASD (through, for example, Social Stories and video modeling) and training peers to help facilitate interactions and foster these skills through their own behavior.

In Chap. 7, Wood, Fujii, and Renno emphasize the importance of addressing comorbid issues that are likely to be the norm rather than the exception in these individuals. Living with a social disability entails virtually constant exposure to one's greatest vulnerability, as just about every context of life involves interaction with another person. For this reason, not only is there heightened anxiety, but repeated failed experiences inevitably result in feelings of helplessness, despair, and, eventually, depression. In severe cases, there can be acting out through aggression, self-injury, or substance abuse as the result of self-medication. With an increasing percentage of individuals with ASD falling into the category of "higher functioning" (as early and intensive intervention is closing the gap of developmental and subsequent cognitive delays), treatment (and ideally preventative) methods such as CBT and psychotherapeutic services will continue to remain a necessary component of intervention, particularly in older, school-aged individuals, adolescents, and most certainly adults. Yet the specific strategies talked about (e.g., using verbally mediated methods to promote conceptual development and generalization, to enhance the ability to solve problem and make inferences) should be incorporated into all treatment methods throughout development. Wood, Fujii, and Renno also state that traditional behavioral methods do not often go beyond explicitly teaching a specific skill to the functional application of that skill. Thus, taking a more cognitive-behavioral approach of teaching problem-solving strategies, for example, becomes imperative. This brings to light the age-old adage about teaching people to fish rather than merely giving them a fish.

Adaptive Behavior as a Measure of Outcome

The assessment of adaptive behavior is critical for understanding profiles of functioning and subsequent planning of interventions for individuals with ASD. Since a defining feature of positive outcome is independence or the translation of abilities and supports into real-life skills, the level of adaptive functioning also represents a fundamental measure of outcome.

Measuring Adaptive Behavior

The Vineland Adaptive Behavior Scales (VABS) (Sparrow et al. 1984) and its second edition, the Vineland-II (Sparrow et al. 2005, 2006, and 2008), are the most widely used instruments to assess adaptive behavior for those studying and working with individuals with developmental disabilities, including autism (Klin et al. 2007). One reason for the wide use of the VABS in ASD is the considerable data suggesting that these individuals exhibit patterns of strengths and weaknesses that differ from their IQ, as well as from age-matched typically developing children and children with intellectual disability. In addition, several investigators report deficits on specific items from the Vineland scales that differentiate children with ASD from these peer groups (Balboni et al. 2001; Klin et al. 1992; Paul et al. 2004). Given the number

of researchers and clinicians using the Vineland scales to study and plan for individuals with autism, a group of investigators across North America developed the normative data for individuals with autism (Carter et al. 1998).

The information obtained from the Vineland scales assesses an individual's adaptive behavior in a semi-structured interview with a parent, caregiver, or teacher. The Vineland scales cover four adaptive behavior domains: communication, daily living skills, socialization, and motor skills (the latter being optional for individuals over 6 years of age). Adaptive behavior is age-based and represents the typical performance of the individual rather than potential ability – what a person actually does as opposed to what a person is capable of doing. Domain and subdomain standard scores and age equivalencies are yielded as well as an overall index of adaptive functioning, the Adaptive Behavior Composite score.

The Vineland Adaptive Behavior Scales (VABS) represented a major revision of the venerable and internationally employed Vineland Social Maturity Scale (VSMS; Doll 1935, 1953). The Vineland-II is the revision of the VABS and has several additional features. The norms were brought up to date and the age range was extended from "birth to 19 years" to "birth to 90+ years." Many items were modified or added to reflect cultural changes and new research knowledge of developmental disabilities since the publication of the Vineland Adaptive Behavior Scales (VABS). In addition, an extensive bias review was carried out by experts in many fields to ensure that the content was as free as possible from cultural or ethnic bias. Data from the standardization suggest that, contrary to IQ testing, adaptive behavior does not demonstrate a "Flynn effect" (Flynn 2007); that is, there does not appear to be a rise in scores over generations. The appendix to this chapter gives more information about the Vineland-II.

Outcomes in ASD

There is no shortage of research demonstrating that many skills can be acquired as a result of early diagnosis and intervention, including developmental abilities and adaptive skills (Chawarska et al. 2009; National Research Council 2001; Rogers and Vismara 2008; Zwaigenbaum et al. 2009). Nevertheless, the rate of skill acquisition may be slower for adaptive skills than for developmental (Saulnier et al. 2008) and cognitive (Klin et al. 2007) abilities despite intensity of intervention. Magiati et al. (2007) conducted a follow-up study on preschoolers with ASD who received early intensive behavioral intervention (EIBI) compared to an autism-specific preschool sample. They reported that the only significant difference found between the groups was on the Vineland daily living skills domain; the standard score was higher in the EIBI group relative to the non-EIBI. However, the daily living skills standard score decreased over time in the EIBI group, suggesting a slowed rate of acquisition of skills relative to age, despite acquiring more than the non-EIBI group.

Recent meta-analyses of EIBI have shown conflicting results with respect to changes in adaptive behavior skills as measured on the Vineland Adaptive Behavior Scales (VABS). Reichow and Wolery (2009) did not perform a statistical analysis of adaptive behavior, but noted small to medium effect sizes with confidence intervals including zero for most of the studies included in their synthesis. Eldevik, Hastings, and their colleagues (2009) performed a statistical analysis of adaptive behavior scores and found a medium effect ($g = .66$). More research is needed to determine what effect, if any, EIBI have on adaptive behavior.

Unfortunately, many investigations stop short of adolescence let alone adulthood. To date, the most consistent factors associated with positive outcome include intact cognitive functioning and functional language by age 5 or 6 (Billstedt et al. 2005; Howlin et al. 2004; Paul and Cohen 1984). Yet, a recent 20-year outcome study on adults that had baseline IQs in the non-impaired range found little evidence to support any childhood factors associated with adult success (Farley et al. 2009). Although long-term outcome for individuals with ASD is variable, current reports indicate that, for at least half of the individuals assessed, independent employment, living, and relationships are problematic (Billstedt et al. 2005; Eaves and Ho 2008; Howlin et al. 2004; Tsatsanis 2003). We are discovering that the needs of adults are likely very different to, and possibly more complex than, even the same individual's needs throughout early development. Not only do adults continue to struggle with the symptoms of the disorder (specifically verbal, nonverbal, and social communication deficits) but they also suffer from other psychiatric conditions – most notably anxiety and depression but also ADHD, learning difficulties, and psychotic features, in some cases (Hofvander et al. 2009; Saulnier and Volkmar 2007). In fact, a recent examination of national data on adults receiving vocational rehabilitation services concluded that adults with ASD were more likely to be rejected services because their disability was deemed too severe to obtain benefit (Lawer et al. 2009).

These findings are extremely concerning considering that the number of adults identified with ASD has increased well over 100% over the past decade despite the field's efforts on effecting change early in development (Cimera and Cowan 2009) and the cost to treat adults with ASD is among the most expensive (Cimera and Cowan 2009; Lawer et al. 2009). Given the field's strong emphasis on early intensive intervention, one would anticipate these outcomes to be more promising. The studies of adults with ASD also serve to remind us that this disorder affects individuals through the lifespan; it is both sensible and essential to emphasize functional outcomes when thinking about how to effect change and optimize potential.

CONCLUSION

In moving toward a broader initiative focusing on adaptive functioning, we suggest a framework that emphasizes the importance of defining goals appropriate to the individual's level of functioning, providing supports based on profiles of strengths and weaknesses, measuring those goals and functional outcomes over time, and transferring the acquired skills to natural life contexts. The following questions are proposed for consideration when thinking about intervention for the individual with ASD as well as larger-scale studies on adaptive functioning in ASD:

- What are the fundamental adaptive behaviors and skills a person needs to function across settings (home, school, work, and in the community)?
- What are the specific deficit areas for individuals with ASD?
- How do the deficit areas relate to variables such as age and level of functioning?
- What are the variables that promote or limit independent functioning in individuals with ASD?
- What are the required environmental and interpersonal supports?
- What is the most suitable method of instruction?
- How is generalization built into the intervention?
- How is the skill defined relative to the individual's level of functioning?
- How is progress measured?
- How is the acquired skill maintained?

It is interesting to note that the measurement of adaptive behavior arose from the assessment of and need to identify individuals with cognitive disability. While a good many individuals with ASD also exhibit cognitive impairment, the striking aspect of this disorder is that there are many very intellectually bright individuals with ASD who have very compromised adaptive functioning. Adaptation may be at the very heart of the disorder.

REFERENCES

Abel, J., Doehring, P., Wagner, B., Lesko, L. R., Peters, K., Myers, K. (2008). Where are the data? Publication profiles of articles on autism in JABA, JADD, and JPBI. Poster presented at the Association for Behavior Analysis – Autism Conference, February, Atlanta, GA.

Ando, H. (1977). Training autistic children to urinate in the toilet through operant conditioning techniques. *Journal of Autism and Childhood Schizophrenia, 7*(2), 151–163.

Balboni, G., Pedrabissi, L., Molteni, M., & Villa, S. (2001). Discriminant validity of the Vineland Scales: score profiles of individuals with mental retardation and a specific disorder. *American Journal on Mental Retardation, 106*(2), 162–172.

Billstedt, E., Gillberg, C., & Gillberg, C. (2005). Autism after adolescence: Population-based 13- to 22-year follow-up study of 120 individuals with autism diagnosed in childhood. *Journal of Autism and Developmental Disorders, 35*(3), 351–360.

Bledsoe, R., Myles, B. S., & Simpson, R. L. (2003). Use of a Social Story intervention to improve mealtime skills of an adolescent with Asperger syndrome. *Autism, 7*(3), 289–295.

Bolte, S., & Poustka, F. (2002). The relation between general cognitive level and adaptive behavior domains in individuals with autism with and without co-morbid mental retardation. *Child Psychiatry and Human Development, 33*(2), 165–172.

Carter, A. S., Volkmar, F. R., Sparrow, S. S., Wang, J., Lord, C., et al. (1998). The Vineland Adaptive Behavior Scales: Supplementary norms for individuals with autism. *Journal of Autism and Developmental Disorders, 28*(4), 287–302.

Chawarska, K., Klin, A., Paul, R., Macari, S., & Volkmar, F. (2009). A prospective study of toddlers with ASD: short-term diagnostic and cognitive outcomes. *Journal of Childhood Psychology and Psychiatry, 50*(10), 1235–45.

Cicero, F. R., & Pfadt, A. (2002). Investigation of a reinforcement-based toilet training procedure for children with autism. *Research in Developmental Disabilities, 23*(5), 319–331.

Cimera, R. E., & Cowan, R. J. (2009). The costs of services and employment outcomes achieved by adults with autism in the US. *Autism, 13*(3), 285–302.

Doll, E. A. (1935). A genetic scale of social maturity. *The American Journal of Orthopsychiatry, 5,* 180–188.

Doll, E. A. (1953). *Measurement of Social Competence.* Circle Pines, MN: American Guidance Service.

Duran, E. (1985). Teaching janitorial skills to autistic adolescents. *Adolescence, 20*(77), 225–32.

Eaves, L. C., & Ho, H. H. (2008). Young adult outcome of autism spectrum disorders. *Journal of Autism and Developmental Disorders, 38*(4), 739–747.

Eldevik, S., Hastings, R. P., Hughes, J. C., Jahr, E., Eikeseth, S., & Cross, S. (2009). Meta-analysis of early intensive behavioral intervention for children with autism. *Journal of Clinical Child and Adolescent Psychology, 38*(3), 439–450.

Farley, M. A., McMahon, W. M., Fombonne, E., Jenson, W. R., Miller, J., et al. (2009). Twenty-year outcome for individuals with autism and average to near-average cognitive abilities. *Autism Research, 2,* 109–118.

Fenton, G., D'Ardia, C., Valente, D., Del Vecchio, I., Fabrizi, A., et al. (2003). Vineland adaptive behavior profiles in children with autism and moderate to severe developmental delay. *Autism, 7*(3), 269–287.

Flynn, J. R. (2007). *What Is Intelligence?: Beyond the Flynn Effect.* Cambridge: Cambridge University Press.

Freeman, B. J., Del'Homme, M., Guthrie, D., & Zhang, F. (1999). Vineland Adaptive Behavior Scale scores as a function of age and initial IQ in 210 autistic children. *Journal of Autism and Developmental Disorders, 29*(5), 379–384.

Harchik, A. E., Sherman, J. A., & Sheldon, J. B. (1992). The use of self-management procedures by people with developmental disabilities: A brief review. *Research in Developmental Disabilities, 13*(3), 211–227.

Hofvander, B., Delorme, R., Chaste, P., Nyden, A., Wentz, E., et al. (2009). Psychiatric and psychosocial problems in adults with normal-intelligence autism spectrum disorders. *BMC Psychiatry, 9,* 35.

Howlin, P., Goode, S., Hutton, J., & Rutter, M. (2004). Adult outcomes for children with autism. *Journal of Autism and Developmental Disorders, 34,* 212–229.

Hume, K., Loftin, R., & Lantz, J. (2009). Increasing independence in autism spectrum disorders: a review of three focused interventions. *Journal of Autism and Developmental Disorders, 39*(9), 1329–1338.

Klin, A., Saulnier, C. A., Sparrow, S. S., Cicchetti, D. V., Volkmar, F. R., et al. (2007). Social and communication abilities and disabilities in higher functioning individuals with autism spectrum disorders: The Vineland and the ADOS. *Journal of Autism and Developmental Disorders, 37*(4), 748–759.

Klin, A., Volkmar, F. R., & Sparrow, S. S. (1992). Autistic social dysfunction: Some limitations of the theory of mind hypothesis. *Journal of Child Psychology and Psychiatry, 33*(5), 861–876.

Koegel, R. L., & Rincover, A. (1976). Some detrimental effects of using extra stimuli to guide learning in normal and autistic children. *Journal of Abnormal Child Psychology, 4*(1), 59–71.

Lawer, L., Brusilovskiy, E., Salzer, M. S., & Mandell, D. S. (2009). Use of vocational rehabilitative services among adults with autism. *Journal of Autism and Developmental Disorders, 39*(3), 487–494.

Liss, M., Harel, B., Fein, D., Allen, D., Dunn, M., et al. (2001). Predictors and correlates of adaptive functioning in children with developmental disorders. *Journal of Autism and Developmental Disorders, 31*(2), 219–230.

Lord, C., Rutter, M., DiLavore, P. C., & Risi, S. (2000). *Autism Diagnostic Observation Schedule.* Los Angeles: Western Psychological Services.

Magiati, I., Charman, T., & Howlin, P. (2007). A two-year prospective follow-up study of community-based early intensive behavioural intervention and specialist nursery provision for children with autism spectrum disorders. *Journal of Child Psychology and Psychiatry, 48,* 803–812.

Mithaug, D. K., & Mithaug, D. E. (2003). Effects of teacher-directed versus student-directed instruction on self-management of young children with disabilities. *Journal of Applied Behavior Analysis, 36*(1), 133–136.

National Research Council. (2001). *Educating Young Children with Autism.* Washington, DC: National Academy Press.

Nelson, D. L., Gergenti, E., & Hollander, A. C. (1980). Extra prompts versus no extra prompts in self-care training of autistic children and adolescents. *Journal of Autism and Developmental Disorders, 10*(3), 311–321.

Paul, C., Williams, K. E., Riegel, K., & Gibbons, B. (2007). Combining repeated taste exposure and escape prevention: an intervention for the treatment of extreme food selectivity. *Appetite, 49*(3), 708–711.

Paul, R., & Cohen, D. (1984). Outcomes of severe disorders of language acquisition. *Journal of Autism and Developmental Disorders*, *14*(4), 405–421.

Paul, R., Miles, S., Cicchetti, D., Sparrow, S., Klin, A., Volkmar, F., et al. (2004). Adaptive behavior in autism and pervasive developmental disorder-not otherwise specified: Microanalysis of scores on the Vineland Adaptive Behavior Scales. *Journal of Autism and Developmental Disorders*, *34*(2), 223–228.

Perry, A., Flanagan, H. E., Dunn Geier, J., & Freeman, N. L. (2009). Brief report: the Vineland Adaptive Behavior Scales in young children with autism spectrum disorders at different cognitive levels. *Journal of Autism and Developmental Disorders*, *39*(7), 1066–1078.

Pierce, K. L., & Schreibman, L. (1994). Teaching daily living skills to children with autism in unsupervised settings through pictorial self-management. *Journal of Applied Behavior Analysis*, *27*(3), 471–481.

Reichow, B., & Wolery, M. (2009). Comprehensive synthesis of early intensive behavioral interventions for young children with autism based on the UCLA Young Autism Project model. *Journal of Autism and Developmental Disorders*, *39*, 23–41.

Rogers, S. J., & Vismara, L. A. (2008). Evidence-based comprehensive treatments for early autism. *Journal of Clinical Child and Adolescent Psychology*, *37*(1), 8–38.

Saulnier, C. A., & Klin, A. (2007). Brief report: Social and communication abilities and disabilities in higher functioning individuals with autism and Asperger syndrome. *Journal of Autism and Developmental Disorders*, *37*, 788–793.

Saulnier, C., & Volkmar, F. (2007). Mental health problems in people with autism and related disorders. In N. Bouras & G. Holt (Eds.), *Psychiatric and behavioral disorders in intellectual and developmental disabilities* (2nd ed., pp. 215–224). New York: Cambridge University Press.

Saulnier, C. A., Chawarska, K., & Klin, A. (2008). The relationship between adaptive functioning and symptom severity in toddlers with ASD. Paper presented at the International Meeting for Autism Research, London, UK.

Sparrow, S. S., Balla, D. A., & Cicchetti, D. V. (1984). *Vineland Adaptive Behavior Scales (Survey Form)*. Circle Pines, MN: American Guidance Service.

Sparrow, S. S., Cicchetti, D. V., & Balla, D. A. (2005). *Vineland Adaptive Behavior Scales: Second Edition (Vineland-II) – Survey Interview Form/ Caregiver Rating Form*. Livonia, MN: Pearson Assessments.

Sparrow, S. S., Cicchetti, D. V., & Balla, D. A. (2006). *Vineland Adaptive Behavior Scales: Second Edition – Teacher Rating Form (Vineland-IITRF)*. Livonia, MN: Pearson Assessments.

Sparrow, S. S., Cicchetti, D. V., & Balla, D. A. (2008). *Vineland Adaptive Behavior Scales: Second Edition (Vineland-II) – Expanded Interview Form*. Livonia, MN: Pearson Assessments.

Szatmari, P., Bryson, S. E., Boyle, M. H., Streiner, D. L., & Duku, E. (2003). Predictors of outcome among high functioning children with autism and Asperger syndrome. *Journal of Child Psychology and Psychiatry*, *44*(4), 520–528.

Tsatsanis, K. D. (2003). Outcome research in Asperger syndrome and autism. *Child and Adolescent Psychiatric Clinics of North America*, *12*(1), 47–63.

Volkmar, F. R., Sparrow, S. S., Goudreau, D., Cicchetti, D. V., Paul, R., & Cohen, D. J. (1987). Social deficits in autism: An operational approach using the Vineland Adaptive Behavior Scales. *Journal of the American Academy of Child and Adolescent Psychiatry*, *26*, 156–161.

Zwaigenbaum, L., Bryson, S., Lord, C., et al. (2009). Clinical assessment and management of toddlers with suspected autism spectrum disorder: Insights from studies of high-risk infants. *Pediatrics*, *123*, 1383–1391.

Appendix: Vineland-II

The Vineland-II provides several assessments of adaptive behavior, which differ in terms of the range of coverage (survey or expanded), the informant (parent or teacher), and the response format (interview or rating form) as listed in Table 11.1.

As with the VABS, the 11 Vineland-II subdomains are grouped into four domain composites (see Table 11.2): communication, daily living skills, socialization, and motor skills. Within each domain, the subdomains yield scaled scores that comprise the domain composite scores. The four domain composite scores comprise the Adaptive Behavior Composite for individuals aged from birth through to 6 years 11 months and 30 days; for individuals aged 7 years and older, three domain composites (communication, daily living skills, and socialization) comprise the Adaptive Behavior Composite. Examiners may choose to administer a single domain or any combination of domains to assess an individual's adaptive functioning in one or more areas. If they choose to administer all the domains required at a given age, they can obtain the Adaptive Behavior Composite.

Three subscales – internalizing, externalizing, and other – comprise the optional maladaptive behavior index, which provides a measure of undesirable behaviors that may interfere with an individual's adaptive behavior. The optional maladaptive critical items do not contribute to a subscale or composite score but provide a brief measure of more severe maladaptive behaviors that examiners may want to consider in the overall assessment of adaptive behavior.

TABLE 11.1   Forms of the Vineland-II

Form	Format	# of Items	Age Range
Survey	Interview	376	Birth to 90+
Parent/Caregiver	Rating Form	376	Birth to 90+
Teacher Report	Rating Form	221	3–21
Expanded Report	Interview	601	Birth to 90+

TABLE 11.2   Vineland-II domains and subdomains

Domain	Subdomain	Description
Communication	Receptive	How the student listens, and pays attention, and what he or she understands
	Expressive	What the individual says, how he or she uses words and sentences to gather and provide information
	Written	What the individual understands about how letters make words, and what he or she reads
Daily Living Skills	Personal	How the student eats, dresses, and practices personal hygiene
	Domestic	What household tasks the individual performs
	Community	How the individual uses time, money, the telephone, the computer and job skills
Socialization	Interpersonal	How the student interacts with others
	Play and Leisure Time	How the student plays and uses leisure time
	Coping Skills	How the student demonstrates responsibility and sensitivity to others
Motor Skills	Gross	How the student uses arms and legs for movement and coordination
	Fine	How the student uses hands and fingers to manipulate objects

Practicing Evidence-Based Practices

Ruth Blennerhassett Eren and Pamela Owen Brucker

ABBREVIATIONS

ABA	Applied behavior analysis
ASDs	Autism spectrum disorders
CEC	Council for Exceptional Children
DSM-IV	Diagnostic and Statistical Manual of Mental Disorders 4th edition
EBP	Evidence-based practice
IDEA	Individuals with Disabilities Education Act
IEP	Individualized education program
NCLB	No child left behind

INTRODUCTION

Public education in the United States has a history of local control in the development of curriculum and instruction. Although notable court decisions have led to more universal applications of educational policy and practices (Brown v. Board of Education 1954, Oberti v. Clementon 1993), it has been federal law that has resulted in significant changes in instruction. The Individuals with Disabilities Education Improvement Act (IDEA; Public Law 108–142), first enacted in Public Law 94–142, guaranteed the right of a free, appropriate public education for all children, regardless of the severity of their disability. The word "appropriate" resulted in the beginning of what we refer to today as differentiated instruction: instructional strategies that allow a child to learn and progress in an educational setting. The federal law, No Child Left Behind (NCLB; Public Law 107-110), enacted in 2001, contributed to this initiative and added a caveat that these differentiated instructional strategies needed to be grounded in scientifically based research. Indeed, the term "scientifically based research" has been noted to appear in NCLB 111 times (Deshler 2002). The federal government, in IDEA 2004, identified 13 eligibility categories. In order to receive special education services, a student

B. Reichow et al. (eds.), *Evidence-Based Practices and Treatments for Children with Autism*,
DOI 10.1007/978-1-4419-6975-0_12, © Springer Science+Business Media, LLC 2011

must, through a multidisciplinary evaluation, meet the eligibility criteria established for one of the 13 categories. Since 1975, when PL94–142 was enacted, educational interventions for students receiving special education have expanded, particularly in disability categories with a high level of incidence such as speech and language disorders and learning disabilities. Low-incidence disabilities, such as mental retardation, visual impairments, and autism, have received less attention.

The fastest growing population of students with disabilities (p. 31, Oller and Oller 2010) is those with autism spectrum disorders (ASDs). Although the federal eligibility category in IDEA is "autistic disorder," this eligibility category may include any one of the five pervasive developmental disorders identified in *Diagnostic and Statistical Manual of Mental Disorders*, fourth edition (*DSM*-IV; APA 1994). ASDs have a spectrum of characteristics in terms of severity. The triad of impairments (social interaction, communication, and repetitive or restricted interests and behaviors) is seen in all individuals meeting these eligibility criteria, yet how these impairments are manifested may be very unique and different from other individuals in this eligibility category. One child's communication difficulties may be manifested in the use of echolalic phrases to indicate wants and needs, while another child's communication difficulties may involve difficulties in pragmatic language. In addition, because ASDs are developmental disorders, symptoms and needs change over time. For example, a teacher may think a child is functioning appropriately in navigating the social environment in fifth grade, but when the child enters middle school the social environment and expectations change and an entire new series of considerations may arise. Consequently, ASDs are complex disorders that require a multidisciplinary team to constantly assess and plan for new challenges

presented at any given time. Indeed, Siegel (2003) refers to the education of children with ASD as a "Sisyphean struggle" in which educators must address the symptoms as they are presented, not the diagnosis in general.

Implementing evidence-based practices (EBP) in public schools is a challenge. The first challenge in public education is to reach agreement in defining the construct. There is not always agreement on the name and definition of EBP. Sometimes called scientifically based research, empirically based practices, research-based intervention, these names have all been used synonymously by educators and vendors, frequently with no qualifying definition or criteria. The reader is referred back to Chap. 1 of this text for the history of EBP. The criteria established by Reichow et al. (2008; see also Chap. 2) has made a significant contribution in clarifying the state of confusion that currently exists. The challenge is for all educators, vendors, etc. to adhere to these rigorous criteria before making claims that an intervention is evidence-based.

Educators must also have access to current research directing them to EBP. Although educators would agree with the importance of knowing which interventions are evidence-based, there is no universally recognized requirement for teachers to search for EBP and then to implement them. In fact, in today's age of standards-based reform, curriculum and methodology are most often determined by central administration and teachers are given little opportunity if any, to digress from the district curriculum or selected methodology. Teachers are teachers first and are responsible for teaching during the workday. They are not given time to engage in research-related activities that would validate the effectiveness of the strategies employed. In fact, even when challenges are made in due process, many hearing/review officers and judges make decisions based on the testimony of expert witnesses, who may or may not have particular expertise and knowledge regarding current best practices in autism eligibility assessment (Fogt et al. 2003).

Despite the absence of a mechanism to identify and implement EBP into teaching by educators, what all educators may be able to agree with are the goals of EBP. As postulated by Reichow et al. (2008), the goal of EBP is to use empirical data to create practice recommendations and guidelines that identify and predict which treatments are most likely to work for certain individuals under specific conditions and circumstances. Taking this one step further, educators will know the treatment or intervention is effective (or not), when systematic data collection is used. This requires ongoing data collection and data-based decision-making by an interdisciplinary team in order to meet the complex, diverse, yet overlapping needs of individuals with ASD.

The first important note that educators must understand is that an intervention that has been deemed "evidence-based" only indicates that it may be an intervention that is more promising to begin with than an intervention that has no evidence. The term "evidence-based" does not automatically ensure success for all children with ASDs. The second important note that educators must keep in mind is that, unlike other disabilities, the recent surge in autism eligibility in public schools has resulted in a plethora of interventions, strategies, "magic bullets", cures, etc., in the market today. Many are worthless and have no evidence even though the claim may be made that they are "research-based." Some, however, may appear to be a promising practice but are so new to the field that enough research has not been completed to deem the intervention "evidence-based." The challenge for educators is to balance the use of EBP interventions while at the same time, validating, through on-

going data collection and evaluation, new and effective procedures for individuals with specific needs or challenges.

On-going data collection and data-based decision-making is not always standard operating procedure in public schools. Although many educators recognize the importance of this practice, the structure of the school program and availability of trained staff is highly variable throughout schools and school districts (McGee and Morrier 2005). Budget constraints in some districts make it almost impossible to train teachers, related service personnel, and paraprofessionals to take data consistently across all settings (i.e., with reliability and validity). As a result, the fidelity of the data may be in question or may not be available in all settings of the school day. In addition to training of staff, availability of staff may be another barrier to data collection. Frequently districts are struggling with high caseloads for their special education teachers due to the continual shortage of teachers in this area. With one teacher for as many as 15 special education students and perhaps one special education paraprofessional assigned to the special education teacher, data collection becomes extremely difficult. Part of this dilemma can be attributed to the lack of understanding of the importance of data collection in order to ensure progress. Administrators, as well as Boards of Education, need to recognize not only the importance of data-based decision-making but also the number of trained staff needed to complete this task effectively. Finally, a barrier often neglected is the time it takes to not only collect data but review it as a team, in order to make multidisciplinary decisions. It is extremely difficult to convene a team of professionals during the school day due to the resulting loss of instructional time with students. After-school planning may be problematic with teacher contracts, conflicting responsibilities of staff, etc. When one considers the importance of parent involvement, the difficulties with teaming become even more complex. Again, district administrators and governing boards need to recognize this barrier and construct dedicated teaming time into the school day or the teacher's daily schedule.

This chapter discusses professional teacher preparation in the areas of pre-service training (undergraduate and graduate level) and then focuses on two critical components necessary for employing EBP in public school settings: additional teacher training and staff teaming.

PROFESSIONAL PREPARATION OR TRAINING FOR TEACHER CERTIFICATION

Initial Teacher Certification (Pre-service Teacher Training)

Given the increase in the number of students with ASD who are being educated in public schools in general education (Oller and Oller 2010), it has become increasingly important that pre-service training for both special education and general education teachers include competencies in teaching students with ASD. Pre-service candidates generally must juggle all university requirements along with the requirements for their teaching certification. The essential questions in pre-service training become "what competencies does an initial educator need?" and "what can be addressed at this level of training?" To date, this question has been only partially answered for teachers of students with ASD by the Council for Exceptional Children (CEC 2010a). These standards are shown in Appendix 1 and are available on the CEC website (http://www.cec.sped.org).

General education candidates. With the rates of students with ASD increasing in the general education classroom, it is essential that

the general education teacher be equipped with knowledge of these students. The Connecticut State Department of Education (2005) noted that there is no standard for training professionals, yet a certain level of knowledge is required for a team to collectively plan and meet the needs of these learners. They further outlined that this knowledge base should include an understanding of early intervention, cooperative planning, curriculum, systematic instruction, evidence-based strategies, social skills, and transition planning. General education teachers need this knowledge despite the presence of a paraprofessional in the classroom to work with the student with ASD (Robertson et al. 2003).

A survey of 35 pre-service teacher candidates who were completing their final student teaching indicated that both elementary education candidates (e.g., general education candidates) and special education candidates had knowledge of ASD, but the quality of their responses to the survey questions varied (Murray 2008). The elementary education candidates tended to have less accurate information and their responses tended to be based more on stereotypes of media images and less on actual data. In general, they did not recognize that ASD was a continuum of disabilities that incorporated a wide range of strengths and weaknesses. Additionally, less than 20% of the general education candidates reported any field experiences that included interaction with students with ASD.

The pre-service elementary education candidates who took this survey received one 37-h, required, overview course in special education that covers all disabilities, disability laws, and instructional accommodations and modifications. This requirement is typical for most general education teacher candidates. This course is taken at the beginning of their coursework for certification. By comparison, special education candidates receive over 300 h of course work. It would appear that more information about ASD, as well as practical experience working with students with ASD in the general classroom is needed and should be offered closer to the time these candidates will actually work with students in a classroom setting.

Special education candidates. Since special education teachers have specific responsibilities for program planning, team consultation, and specialized instruction, pre-service special education candidates need a higher level of knowledge and skill in working with students with ASD. Consequently, special education pre-service candidates take additional coursework in these areas. But does this additional pre-service coursework prepare the initial special educator to meet the needs of the ASD student?

In the Murray (2008) survey, special education candidates received an additional seven courses in teaching students with disabilities. On the survey questions, they demonstrated higher levels of scientifically-based information about ASD. For instance, 100% of the candidates in this group were able to list common characteristics of ASD and to name common strategies to be used with students with ASD. However, this group was less clear on who has the responsibility to identify student's eligibility and they continued to harbor some stereotypic myths, although at a lower level than their general education peers. Although special education candidates reported more interaction with students with ASD in field experiences, less than 50% of the special education candidates reported having two or more field experiences with students with ASD.

Why is this important? Practical experience and fieldwork are essential to develop skills in working with students with disabilities. Research has shown that, when well-supervised field experiences replace some classroom lectures, candidates can actually master the course content at a higher level than those who have only had

the classroom teaching (Spear-Swerling and Brucker 2004). Additionally, candidates' self-perceptions of their content knowledge acquisition was increased (Fang and Ashley 2004; Spear-Swerling et al. 2005). Likewise, working with a variety of students on the spectrum can help to dispel myths and stereotypes associated with individuals with ASD (see Case Study 12.1).

Case Study 12.1:

Mark and Robert

Mark is in his final year of a pre-service certification program that prepares him to teach both elementary and special education students. Next semester, he will student teach in general education and special education classrooms for a total of 16 weeks. This semester, in preparation for student teaching he is taking a required field experience that requires him to work with students at an urban K-8 school 3 h per week for 16 weeks. The field experience is supervised by two faculty members. Mark's time is split between assessing and providing remedial instruction for a student and teaching a science unit in the general education classroom with three other candidates. The first week, Mark was assigned to do his individual work with Robert, a student with ASD. Robert is also in the first-grade classroom where Mark is teaching science with his group. Last year, in kindergarten, Robert did not speak all year. This year, he has established a relationship with his first-grade teacher and uses limited language within the classroom. He likes anything red and carries a red footstool wherever he goes in the school.

Mark's initial reaction to working with Robert was panic. He indicated to the faculty supervisors that he did not know how to teach children with autism. In the first session, Robert had not responded verbally to any of Mark's assessment questions, although Robert did write a sentence. After the first session, Mark consulted with the faculty supervisors and, using his knowledge from his coursework, developed a plan for assessment that would build on pointing to choices and reward any attempt Robert made to comply with Mark's request. Mark added visuals to his instruction and, through consultation with the classroom teacher, he began to use Robert's favorite white board and a red marker. Mark also observed Robert in the classroom and determined which strategies the teacher used to work effectively with Robert. By the second week, Robert was complying with all of Mark's directions. By the third week, he was answering Mark in one- or two-word responses. At the end of the ninth week, Robert was responding verbally, writing dictated words and sentences on his white board, and remaining focused. He was tolerating the supervisors' observation of his sessions and the red footstool was left in the classroom for the first time this semester. Mark noted that he was fortunate to have this field experience because it helped him to recognize what he already knew and how he could use consultation with other professionals to work with students with ASD. It also dispelled some misconceptions he had about ASD. His confidence level in working with these students is very high.

Conclusions. It is apparent that both general education and special education pre-service teacher candidates need additional knowledge of and exposure to students with ASD, as opposed to generalized knowledge about students with disabilities. General education candidates need a basic knowledge to work with students with disabilities, including students with ASD in their classrooms and the skills to team with other professionals. Special education candidates need more scientifically-based information and skills in order to make appropriate instructional decisions for these students. If it is not possible to add coursework into candidate programs, topic specific seminars on ASD should be required. Both groups need consistent, well-supervised

field experiences to increase pre-service knowledge and skills as well as to increase candidates' self-perceptions about working with students with ASD. Appropriate field experiences can also help to dispel stereotypes of students with ASD.

Given the nature and needs of students with ASD, a generalized special education pre-service program that prepares students to teach a broad variety of students with disabilities may not be sufficient to equip initial educators with the competencies to program, manage, assess, and provide specialized instruction to students with ASD. If this is the case, both advanced instruction at the graduate level and well-developed in-service programs may be needed before competencies can be fully developed.

Advanced Certification (Graduate Level)

Given the amount of information, training and experience required for initial certification, it is no wonder that advanced training is required to fully understand ASD and appropriate interventions for this population. It is at the graduate level that educators have the opportunity to study a disability category in depth and develop more disability specific knowledge and understanding. Many teacher preparation universities therefore provide graduate programs in which students may earn a master's or other advanced degree in a specific disability category. The CEC has developed standards for teachers of specific disabilities that university programs may use as a framework in developing their graduate program (CEC 2010b). These guidelines are shown in Appendix 2 and are available from the CEC website.

Due to the low incidence of autistic disorder in the past and its current rapid growth (Oller and Oller 2010), the CEC standards have only recently been developed. This action again reflects the rapid rise in the identification of children under IDEA as eligible for special education under the educational disability category of autism. The ten professional standards addressed in the Initial Skill Set are foundations, development and characteristics of learners, individual learning differences, instructional strategies, learning environments/social interactions, language, instructional planning, assessment, professional and ethical practice, and collaboration. The six standards addressed in the Advanced Knowledge Skill Set are leadership and policy, program development and organization, research and inquiry, individual and program evaluation, professional development and ethical practice, and collaboration. Hopefully, these standards will be addressed in the course work requirements at graduate level for students pursing advanced degrees in ASD.

As important as course work is in advanced levels of teacher preparation, nothing enhances a student's program more than supervised clinical experience with children with ASD. A clinical experience in a controlled setting conducted under the direction of professors allows the graduate student to acquire the ability to translate knowledge into practice. Indeed, there is a large body of research that speaks to the effectiveness of supervised clinical experiences. For instance, research has shown that having a longer student teaching experience, especially when it is concurrent with theoretical coursework, is associated with stronger outcomes for teachers in terms of ability to apply learning to practice. Program designs that include more practicum experiences and student teaching, integrated with coursework, appear to make a difference in teacher's practices, confidence, and long-term commitment to teaching (Darling-Hammond and Bransford 2005).

Given the combination of course work and clinical practice, institutions in higher education have the opportunity today to fully prepare students in advanced degree programs to be competent in delivering appropriate services to individuals with ASD in the public schools. In fact, these individuals would be expected to be the leaders in their district for the ASD population and, because of their solid knowledge and understanding of the disorder, would be expected to engage in identifying evidence-based or at least promising practices for children with ASD. When these students leave their graduate programs and engage in teaching in the public schools, it is then the responsibility of the school districts' professional development initiatives to address the dissemination of newly identified EBP information and to conduct on-going training in the implementation of such practices.

In-service Training

In addition to being a Sisyphean effort to constantly identify and address the changing needs of an individual with ASD, it is an equally Herculean effort for districts to stay abreast of the most recent knowledge and practices for this population. It becomes a moving target, as research into this disability increases and more and more interventions are identified. How are districts to stay on top of this constant flow of information? How can they distinguish best practice from popular practice from ineffective practice? Another hurdle districts encounter with in-service training is staff turnover. A district might carefully and thoughtfully craft a series of in-service workshops on ASD but if those teachers leave for any reason, the district needs to retrain or at least re-visit their in-service program for teachers of students with ASD. All of these issues can be very costly in an age where many district Boards of Education are looking for cost effectiveness.

Public school personnel engage in on-going training through their district's professional development activities, activities that are mandated under NCLB. Much has been written about teacher training after certification, which has its roots in the educational theory of situated learning. This theory believes that learning needs to take place within the context and culture of real situations, as opposed to presentations of abstract concepts (Lave and Wenger 1991).

In the area of ASD, it has become the mission of many districts to give knowledge to both parents and professionals in order to support individuals with ASD in the inclusive classroom, the community, and their special education program. Challenges in doing this involve the complexity of ASDs, the number of individuals with ASD in the general education classroom, and the specialized treatment and services that may be needed by these individuals. States face the challenge of possible inequity of service if there is not a statewide plan for this type of professional development and it may result in not only inequity of services but inadequate knowledge of the spectrum disorders and the implementation of only those methodologies that someone in the district is aware of despite lack of evidence of effectiveness or appropriateness for all individuals with ASD in the district. For example, many districts have a centralized preschool program that has a comprehensive program for young children with ASD but have many elementary and several middle schools and high schools to which this population transitions as they advance in age. These receiving schools may frequently be unprepared and ill-advised regarding programs and supports for this population. This may then lead to parental frustration, staff anxiety, and inappropriate programming for these children. School districts often find themselves employing a variety of consultants to support staff in the various buildings resulting in inequity of service, disconnected programs, lack of ownership by the district staff, and no internal level of expertise. This inefficient model can become costly and difficult to maintain (Eren and Cook 2009).

In order to begin the process of developing comprehensive programming for all individuals with ASD in a district and employing EBP to meet their complex needs, a district must have the internal expertise in ASD and the ability to assign people to create a comprehensive school district program or it must engage a consultant with expertise in ASD to coordinate the program development process in the district to ensure that the district develops the capacity to serve all children on the spectrum at all grade levels. Through a consultative model, a district can develop and assume ownership of all of their children on the spectrum, have appropriate training and guidance in assessment, educational intervention, and transition for children with this disability. Only then will a district be able to avoid limiting itself to one methodology and be able to address the totality of district program development through in-service training.

In order to be comprehensive, effective, and long lasting, an in-service plan for educators who are working with individuals with ASD must, to some degree, parallel the training provided in advanced teacher preparation programs. The graduate program design can be reconfigured into three phases of training, again basing the training on the development of a teacher's competency as indicated in the CEC standards. All three phases of training would include traditional, didactic instructional workshops as well as hands-on follow-up in the form of demonstrations, modeling and guided practice by the trainers with the actual children the teachers are currently teaching. Supervision would also occur by targeting specific competencies taught in the training workshops and follow-up and objectively measuring the teacher's performance in their implementation.

The follow up demonstrations, modeling, guided practice and supervision are critical for successful implementation of EBP. McGee and Morrier (2005) point out that numerous studies have provided repeated documentation of the failure of traditional training workshops to develop new skills. This is especially true when outcomes of workshop training were compared with hands-on training.

Phase 1 of in-service teacher training would be available to and required of all teachers in the district. This training would incorporate general knowledge of the characteristics of individuals with ASD and the challenges they face in the areas of communication, behavior, and social interaction. General strategies and positive behavioral supports would be emphasized on this level as well as a deep understanding of the ASD perspective or limited understanding of theory of mind, central coherence, and executive functioning. Only by having this basic knowledge would a teacher be expected to understand why one intervention might be more appropriate and effective over another suggested intervention. For example, understanding that many individuals with ASD also have an intellectual disability and poor motor planning skills would allow a teacher or therapist to possibly rule out the use of sign language as a long-range communicative strategy and suggest that the team look at alternative long-range plans in communication development for this particular child. Competency at this level would ensure that the professional educator would be able to understand the need for and to provide for appropriate visual supports, organizational supports, task analysis support, communicative supports, and behavioral supports in the general education setting. Educators would not be making excuses for the individual with ASD and modifying all work, requiring less work, and relaxing behavioral standards, but rather they would better understand why the student is engaging in the behavior he is currently engaging in and support him in the development of more appropriate behavior and self-initiated strategies. On a larger, systemic scale, phase 1 would provide basic information about ASD and assist the district in developing guiding principles for supporting students with ASD within a sound philosophical structure and support. Phase 1 would also emphasize the importance of a multidisciplinary team approach for planning, implementing, and tracking program success through on-going data collection.

Phase 2 of in-service teacher training would focus on the training of specific methodologies for specific populations with ASD. For example, a preschool program staff might be given intensive training in the methodology of applied behavior analysis (ABA), including discrete trial instruction, while a high school staff training might focus on intensive training in the use of video modeling and peer buddy systems to enhance social competency at that level. In this phase, it would be critical for the district to identify current evidence-based strategies and develop a plan to ensure that training is given in these specific strategies or methodologies to the appropriate personnel in the district. In this phase, professional staff in the district would also be given the directive and training to review research on a proposed intervention and together, as a multidisciplinary team, decide if it might be a promising practice for an individual child.

Phase 3 of in-service teacher training would be specific to the area of assessment and eligibility determination. According to IDEA, a multidisciplinary team must conduct a multidisciplinary assessment in order to determine eligibility and specific program goals and objectives for each child referred to special education for services. In the area of assessment, there are specific instruments that are used to identify/diagnose ASD and specific instruments to test specific domains related to the triad of disabilities in this population (social, communication, and behavior). For example, in the area of communication, it is critical to assess pragmatic language in an individual suspected of having an ASD although pragmatic language assessment is not always required or needed in a communication assessment with other suspected populations. Much has been written about assessment in ASD and the importance of an in-depth knowledge of the disability and knowledge of and training in specific instruments. Volkmar et al. (2005) discuss issues related to the assessment of individuals with ASD. It is highly unlikely to have everyone in a district trained comprehensively, even within their discipline, in assessment of individuals with ASD. Therefore, it may be more prudent for a district to have a highly trained, multidisciplinary assessment team that is responsible for assessing and determining eligibility for autistic disorder under IDEA along with the child's home school team. This specialized team would have extensive training in instruments within their domain of expertise as well as extensive training and experience in assessing individuals with ASD. This level of training would be ongoing as new information and assessments become available.

Finally, Phase 3 would include ongoing, intensive, hands-on training across all schools and with all staff working with the ASD population, in all settings, in measures of on-going assessment, data collection, and data-based decision-making. School districts cannot assume that anyone and everyone can take data if they are given paper and pencil. In order to ensure fidelity of data, all individuals must be trained in the type of data they are expected to take and teams will need guided training in reviewing data on a regular basis and making decisions based on the data. Data-driven instruction is not a new concept for educators but it is not always addressed in in-service training modules other than modules grounded in ABA.

The Teaming Process

Teaming, sometimes referred to as *collaborative teaming*, is a dynamic process in which teachers, parents, related service providers and other individuals working with a child, come together to troubleshoot problems a child might be experiencing in his or her educational program. The ultimate goal of collaboration is to improve teaching and learning (Turnbull et al. 2004).

Mandates for Teams

As previously discussed, IDEA has a clear mandate for a multidisciplinary team to not only assess but also plan and implement educational programs for children with ASD. The National Research Council (2001) states the domains that need to be addressed in a comprehensive program for a child with ASD. These domains are social development, cognitive development, verbal and non-verbal communication, adaptive skills, motor skills, and behavior. In young children, the pivotal skills that need to be addressed include joint attention, symbolic play, and receptive language. Given the variety of domains, it is clear that no one team member will have a high level of expertise in all domains. Yet a team, collectively, should have the breadth and depth of knowledge about ASD in all of the domains required for program decision-making and planning (Connecticut State Department of Education 2005). In addition, NCLB requires that all children have access to the general education curriculum. For a student with ASD to achieve these goals, a teacher who knows the general education curriculum will need to be involved in program planning and intervention. Finally, a parent, under IDEA, is a member of their child's educational team and must also be included to ensure a comprehensive picture of a child across all settings. Without these representatives, errors in decision-making can and will occur (see Case Study 12.2).

Case Study 12.2:

Special Education Eligibility

A team was discussing continuing eligibility for special education services under IDEA for a child who had been given a diagnosis of high-functioning autism by a private, clinical psychologist. The school psychologist believed the child no longer qualified based on his score on the Childhood Autism Rating Scale (CARS; Schopler et al. 1988). When the consultant asked who completed the CARS, the school psychologist replied that she did with the help of the child's teacher. The parent had not been consulted.

As the team reviewed the CARS results with the parent, the parent was able to give very clear examples of John's inability to adapt to change (new environments) while the school staff stated they did not see any difficulty at all with this. The team was asked to consider that it was June and John was very familiar with his current schedule and routine and transitioned without difficulty at this time, as opposed to significant transition issues at the beginning of the school year. The mother requested that the team take her son to McDonald's and sit at a table other than the one right next to the door and see how he adjusted! She was also able to give additional examples to illustrate John's abnormal fears, object use, and emotional response.

As the parent gave these examples, other members of the team thought of some related school examples to which they had not previously given much thought. For example, the teacher stated that John showed abnormal fear during storybook week when adults visited the building dressed as storybook

characters. John would get very upset and cry if he encountered one of these characters in the hall. The paraprofessional stated that John would also get upset if his seat was taken at the lunch table. He would always rush into the lunchroom to be sure he was first so that he could take "his" seat.

These comments, when considered, changed the CARS overall rating significantly. With this new information and perspective, the team decided that this child continued to have characteristics consistent with autism that impacted his educational progress (both academic and social). It was decided he did indeed continue to qualify for services under the IDEA eligibility category of autistic disorder.

Another initiative in education across all states is inclusive education, first discussed in IDEA (Public Law 94-142) as it relates to the least restrictive environment (LRE) and further supported by NCLB, which requires all but 1% of the total special education population to participate in district-wide mastery testing that is based on the general education curriculum. Again, it would be difficult to include a child with ASD for any part of the day in the general education environment without a team of educators representing special education, related services, and general education involved in the planning of his program. This becomes even more imperative at the secondary level where multiple general education teachers would be involved in addressing goals and objectives and generalizing academic, communication, behavior, and social skills across all settings. It is less likely that educators who received training 10 or more years ago learned strategies for supporting students with significant disabilities to fully participate and learn within the general education curriculum (Sonnenmeier et al. 2005).

Finally, to further support the importance of the teaming process one only has to look at the complexity of a child on the autism spectrum. In addition to the academic domains that would be addressed for all children, children with ASD may have needs that are not specifically included in the standards for a given district or state. For example, toileting, dressing, and eating skills would not be part of the educational standards in the general education curriculum yet they are clearly areas that may need to be directly addressed with some individuals with ASD. One would likely not find social competency skills listed in the standards for secondary education, yet many individuals with ASD need specific instruction in social skills, such as answering the telephone and personal grooming. In short, the uniqueness and complexity of ASD requires a multidisciplinary team with individual expertise in multiple disciplines, to fully address all program components required for a comprehensive program for a child with ASD.

Theoretically, many can agree on the importance of a multidisciplinary team with individual expertise in each of the many areas that need to be addressed in a program for an individual with an ASD. However, teaming itself can be a very complex process and can result in a dysfunctional teaming process that is ineffective in program planning and delivery. Strong team relationships are based on trust, cooperation, and open communication and positively impact outcomes for the individual (Connecticut State Department of Education 2005).

Differing Philosophical Perspectives of Team Members

Each team member will often come to a team meeting with their own perspective and philosophy regarding effective intervention, their own level of knowledge about ASDs,

and their own level of knowledge of EBP within their discipline (Swiezy et al. 2008). Mallory (1992) discussed the three theoretical models of early intervention practice in order to identify the common values that characterize them: the developmental perspective, the biological perspective, and the functional (or behavioral) perspective. These theoretical models are still evident today and are reflected in the training of the professionals involved in program planning and implementation for individuals with ASD. Each theoretical foundation has value and deserves respect and consideration when looking at a child's needs.

Developmental model. This model is most often represented on the team by the general education teacher, especially if we are discussing a child at the elementary level. The individual trained in the developmental model is often concerned with the concept of "readiness." If the student is not ready to learn something, we need to wait until he is developmentally ready to achieve this skill. The assumption is, according to Mallory (1992), that developmental principles can guide intervention practice. The educator trained within a developmental philosophy would most likely be child-centered, emotionally supportive, and value play and problem solving activities in the educational process.

Biological model. This model is an outreach from the medical model. It seeks biological explanations for development and behavior. Frequently the biological perspective is represented by the occupational therapist or physical therapist on the team. Their philosophy focuses on goodness of fit. They recognize and respect individual differences and focus on helping the individual adapt to or cope with the environment. The child's biological constitution is respected and addressed in the educational environment in the form of sensory integration activities and adaptive equipment and materials. According to Mallory (1992), progress is seen in this model as children become able to self-regulate when presented with complex environmental stimuli.

Behavioral model. This model (the functional model, defined by Mallory (1992)) has its roots in the philosophy of John Watson and B. F. Skinner. These two individuals have contributed to our understanding of the operant conditioning model for explaining, predicting and changing human behavior (Alberto and Troutman 2009). All behavior is learned and behavior that is reinforced will increase, while behavior that is ignored or punished will decrease. Over time, contingent responses become internalized. Typically, the individual on the team most closely grounded in the behavioral philosophy is the special education teacher. Their training often involves direct, systematic instruction based upon individualized, measurable goals and objectives. Task analysis, shaping, chaining, teacher-directed instruction, and positive reinforcement are part of this perspective, along with the recognition and importance of data collection.

Summary. Each of these philosophies has value and merit when making program decisions. The three philosophies can at times converge and help to guide professional practice. The teacher with the developmental background will know what is an age-appropriate task for an individual; the behaviorist will be most adept at data collection and functional behavior assessments; and the biologically based interventionist will have creative ways to adapt the environment in order for the child to participate in activities and develop skills. The challenge in the teaming process is to decide which lens or perspective is the appropriate one for any given situation at any given time in the child's life and what EBP can be implemented related to this perspective.

In Case Study 12.3, each team member had a valid opinion based on their philosophical training and the team could have argued the strategy for hours. Is there an

---

Case Study 12.3:

Multiple Philosophical Perspectives in the Teaming Process

A team meeting was held for Bryan, who is 12 years old, diagnosed with autism, nonverbal and intellectually impaired. His mother came to the meeting and requested that the team teach him to tie his shoes. He was a large youngster and she felt it was stigmatizing and embarrassing for her to have to tie his shoes in public places (such as the mall or church). The general education teacher immediately explained to the mother that her son had a cognitive disability and was not ready to comprehend the complicated task of tying his shoes. Mentally he was very much like a 5 year old and most 5 year olds do not tie their shoes independently. The occupational therapist explained to the parent that her son had significant fine motor problems and would not be able to perform the fine motor movements required to tie one's shoes, therefore she should buy him shoes with Velcro. The special education teacher stated that this youngster needed to develop more independence and since shoe-tying instruction had not been attempted, it was worth a try. She would use a task analysis, take data on the mastery of each step and the team could evaluate Bryan's progress based on the data in one month.

EBP for shoe tying? Not that we are aware of, but task analysis is an evidence-based strategy and therefore might be a promising place to begin with in addressing this issue. The fact that data collection would occur meant that the team was comfortable in trying this intervention and revisiting their decision based on the data presented at the next team meeting. If the data showed no progress in 1 month of consistent instruction, then the use of Velcro might be reconsidered for this issue. Effective teaming must be in place in order for a multidisciplinary team to explore and discuss options that represent different philosophical models.

Communication in the Teaming Process

Communication among team members is essential for implementing EBP. Typically, the individualized education program (IEP) meeting is the only time the entire team comes together to discuss issues or challenges in program planning and implementation. This is not necessarily the most effective vehicle to promote communication among team members. IEP meetings have a regulatory purpose and must cover specific topics, lengthy paperwork needs to be completed, and discussion and decisions must be documented. It is a formal process that is not always a comfortable one for parents to participate in and may result in one-way communication, with the school personnel telling a parent what the issues are and what will be done to address them. Research on the IEP process has generally reported that the traditional process has been more of legal compliance in the form of documentation in paperwork rather than a problem-solving, dynamic process (Turnbull et al. 2004).

A team meeting process is suggested in addition to the federally required IEP process. Teams that function collaboratively and meet on a regular basis provide a successful mechanism for proactively developing, implementing, and monitoring the effectiveness of programs and interventions for children with ASD throughout the school year (Connecticut State Department of Education 2005). A team meeting is less formal, can include everyone working with the child, and has an agenda established by the team members beforehand. It can be an effective mechanism in decision-making for program planning and implementation of EBP. Parents may feel more comfortable with this process and teachers and related service providers can be involved in collaborative problem solving instead of simply reporting current levels of functioning. An effective team meeting has an agenda developed prior to the meeting, with everyone invited to submit a topic to be discussed; is time limited; and results in notes, given to all participants, that identifies what topics were discussed, who will be doing what to address each issue, and when this action will occur. A sample of team meeting notes can be found in Appendix 3.

Team meetings can be held as frequently as every month or as infrequently as twice a year. The team meeting process allows team members to review current data, discuss progress, and make recommendations for changes in program implementation to ensure progress. The number of team members at the meeting allows many different disciplines to suggest possible EBP solutions for issues that are raised (see Case Study 12.4). Waiting for an IEP meeting to be scheduled and held can often result in weeks of wasted time in pursuing a strategy that is not working or allowing a strategy to continue that can be harmful to the student.

Case Study 12.4:

Team Meetings

A high school student, Susie, was having difficulties during her free period in the Media Center. Every day, loud arguments occurred at her table until the Media Center librarian separated the students. A team meeting was requested by the parent and held within a week.

At the team meeting, the psychologist reported that the meeting was not necessary, everything in the Media Center during Susie's free period was fine. The students were all sitting together again and there were no arguments or disruptions. The parent contributed the following information to the team. When she asked her daughter how things were going during her free period in the Media Center, her daughter innocently replied, "Oh fine, I just give Katie a dollar everyday and I can sit at the table with all of my friends."

Clearly, this information uncovered a bullying situation and led the team in deciding to implement a peer buddy system suggested by the social worker as an evidence-based practice to improve social interaction. The special education teacher also suggested video modeling as another evidenced-based strategy to use to help this youngster recognize and appropriately respond to a bullying situation. Without this team communication and discussion, the bullying would most likely have continued.

Curriculum matrix. Communication among team members allows the team to engage in on-going evaluation of chosen strategies and the opportunity to discuss new evidence-based strategies for different situations throughout the day. Other ways to facilitate communication among team members include the curriculum matrix (see Appendix 4), which allows all teachers to see which goals and objectives may be addressed in their educational setting. The team can help decide which EBP is appropriate for each setting or, if one has been identified for all settings, training can occur for all team members at the meeting.

Curriculum template. Another way to promote communication among team members and to facilitate discussion among team members in implementing EBP is the curriculum template. The curriculum template (see Appendix 5) gives all team members the unit of study in any given subject area, the key concepts to be covered in the unit, the key vocabulary to be understood, the specific teaching methods, and the evaluation methods the teacher will employ in the class. The team can then review the template for any given subject area and various professionals may make suggestions regarding evidence-based instructional strategies. For example, the special education teacher may suggest priming, an evidence-based strategy that essentially pre-teaches some of the more difficult concepts. Perhaps the speech and language

pathologist will be able to prime the vocabulary in the unit prior to the unit starting in the general education classroom.

Ecological inventory. A final strategy to promote team communication so that the team can discuss and suggest EBP to support a student is an ecological inventory. An ecological inventory is intended to delineate the types of performance and skills that would be expected by a person without a disability in the environment (Westling and Fox 2004). It is helpful for a collaborative team to have an inventory of the behavioral expectations for an individual in the educational environment in which they are to be included. For example, when a student is in fifth grade and transitioning to sixth grade, an ecological inventory of the sixth grade environment can be very helpful to the team in determining what skills might be primed to make the transition easier for the student. An example of an ecological inventory for a student entering middle school can be found in Appendix 6. Using this example, a team might decide that the evidence-based practice of priming be used to teach the student how to open a combination lock, a behavior that was not expected in the elementary school. The special education teacher could create a task analysis to open a combination lock and the student could practice the steps at home during the summer prior to the opening of school.

Other Examples of Implementing EBP Using the Teaming Process

- The preschool special education teacher was working on the development of joint attention during circle time with Katie. Through a team discussion, the speech and language pathologist suggested several games to promote joint attention on the child's developmental level, including Peek-A-Boo and joint activity routines.
- John was a nonverbal, 3 year old who screamed throughout the day. The school

psychologist on the team suggested that she do an assessment to determine the function of the behavior. When the data was reviewed by the team, it was determined that the function of the screaming was to refuse a task. The speech and language pathologist suggested the development of a functional communication program beginning with teaching John a way to say no in an appropriate way. The team decided on using a head nod for no and the special education teacher suggested she teach the head nod for no in a discrete trial format until it was understood by John.

- Lizzy, for no apparent reason, became frightened by people who entered her second-grade classroom wearing eyeglasses. Even the speech and language teacher who had previously had a positive working rapport with Lizzy was met with a scream when she entered the room wearing her much needed eyeglasses. Since the function of the behavior was obvious, the team meeting focused on deciding on an evidence-based practice to extinguish the screaming. The psychologist suggested a behavior plan for Lizzy. Simply ignore the behavior and reinforce Lizzy when she stops screaming. Since this was an evidence-based practice, the team decided to try this intervention. After 2 weeks of implementation, the data showed that this intervention was not at all effective. The screaming could not be ignored. Lizzy kept screaming until the person with the eyeglasses left the room. The team met again to discuss other options. The special education teacher suggested a Social Story (Gray 2000) to explain why people wear eyeglasses. Given Lizzy's cognitive ability, the team felt this evidence-based strategy might be effective. The Social Story was written and reviewed with Lizzy prior to the arrival of the speech pathologist. The Social Story effectively gave Lizzy the reason for the eyeglasses (people wear glasses so they can see) as well as a strategy to replace screaming (I will try not to scream and tell the person to remove their glasses). After 3 days, Lizzy did not

scream when the SLP entered the room but immediately said, "Please remove your glasses." Once the SLP removed the glasses, Lizzy was heard to reply, "Oh there you are!"

Conclusion

More research and exploration into effective teaming practices to enhance the implementation of EBP is certainly warranted. The Ziggurat Model developed by Aspy and Grossman (2008) is one such program that might be reviewed and evaluated as an evidence-based teaming process for evidence-based practice decision-making. This model, according to the authors, provides a process and a framework for designing individualized, comprehensive intervention plans for individuals with ASD and promotes collaboration and communication among team members throughout the stages of the intervention process. This model is further supported by the Comprehensive Autism Planning System (CAPS) for individuals with Asperger syndrome, autism, and related disabilities (Henry and Smith Myles 2007). The CAPS assists a team in organizing a student's day and incorporating needed supports.

In conclusion, practicing evidence-based practices can be a daunting challenge in public schools. Effective implementation of EBP requires adequate training and team collaboration. Training begins with pre-service teacher candidates and progresses through advanced training at the university level. Content at these levels should be carefully selected to address not only EBP but also skills related to teaming with other professionals and parents, and to dispel myths related to ASDs. Additionally, well-supervised field experiences with students with ASD need to be incorporated into pre-service and advanced level courses. Recently developed professional standards for teacher competencies are helpful in developing course content.

Course content at the pre-service and advanced levels can be controlled to include the important components and candidates can be supervised to ensure that practices are implemented with fidelity. It may be more of a challenge to ensure that adequate training and implementation are effected at the in-service level in public schools. Careful crafting of the training process for each school or district must include the necessary competencies for the level of exposure each teacher has to students with ASD and the training needs to include both didactic workshops and hands-on, follow-up experiences. Teachers and related service personnel also need to be carefully trained in the teaming process and the implementation of EBP recommendations resulting from this teaming process must be carefully monitored. Although this becomes difficult with the complexity of training and experience of school personnel, it is the final crucial step to ensure the effective practice of EBP. Through careful pre-service, advanced, and in-service training and teaming, we can ensure that students with ASD receive the most effective interventions.

References

Alberto, P. A., & Troutman, A. C. (2009). *Applied behavior analysis for teachers* (8th ed.). Upper Saddle River, NJ: Pearson Education.

APA. (1994). *Diagnostic and statistical manual of mental disorders* (4th ed.). Washington, DC: American Psychiatric Association.

Aspy, R., & Grossman, B. G. (2008). *Designing comprehensive interventions for individuals with high functioning autism and Asperger syndrome: The Ziggurat model.* Shawnee Mission, Kansas: Autism Asperger Publishing.

Brown v. Board of Education (1954) 347 U.S. 483.

CEC. (2010a). *Professional Standards: Initial knowledge and skill set: Teachers of individuals with developmental disabilities/autism.* Council for Exceptional Children. Obtained 5 Jan 2010 from http://www.cec.sped.org/Content/

NavigationMenu/ProfessionalDevelopment/ProfessionalStandards/Initial_DD&A_K&S_set_NEW.doc.

CEC. (2010b). *Professional standards: Advanced knowledge and skill set for teachers of individuals with developmental disabilities/autism.* Council for Exceptional Children. Obtained 5 Jan 2010 from http://www.cec.sped.org/Content/NavigationMenu/ProfessionalDevelopment/ProfessionalStandards/DD&A_Specialist.doc.

Connecticut State Department of Education. (2005). *Guidelines for Identification and Education of Children and Youth with Autism.* Division of Teaching and Learning Programs and Services, Bureau of Special Education (eds). Hartford, CT.

Darling-Hammond, L., & Bransford, J. (Eds.). (2005). *Preparing teachers for a changing world.* San Francisco, CA: John Wiley & Sons.

Deshler, D. D. (2002) *Intervention research and bridging the gap between research and practice.* Testimony to the President's Commission on Excellence in Special Education Research Task Force, Nashville, TN. Obtained 5 Jan 2010 from http://www.kucrl.org/images/presentations/deshler.pdf.

Education of All Handicap Children Act, Pub. L. No. 94-142. (1975).

Eren, R., and Cook, B. (2009). *Building School District Capacity for Servicing Individuals with ASD.* Presentation at Ocali Conference and Exposition, November, Columbus, Ohio.

Fang, Z., & Ashley, C. (2004). Preservice teachers' interpretations of a field-based reading block. *Journal of Teacher Education, 55*(1), 39–54.

Fogt, J. B., Miller, D. N., & Zirkel, P. A. (2003). Defining autism: Professional best practices and published case law. *Journal of School Psychology, 41*, 201–216.

Gray, C. (2000). *The new Social Story book.* Arlington TX: Future Horizons.

Henry, S., & Smith Myles, B. (2007). *The Comprehensive Autism Planning System (CAPS) for individuals with Asperger syndrome, autism, and related disabilities.* Shawnee Mission, Kansas: Autism Asperger Publishing.

Individuals with Disabilities Education Improvement Act of 2004, Pub. L. No. 108-446, § 118, Stat. 2647 (2004).

Lave, J., & Wenger, E. (1991). *Situated learning and legitimate peripheral participation.* New York: Cambridge University Press.

Mallory, B. L. (1992). Is it always appropriate to be developmental? Convergent models for early intervention practice. *Topics in Early Childhood and Special Education, 11*, 1–12.

McGee, G. G., & Morrier, M. J. (2005). Preparation of autism specialists. In F. R. Volkmar, R.

Paul, A. Klin, & D. Cohen (Eds.), *Handbook of autism and pervasive developmental disorders* (3rd ed., pp. 1123–1160). Hoboken, NJ: Wiley.

Murray, S. (2008). *Preservice Teacher's Perceptions of Students with Autism Spectrum Disorders* (Unpublished master's thesis). Southern Connecticut State University, New Haven, CT.

National Research Council. (2001). *Educating young children with autism*. Washington, DC: National Academy Press.

No Child Left Behind Act of 2001, Pub. L. No. 107-110, § 115, Stat. 1425 (2002).

Oberti v. Clementon (1993) 995F.2nd 1204.

Oller, J. W., Jr., & Oller, S. D. (2010). *Autism: the diagnosis, treatment & etiology of the undeniable epidemic*. Sudbury, MA: Jones and Bartlett.

Reichow, B., Volkmar, F. R., & Cicchetti, D. V. (2008). Development of an evaluative method for determining the strength of research evidence in autism. *Journal of Autism and Developmental Disorders, 38,* 1311–1319.

Robertson, K., Chamberlin, B., & Kasari, C. (2003). General education teachers' relationships with students with autism. *Journal of Autism and Developmental Disorders, 33,* 123–130.

Schopler, E., Reichler, R. J., & Renner, B. R. (1988). *The childhood autism rating scale (CARS)*. Los Angeles, CA: Western Psychological Services.

Siegel, B. (2003). *Helping children with autism learn*. New York: Oxford University Press.

Sonnenmeier, R. M., McSheehan, M., & Jorgensen, C. M. (2005). A case study of team supports for a student with autism's communication and engagement within the general education curriculum: Preliminary report of the Beyond Access Model. *Augmentative and Alternative Communication, 21,* 101–115.

Spear-Swerling, L., & Brucker, P. (2004). Preparing novice teachers to develop basic reading and skills in children. *Annals of Dyslexia, 54,* 332–364.

Spear-Swerling, L., Brucker, P., & Alfano, M. (2005). Teacher's literacy-related knowledge and perceptions in relation to preparation and experience. *Annals of Dyslexia, 55,* 266–296.

Swiezy, N., Stuart, M., & Korzekwa, P. (2008). Bridging for success in autism: training and collaboration across medical, educational, and community systems. *Child and Adolescent Psychiatric Clinics of North America, 17*(4), 907–922.

Turnbull, R., Turnbull, A., Shank, M., & Smith, S. J. (2004). *Exceptional lives: Special education in today's schools* (4th ed.). Upper Saddle River, NJ: Pearson.

Volkmar, F. R., Paul, R., Klin, A., & Cohen, D. (Eds.). (2005). *Handbook of autism and pervasive developmental disorders* (3rd ed.). Hoboken, NJ: Wiley.

Westling, D. L., & Fox, L. (2004). *Teaching students with severe disabilities* (3rd ed.). Upper Saddle River, NJ: Pearson Education.

Appendix 1:
Initial Knowledge and Skill Set:
Teachers of Individuals with Developmental Disabilities/Autism (Reprinted with permission from the Council for Exceptional Children)

Standard 1: Foundations

Knowledge

ICC1K1	Models, theories, philosophies, and research methods that form the basis for special education practice
ICC1K2	Laws, policies, and ethical principles regarding behavior management planning and implementation
ICC1K3	Relationship of special education to the organization and function of educational agencies
ICC1K4	Rights and responsibilities of students, parents, teachers, and other professionals, and schools related to exceptional learning needs
ICC1K5	Issues in definition and identification of individuals with exceptional learning needs, including those from culturally and linguistically diverse backgrounds
ICC1K6	Issues, assurances and due process rights related to assessment, eligibility, and placement within a continuum of services
ICC1K7	Family systems and the role of families in the educational process
ICC1K8	Historical points of view and contribution of culturally diverse groups
ICC1K9	Impact of the dominant culture on shaping schools and the individuals who study and work in them
ICC1K10	Potential impact of differences in values, languages, and customs that can exist between the home and school
DDA1.K1	Definitions and issues related to the identification of individuals with developmental disabilities/autism spectrum disorders
DDA1.K2	Continuum of placement and services available for individuals with developmental disabilities/autism spectrum disorders
DDA1.K3	Historical foundations and classic studies of developmental disabilities/autism spectrum disorders
DDA1.K4	Trends and practices in the field of developmental disabilities/autism spectrum disorders
DDA1.K5	Theories of behavior problems of individuals with developmental disabilities/autism spectrum disorders
DDA1.K6	Perspectives held by individuals with developmental disabilities/autism spectrum disorders
DDA1.K7	Concepts of self-determination, self-advocacy, community and family support and impact in the lives of individuals with developmental disabilities/autism spectrum disorders

Skills

ICC1S1	Articulate personal philosophy of special education

Standard 2: Development and Characteristics of Learners

Knowledge

ICC2K1	Typical and atypical human growth and development
ICC2K2	Educational implications of characteristics of various exceptionalities
ICC2K3	Characteristics and effects of the cultural and environmental milieu of the individual with exceptional learning needs and the family
ICC2K4	Family systems and the role of families in supporting development
ICC2K5	Similarities and differences of individuals with and without exceptional learning needs
ICC2K6	Similarities and differences among individuals with exceptional learning needs
ICC2K7	Effects of various medications on individuals with exceptional learning needs
DDA2.K1	Medical aspects and implications for learning for individuals with developmental disabilities/autism spectrum disorders
DDA2.K2	Core and associated characteristics of individuals with developmental disabilities/autism spectrum disorders
DDA2.K3	Co-existing conditions and ranges that exist at a higher rate than in the general population
DDA2.K4	Sensory challenges of individuals with developmental disabilities/autism spectrum disorders
DDA2.K5	Speech, language, and communication of individuals with developmental disabilities/autism spectrum disorders
DDA2.K6	Adaptive behavior needs of individuals with developmental disabilities/autism spectrum disorders

Skills

None in addition to the Common Core

Standard 3: Individual Learning Differences

Knowledge

ICC3K1	Effects an exceptional condition(s) can have on an individual's life
ICC3K2	Impact of learners' academic and social abilities, attitudes, interests, and values on instruction and career development
ICC3K3	Variations in beliefs, traditions, and values across and within cultures and their effects on relationships among individuals with exceptional learning needs, family, and schooling
ICC3K4	Cultural perspectives influencing the relationships among families, schools, and communities as related to instruction
ICC3K5	Differing ways of learning of individuals with exceptional learning needs, including those from culturally diverse backgrounds and strategies for addressing these differences
DDA3.K1	Impact of theory of mind, central coherence, and executive function on learning and behavior
DDA3.K2	Impact of neurological differences on learning and behavior
DDA3.K3	Impact of self-regulation on learning and behavior

Standard 4: Instructional Strategies

Knowledge

ICC4K1	Evidence-based practices validated for specific characteristics of learners and settings
DDA4K1	Specialized curriculum designed to meet the needs of individuals with developmental disabilities/autism spectrum disorders

Skills

ICC4S1	Use strategies to facilitate integration into various settings
ICC4S2	Teach individuals to use self-assessment, problem-solving, and other cognitive strategies to meet their needs
ICC4S3	Select, adapt, and use instructional strategies and materials according to characteristics of the individual with exceptional learning needs
ICC4S4	Use strategies to facilitate maintenance and generalization of skills across learning environments
ICC4S5	Use procedures to increase the individual's self-awareness, self-management, self-control, self-reliance, and self-esteem
ICC4S6	Use strategies that promote successful transitions for individuals with exceptional learning needs
DDA4.S1	Match levels of support to changing needs of the individual
DDA4.S2	Implement instructional programs that promote effective communication skills using verbal and augmentative/alternative communication systems for individuals with developmental disabilities/autism spectrum disorders
DDA4.S3	Provide specialized instruction for spoken language, reading and writing for individuals with developmental disabilities/autism spectrum disorders
DDA4.S4	Use instructional strategies that fall on a continuum of child-directed to adult-directed in natural and structured context
DDA4.S5	Consistently use of proactive strategies and positive behavioral supports
DDA4.S6	Involve individuals with developmental disabilities/autism spectrum disorders in the transition planning process
DDA4.S7	Plan for transition needs including linkages to supports and agencies focusing on lifelong needs

Standard 5: Learning Environments/Social Interactions

Knowledge

ICC5K1	Demands of learning environments
ICC5K2	Basic classroom management theories and strategies for individuals with exceptional learning needs
ICC5K3	Effective management of teaching and learning
ICC5K4	Teacher attitudes and behaviors that influence behavior of individuals with exceptional learning needs
ICC5K5	Social skills needed for educational and other environments
ICC5K6	Strategies for crisis prevention and intervention
ICC5K7	Strategies for preparing individuals to live harmoniously and productively in a culturally diverse world
ICC5K8	Ways to create learning environments that allow individuals to retain and appreciate their own and each other's respective language and cultural heritage

| ICC5K9 | Ways specific cultures are negatively stereotyped |
| ICC5K10 | Strategies used by diverse populations to cope with a legacy of former and continuing racism |

Skills

ICC5S1	Create a safe, equitable, positive, and supportive learning environment in which diversities are valued
ICC5S2	Identify realistic expectations for personal and social behavior in various settings
ICC5S3	Identify supports needed for integration into various program placements
ICC5S4	Design learning environments that encourage active participation in individual and group activities
ICC5S5	Modify the learning environment to manage behaviors
ICC5S6	Use performance data and information from all stakeholders to make or suggest modifications in learning environments
ICC5S7	Establish and maintain rapport with individuals with and without exceptional learning needs
ICC5S8	Teach self-advocacy
ICC5S9	Create an environment that encourages self-advocacy and increased independence
ICC5S10	Use effective and varied behavior management strategies
ICC5S11	Use the least intensive behavior management strategy consistent with the needs of the individual with exceptional learning needs
ICC5S12	Design and manage daily routines
ICC5S13	Organize, develop, and sustain learning environments that support positive intracultural and intercultural experiences
ICC5S14	Mediate controversial intercultural issues among students within the learning environment in ways that enhance any culture, group, or person
ICC5S15	Structure, direct, and support the activities of paraeducators, volunteers, and tutors
ICC5S16	Use universal precautions
DDA5.S1	Provide instruction in community-based settings
DDA5.S2	Demonstrate transfer, lifting and positioning techniques
DDA5.S3	Structure the physical environment to provide optimal learning for individuals with developmental disabilities/autism spectrum disorders
DDA5.S4	Provide instruction in self-regulation
DDA5.S5	Utilize student strengths to reinforce and maintain social skills

Standard 6: Language

Knowledge

ICC6K1	Effects of cultural and linguistic differences on growth and development
ICC6K2	Characteristics of one's own culture and use of language and the ways in which these can differ from other cultures and uses of languages
ICC6K3	Ways of behaving and communicating among cultures that can lead to misinterpretation and misunderstanding
ICC6K4	Augmentative and assistive communication strategies

Skills

| ICC6S1 | Use strategies to support and enhance communication skills of individuals with exceptional learning needs |

ICC6S2	Use communication strategies and resources to facilitate understanding of subject matter for students whose primary language is not the dominant language
DDA6.S1	Provide pragmatic language instruction that facilitates social skills
DDA6.S2	Provide individuals with developmental disabilities/autism spectrum disorders strategies to avoid and repair miscommunications

Standard 7: Instructional Planning

Knowledge

ICC7K1	Theories and research that form the basis of curriculum development and instructional practice
ICC7K2	Scope and sequences of general and special curricula
ICC7K3	National, state or provincial, and local curricula standards
ICC7K4	Technology for planning and managing the teaching and learning environment
ICC7K5	Roles and responsibilities of the paraeducator related to instruction, intervention, and direct service
DDA7.K1	Evidence-based career/vocational transition programs for individuals with developmental disabilities/autism spectrum disorders

Skills

ICC7S1	Identify and prioritize areas of the general curriculum and accommodations for individuals with exceptional learning needs
ICC7S2	Develop and implement comprehensive, longitudinal individualized programs in collaboration with team members
ICC7S3	Involve the individual and family in setting instructional goals and monitoring progress
ICC7S4	Use functional assessments to develop intervention plans
ICC7S5	Use task analysis
ICC7S6	Sequence, implement, and evaluate individualized learning objectives
ICC7S7	Integrate affective, social, and life skills with academic curricula
ICC7S8	Develop and select instructional content, resources, and strategies that respond to cultural, linguistic, and gender differences
ICC7S9	Incorporate and implement instructional and assistive technology into the educational program
ICC7S10	Prepare lesson plans
ICC7S11	Prepare and organize materials to implement daily lesson plans
ICC7S12	Use instructional time effectively
ICC7S13	Make responsive adjustments to instruction based on continual observations
ICC7S14	Prepare individuals to exhibit self-enhancing behavior in response to societal attitudes and actions
ICC7S15	Evaluate and modify instructional practices in response to ongoing assessment data
DDA7.S1	Plan instruction for independent functional life skills and adaptive behavior
DDA7.S2	Plan and implement instruction and related services for individuals with developmental disabilities/autism spectrum disorders that is both age-appropriate and ability-appropriate
DDA7.S3	Use specialized instruction to enhance social participation across environments
DDA7.S4	Plan systematic instruction based on learner characteristics, interests, and ongoing assessment

Standard 8: Assessment

Knowledge	
ICC8K1	Basic terminology used in assessment
ICC8K2	Legal provisions and ethical principles regarding assessment of individuals
ICC8K3	Screening, prereferral, referral, and classification procedures
ICC8K4	Use and limitations of assessment instruments
ICC8K5	National, state or provincial, and local accommodations and modifications
DDA8.K1	Specialized terminology used in the assessment of individuals with developmental disabilities/autism spectrum disorders
DDA8.K2	Assessments of environmental conditions that promote maximum performance of individuals with developmental disabilities/autism spectrum disorders
DDA8.K3	Components of assessment for the core areas for individuals with developmental disabilities/autism spectrum disorders
DDA8.K4	Individual strengths, skills and learning styles
Skills	
ICC8S1	Gather relevant background information
ICC8S2	Administer nonbiased formal and informal assessments
ICC8S3	Use technology to conduct assessments
ICC8S4	Develop or modify individualized assessment strategies
ICC8S5	Interpret information from formal and informal assessments
ICC8S6	Use assessment information in making eligibility, program, and placement decisions for individuals with exceptional learning needs, including those from culturally and/or linguistically diverse backgrounds
ICC8S7	Report assessment results to all stakeholders using effective communication skills
ICC8S8	Evaluate instruction and monitor progress of individuals with exceptional learning needs
ICC8S9	Create and maintain records
DDA8.S1	Select, adapt and use assessment tools and methods to accommodate the abilities and needs of individuals with developmental disabilities/autism spectrum disorders
DDA8.S2	Develop strategies for monitoring and analyzing challenging behavior and its communicative intent
DDA8.S3	Conduct functional behavior assessments that lead to development of behavior support plans

Standard 9: Professional and Ethical Practice

Knowledge	
ICC9K1	Personal cultural biases and differences that affect one's teaching
ICC9K2	Importance of the teacher serving as a model for individuals with exceptional learning needs
ICC9K3	Continuum of lifelong professional development
ICC9K4	Methods to remain current regarding research-validated practice
Skills	
ICC9S1	Practice within the CEC Code of Ethics and other standards of the profession
ICC9S2	Uphold high standards of competence and integrity and exercise sound judgment in the practice of the professional
ICC9S3	Act ethically in advocating for appropriate services
ICC9S4	Conduct professional activities in compliance with applicable laws and policies

ICC9S5	Demonstrate commitment to developing the highest education and quality-of-life potential of individuals with exceptional learning needs
ICC9S6	Demonstrate sensitivity for the culture, language, religion, gender, disability, socio-economic status, and sexual orientation of individuals
ICC9S7	Practice within one's skill limits and obtain assistance as needed
ICC9S8	Use verbal, nonverbal, and written language effectively
ICC9S9	Conduct self-evaluation of instruction
ICC9S10	Access information on exceptionalities
ICC9S11	Reflect on one's practice to improve instruction and guide professional growth
ICC9S12	Engage in professional activities that benefit individuals with exceptional learning needs, their families, and one's colleagues
ICC9S13	Demonstrate commitment to engage in evidence-based practices

Standard 10: Collaboration

Knowledge

ICC10K1	Models and strategies of consultation and collaboration
ICC10K2	Roles of individuals with exceptional learning needs, families, and school and community personnel in planning of an individualized program
ICC10K3	Concerns of families of individuals with exceptional learning needs and strategies to help address these concerns
ICC10K4	Culturally responsive factors that promote effective communication and collaboration with individuals with exceptional learning needs, families, school personnel, and community members
DDA10.K1	Services, networks, and organizations for individuals, professionals, and families with developmental disabilities/autism spectrum disorders

Skills

ICC10S1	Maintain confidential communication about individuals with exceptional learning needs
ICC10S2	Collaborate with families and others in assessment of individuals with exceptional learning needs
ICC10S3	Foster respectful and beneficial relationships between families and professionals
ICC10S4	Assist individuals with exceptional learning needs and their families in becoming active participants in the educational team
ICC10S5	Plan and conduct collaborative conferences with individuals with exceptional learning needs and their families
ICC10S6	Collaborate with school personnel and community members in integrating individuals with exceptional learning needs into various settings
ICC10S7	Use group problem-solving skills to develop, implement, and evaluate collaborative activities
ICC10S8	Model techniques and coach others in the use of instructional methods and accommodations
ICC10S9	Communicate with school personnel about the characteristics and needs of individuals with exceptional learning needs
ICC10S10	Communicate effectively with families of individuals with exceptional learning needs from diverse backgrounds
ICC10S11	Observe, evaluate, and provide feedback to paraeducators
DDA10S1	Collaborate with team members to plan transition to adulthood that encourages full community participation

Appendix 2:
Advanced Knowledge and Skill Set: Developmental Disabilities/Autism Specialist (Reprinted with permission from the Council for Exceptional Children)

Standard 1: Leadership and Policy

Knowledge

ACC1K1	Needs of different groups in a pluralistic society
ACC1K2	Evidence-based theories of organizational and educational leadership
ACC1K3	Emerging issues and trends that potentially affect the school community and the mission of the school
ACC1K4	National and State education laws and regulations
ACC1K5	Current legal, regulatory, and ethical issues affecting education
ACC1K6	Responsibilities and functions of school committees and boards
DDA1K1	Electronic print and organizational resources on developmental disabilities/autism spectrum disorders

Skills

ACC1S1	Promote a free appropriate public education in the least restrictive environment
ACC1S2	Promote high expectations for self, staff, and individuals with exceptional learning needs
ACC1S3	Advocate for educational policy within the context of evidence-based practices
ACC1S4	Mentor teacher candidates, newly certified teachers and other colleagues
DDA1.S1	Prepare personnel and community members for interaction with individuals with developmental disabilities/autism spectrum disorders
DDA1.S2	Promote high expectations for self, staff, and individuals with exceptional learning needs
DDA1.S3	Provide structure, on-going training, and support to families, professionals, and paraprofessionals
DDA1.S4	Oversee and monitor routines, schedules, and sequences of events and activities
DDA1.S5	Act as a positive role model for the acceptance, treatment and interaction with individuals with developmental disabilities/autism spectrum disorders and their families

Standard 2: Program Development and Organization

Knowledge

ACC2K1	Effects of the cultural and environmental milieu of the individual and the family on behavior and learning
ACC2K2	Theories and methodologies of teaching and learning, including adaptation and modification of curriculum
ACC2K3	Continuum of program options and services available to students with exceptional learning needs
ACC2K4	Prereferral intervention processes and strategies
ACC2K5	Process of developing individualized education plans
ACC2K6	Developmentally appropriate strategies for modifying instructional methods and the learning environment

DDA2.K1	General education curriculum and supports to facilitate the success of individuals with developmental disabilities/autism spectrum disorders
DDA2.K2	Range of environmental supports that maximize learning for individuals with developmental disabilities/autism spectrum disorders
DDA2.K3	Modify the verbal and non-verbal communication and instructional behavior in accord with the needs of individuals with developmental disabilities/autism spectrum disorder
DDA2.K4	Activities and techniques for developing independent living skills

Skills

ACC2S1	Develop programs including the integration of related services for individuals based on a thorough understanding of individual differences
ACC2S2	Connect educational standards to specialized instructional services
ACC2S3	Improve instructional programs using principles of curriculum development and modification, and learning theory
ACC2S4	Incorporate essential components into individualized education plans
DDA2.S1	Apply inclusive principles in the education of individuals with developmental disabilities/autism spectrum disorder
DDA2.S2	Develop and implement program plans to transition individuals with developmental disabilities/autism spectrum disorder between settings across the life-span
DDA2.S3	Identify match between job requirements and individual's skills, preferences, and characteristics
DDA2.S4	Provide individuals with multiple job experiences
DDA2.S5	Implement instructional strategies that promote the generalization of skills across domains and settings
DDA2.S6	Arrange program environments to facilitate spontaneous communication
DDA2.S7	Design and implement instruction that promote effective communication and social skills for individuals with developmental disabilities/autism spectrum disorders
DDA2.S8	Provide varied instruction and opportunity to learn play and leisure skills
DDA2.S9	Create opportunities and provide supports for individuals to organize and maintain personal materials across environments
DDA2.S10	Organize the curriculum to integrate individuals' special interests and materials, activities and routines across curriculum
DDA2.S11	Identify evidence based strategies to increase self-awareness, and ability to self-regulate
DDA2.S12	Identify evidence based strategies to increase an individual's self-determination of activities, services and preferences
DDA2.S13	Design and implement program activities and techniques for developing independent-living skills
DDA2.S14	Plan and implement individualized and intensive programming that matches the individual's needs

Standard 3: Research and Inquiry

Knowledge

ACC3K1	Evidence based practices validated for specific characteristics of learners and settings
DDA3.K1	Current etiology and practice based research specific to developmental disabilities/autism spectrum disorders

Skills

ACC3S1	Identify and use the research literature to resolve issues of professional practice
ACC3S2	Evaluate and modify instructional practices in response to ongoing assessment data
ACC3S3	Use educational research to improve instruction, intervention strategies, and curricular materials
DDA3.S1	Interpret and relay research findings in layperson terms or jargon free language
DDA3.S2	Remain informed of current research, legislation and debate concerning developmental disabilities/autism spectrum disorders

Standard 4: Individual and Program Evaluation

Knowledge

ACC4K1	Evaluation process and determination of eligibility
ACC4K2	Variety of methods for assessing and evaluating students' performance
ACC4K3	Strategies for identifying individuals with exceptional learning needs
ACC4K4	Evaluate a student's success in the general education curriculum
DDA4.K1	Criteria used to diagnose or identify the continuum of developmental disabilities/autism spectrum disorders as defined by the most current version of the *Diagnostic and Statistical Manual of Mental Disorders*
DDA4.K2	Ethical implications and obligations related to diagnosis and identification of an individual suspected of having developmental disabilities/autism spectrum disorders
DDA4.K3	Comprehensive assessment including specialized terminology and assessment tools
DDA4.K4	Importance of ongoing evaluation of strengths and needs in varied contexts
DDA4.K5	Conditions for individuals who are dually diagnosed with developmental disabilities/autism spectrum disorders and mental health
DDA4.K6	Comprehensive transition assessment including identification of external agency assessment sharing

Skills

ACC4S1	Design and use methods for assessing and evaluating programs
ACC4S2	Design and implement research activities to examine the effectiveness of instructional practices
ACC4S3	Advocate for evidence based practices in assessment
ACC4S4	Report the assessment of students' performance and evaluation of instructional programs
DDA4.S1	Describe the core and associated characteristics of individuals with developmental disabilities/autism spectrum disorders
DDA4.S2	Describe the distinguishing features of disorders on the autism spectrum
DDA4.S3	Identify conditions that co exist between developmental disabilities and autism spectrum disorders
DDA4.S4	Conduct non biased assessment
DDA4.S5	Use information from assessments and educational records to design instruction
DDA4.S6	Collect, interpret and use data to document outcomes for individuals with developmental disabilities/autism spectrum disorders, and change programming as indicated with family and team
DDA4.S7	Share a thorough profile of the individuals with developmental disabilities/autism spectrum disorders with their family and the current and future educational team(s)

DDA4.S8	Conduct functional behavioral assessments (FBA) to determine what initiates and maintains a challenging/interfering behavior
DDA4.S9	Uses assessments information from a variety of school and external agency resources to make transition recommendations
DDA4.S10	Articulate awareness of and the impact of mental health disorders on individuals with developmental disabilities/autism spectrum disorders in collaborating with family and colleagues

Standard 5: Professional Development and Ethical Practice

Knowledge

ACC5K1	Legal rights and responsibilities of students, staff, and parents/guardians
ACC5K2	Moral and ethical responsibilities of educators
ACC5K3	Human rights of individuals with exceptional learning needs and their families
DDA5.K1	Benefits of low- to high-technology across all areas of development
DDA5.K2	Criteria for evaluating effectiveness of interventions and strategies with individuals with developmental disabilities/autism spectrum disorders
DDA5.K3	Impact of core and associated characteristics of developmental disabilities/autism spectrum disorders on family dynamics and functioning
DDA5.K4	Critical social and ethical issues that impact the education of individuals with developmental disabilities/autism spectrum disorders, families and professionals

Skills

ACC5S1	Model ethical behavior and promote professional standards
ACC5S2	Implement practices that promote success for individuals with exceptional learning needs
ACC5S3	Use ethical and legal discipline strategies
ACC5S4	Disseminate information on effective school and classroom practices
ACC5S5	Create an environment which supports continuous instructional improvement
ACC5S6	Develop and implement a personalized professional development plan
DDA5.S1	Teach others to actively engage individuals with developmental disabilities/autism spectrum disorders in individualized education and life planning
DDA5.S2	Teach others to use individual strengths to reinforce and maintain skills
DDA5.S3	Model use of and implementation of assistive technology and augmentative alternative communication to aid in individual's comprehension and level of engagement
DDA5.S4	Mentor others to teach unstated rules and customs that govern social behavior
DDA5.S5	Provide professional service through leadership in the field of developmental disabilities/autism spectrum disorders
DDA5.S6	Provide service to the profession through leadership activities in professional organizations

Standard 6: Collaboration

Knowledge

| ACC6K1 | Methods for communicating goals and plans to stakeholders |
| ACC6K2 | Roles of educators in integrated settings |

Skills

| ACC6S1 | Collaborate to enhance opportunities for learners with exceptional learning needs |

ACC6S2	Apply strategies to resolve conflict and build consensus
DDA6.S1	Coordinate processes that encourage collaboration needed for transition between settings
DDA6.S2	Provide leadership in collaborating with individuals and families around the issues of sexuality
DDA6.S3	Collaborate with families and other team members in non-judgmental ways to make informed decisions about interventions and life planning
DDA6.S4	Promote collaborative practices that respect the family's culture, dynamics, and values and the impact the diagnosis may have on the family
DDA6.S5	Connect families and professionals to educational and community resources

APPENDIX 3:
SAMPLE TEAM MEETING NOTES

TEAM MEETING NOTES

DATE: January 5, 2009
FOR: Elizabeth
ATTENDEES: Parent, special ed. teacher, classroom teacher, consultant, speech/language teacher

_____ AGENDA

_____X_____ MEETING NOTES

Agenda/Issues	Decision/Action	Who	When	Where
1. Spelling will be increased to 12 words per week and include words from science and social studies	Parent will reinforce meaning when doing homework sentences.	Parent	Weekly	
	Speech/Language pathologist will integrate words into stories during SLP time	SLP	Weekly	SLP room
2. Difficulty with addition and subtraction since September, previously suggested strategies not working	Probe new program: Touch Math	Consultant will train teacher	Next week	Staff room
		Classroom teacher will take data on progress	Daily data	
3. Show and Tell: Elizabeth would like to participate in class	Develop Show and Tell script	Special ed. teacher	This week	
	Practice script	SLP	This week during speech time	

APPENDIX 4:
SAMPLE EDUCATIONAL MATRIX

Subject	Staff	Objectives	Modifications or accommodations
Physical Education	PE Teacher with Sp Ed Support	1. Student will choose appropriate dress for a particular event. 2. Student will be able to engage in cooperative group activities to complete a task. 3. Student's conversations with others will include yes/no questions, use of 2–3 word responses to answer simple questions and use of appropriate declarative statements. 4. Student will consistently respond in a socially appropriate manner when approached by others.	See modification and accommodations summary page on IEP
World History	General Ed Teacher with Sp Ed Support	1. Student will be able to read and follow directions to complete a task. 2. Student will apply the concepts of time to critical thinking. 3. Student will identify cause/effect in a reading passage on his instructional level with visual supports. 4. Given a passage at his instructional reading level, student will answer an inferential or evaluative question with visual supports. 5. Student will compare/contrast two characters in a reading passage on his instructional level with visual supports. 6. Student will demonstrate perspective taking of a character in a reading passage at his instructional level by explaining why a character engaged in deceitful behavior with visual support. 7. Given a short passage or story at his instructional reading level, student will identify the sequential order of events with visual support 8. Student will increase use of descriptors (adjectives, adverbs) in his written language. 9. Student will independently select and organize the necessary materials on his desk in order to participate in classroom activities. 10. Student will demonstrate the ability to follow written and oral directions of assignments.	See modification and accommodations summary page on IEP

(Continued)

Appendix 4: (Continued)

Subject	Staff	Objectives	Modifications or accommodations
Lunch	Para Support	1. Student's conversations with others will include yes/no questions, use of 2–3 word responses to answer simple questions and use of appropriate declarative statements. 2. Student will consistently respond in a socially appropriate manner when approached by others. 3. Student will demonstrate pragmatic language skills by responding appropriately in social situations (i.e., eye contact; body posture, gestures, proximity; voice volume, tone; facial expressions, timing, manners).	See modification and accommodations summary page on IEP

Appendix 5:
Sample Curriculum Template

Unit of Study	Animals
Key Concepts	• State five things animals need to survive • Define and give examples of animal camouflage • Explain how body shape can hide an animal in its environment • Explain how mimicry is an adaption • Define behavior • State at least four behaviors that can help some animals survive in winter
Key Vocabulary	• Behavior • Inborn behavior • Camouflage • Mimicry • Environment
Teaching Strategies/ Methods	• Pictures/visuals • Diagrams • Worksheets • Picture books
Materials	A list of materials will be given to the special education teacher from the general education teacher each Friday for the following week of lessons. The special education teacher will adapt the materials as needed for the student prior to the lesson presentation in class.

(Continued)

Appendix 5: (Continued)

Unit of Study	Animals
Assignments in Class/ Homework	Both in-class and homework assignments will be discussed by the general education teacher and the special education teacher the Friday before so that they can be modified by the special education teacher before the class assignment is given.
Assessment Methods	• Multiple choice tests • Close format tests • Short answer tests • Drawings • Teacher observation • Habitat brochure project

Appendix 6: Sample Ecological Inventory

Enter School

1. Walk in the hallway as you enter the building.
2. Go to the cafeteria, sit at a table and wait for assistant to tell sixth graders to go to homeroom.

Homeroom

1. Walk in the hallway to your locker.
2. Open combination lock.
3. Place coat, lunch and backpack in locker.
4. Get books, notebooks, pencils and other needed materials out of backpack.
5. Sit at your desk in homeroom while attendance is taken.
6. Check schedule and identify first period class.
7. When bell rings, walk to first period class.

Lunch

1. When bell rings, go to locker and get lunch, place all other materials in locker.
2. Walk down the hall to the cafeteria.
3. Wait in line for your turn to buy a drink.
4. Tell the lunch lady the drink you would like to buy.
5. Pay the lunch lady for your drink.
6. Choose a table and sit down and eat your lunch.
7. When finished eating, take trash to trash can.
8. Return to the table and wait for recess bell.

Recess

1. When recess bell rings, go outside to the blacktop and fields.
2. Locate a friend.
3. Choose an activity to join, participate in the activity with your friend.
4. When bell rings, line up and walk to locker.
5. Get materials out of your locker for next class.
6. Walk to class.

CHAPTER 13

The Implementation of Evidence-Based Practices in Public Schools

Peter Doehring and Vincent Winterling

ABBREVIATIONS

ASDs Autism spectrum disorders
DAP   Delaware Autism Program
EBP   Evidence-based practice

INTRODUCTION

Educators have sometimes been chided for the enthusiasm with which they embrace new trends and concepts. Their enthusiasm regarding evidence-based practice (EBP) is crucial, however, as it will be key to the movement of EBP from the laboratory to real-world settings, such as public schools. Generalizing from the laboratory to public schools is essential if EBP are to ever reach a meaningful proportion of individuals affected by autism spectrum disorders (ASD). Public schools remain the primary mechanism by which the majority of children with ASD receive highly specialized interventions until adulthood. The quality of public education is arguably the single greatest factor in our control for improving the quality of life and mitigating the overall cost of adults with ASD, until there is a significant shift in the extent and quality of support available to them. The impact of EBP can be magnified by the educational infrastructure, to the extent that EBP are embedded in special education laws, emphasized in teacher training programs, and encouraged via funding and oversight at the local, state, and federal levels. Though public schools rarely have the resources to develop new EBPs, they are well placed to implement them. Yet most research to date demonstrating the effectiveness of interventions has been conducted in university-based or university-affiliated programs, with relatively limited effort to demonstrate generalization to public school settings.

In this chapter, we describe how one public school program – the Delaware Autism Program (DAP) – sought to implement

B. Reichow et al. (eds.), *Evidence-Based Practices and Treatments for Children with Autism*,
DOI 10.1007/978-1-4419-6975-0_13, © Springer Science+Business Media, LLC 2011

EBP. We begin by briefly describing some of the mechanisms for statewide training and oversight that are unique to DAP and facilitate the adoption of EBP. We seek to draw some lessons for educators and researchers for defining EBP, identifying broad and specific EBP, and implementing EBP. We conclude by discussing some directions for future research.

THE DELAWARE AUTISM PROGRAM

Established more than 30 years ago, DAP is a statewide network of public school programs designed to provide highly specialized, full-time, and year-round educational services to the full spectrum of persons with ASD until 21 years of age. Students are served in a variety of settings ranging from self-contained, center-based programs operated by a designated school district for the benefit of students in multiple districts, as well as smaller programs that only serve students within that district. In addition to favorable teacher- and specialist-to-student ratios, students enrolled in one of DAP's affiliated school districts become automatically eligible for an extended school year and a full-time program as soon as they are identified, from birth through 21 years of age.

In 2008, DAP served almost 700 students across six school districts, with the support of more than 400 staff. Assuming a prevalence of one in 150, about 52% of the total projected number of children with ASD had been identified with an educational classification of ASD in Delaware's public schools, with more than 90% of these receiving services through one of DAP's programs. Some of those not educationally identified with ASD may have ASD as a secondary diagnosis or may require relatively less intensive and specialized services that those provided by DAP (Doehring 2008).

In addition to programs in affiliated school districts, DAP also provides unique services and oversight under the leadership of the Statewide Director, and as mandated by state law in 2009, state regulations, and interagency agreements. The Statewide Monitoring Review Board, chaired by the Statewide Director and with members from across the state, provides general oversight with an emphasis on research-based practices. An independent peer review committee (PRC) that includes three experts in ASD, applied behavior analysis (ABA), special education, and functional behavioral assessment conducts monthly reviews of all behavior support plans that address potentially dangerous behaviors, necessitate intrusive procedures, or result in a recommendation for a more restrictive placement. The Statewide Director also delivers or coordinates a wide range of training activities statewide and is the primary liaison with Delaware Universities that provide the coursework needed by teachers to complete a required 15 credit post-graduate certificate in ASD. The Statewide Director oversees Extended Educational Services unique in the United States: three off-campus, home-like environments within which students can be provided with a range of education-based services that cannot be easily or effectively taught in a typical classroom setting. This program is available to students approximately 335 days per year. In addition, the Director oversees a program of Extended Support Services that offers respite to DAP students through a network of providers drawn from DAP's affiliated school programs.

DAP has traditionally adopted an educational model based in ABA (Bondy and Sulzer-Azaroff 2000) and the Picture Exchange Communication System (PECS; Bondy and Frost 2001; Frost and Bondy 2000). This has been supplemented by a much more diverse range of strategies addressing the social, language, and other unique learning needs of all students, including the increasing population of students with high-functioning autism (HFA) or Asperger syndrome. The specific combination of elements has also varied somewhat from site to site (Battaglini and Bondy 2006).

As might be expected by the increased numbers of students requesting service and the increasing prominence of the internet as a source for information regarding interventions for autism, DAP administration has received many requests to adopt new practices over the past decade. For example, parents approached state legislators in 2000 to advocate that the state public schools adopt the Son-Rise, or Options Program. Son-Rise was originally described through a series of books (Kaufman 1982, 1994) recounting the progress of Raun Kaufman from his initial diagnosis of autism to his full recovery, using a program designed by his parents.

Whenever we were presented with such requests, we sought to evaluate whether there was sufficient scientific data to support the use of the practice, but found that existing reviews of EBP were of limited use. The standards developed by the New York State Department of Health (1999) provided one approach to evaluating the data but the recommendations did not address school-aged children. The guidelines from the National Research Council (2001) tended to outline broad principles rather than provide clear recommendations about specific practices. In the case of Son-Rise, we invited the interested parents, as well as the proponents of the program, to offer data to support the broad claim of success they made regarding the program's effectiveness. When they were unable to provide data that rose to these early standards of EBP (e.g., more than testimonials, reports of parental satisfaction, or general ratings by parents of behavior changes), we concluded that we lacked data to support the adoption of all or part of Son-Rise.

Nevertheless, the intelligent and insightful questions that parents, legislators, and other professionals asked when making these and other requests, and our responsibility to a provide high-quality education to our students, motivated us to frankly reexamine the status quo: How much – and what kind of – data are needed to say that something is a "best practice?" What are the data supporting the practices traditionally used by DAP? Is there an assumption that "one size fits all" or is the choice of a specific method or goal driven by the individual needs of a student? Does the program itself gather data to support the use of a particular practice? We asked these questions of our public school program but they are applicable to any educational or clinical practice. We outline below some of the steps we took to seek answers and some of the findings that supported our approach.

Defining EBP for Educators

Achieve Consensus Among Researchers

Researchers must agree on – and objectively apply – a clear standard for evaluating EBP. The rubric used in this volume and others developed over the past 5 years represent significant steps forward for several reasons that should encourage practitioners. First, there is convergence among researchers regarding the general characteristics of high-quality research studies, as well as the number and quality of such studies to constitute EBP. We are optimistic that researchers will objectively apply the standard to all interventions, perhaps resulting in converging recommendations in regards to specific practices.

Second, researchers have recognized that it is both unnecessary and unrealistic to apply the traditional gold standard of clinical research – the randomized, double-blind, placebo-controlled, clinical trial – to psychosocial intervention and instead advocate a randomized, controlled trial (National Center for Education Evaluation and Regional Assistance 2003). An innovative adaptation of the randomized clinical trial was used by Mandell (2009) to compare a program based in ABA with a more traditional model based on structured teaching methods and the environment, as implemented by teachers in Philadelphia public classrooms serving children with ASD. This design balances both the desire for experimental control (by randomly assigning teachers to the ABA program or to "teaching as usual" in year 1) and the desire to quickly implement practices with proven effectiveness (by training all teachers in year 2 in the more effective of the two practices as based on analysis of year 1 data). It also tests the program in a real-world setting, so that effectiveness, rather than efficacy, can be measured.

Third, virtually all of the reviewers in this area now agree that well-controlled, single subject experimental designs (SSEDs) represent valid and important forms of evidence that complement evidence gained via group designs. While group designs may establish broad patterns of improvement that can help to establish overall priorities for training, SSEDs provide methods and yield data that can shape individualized educational planning, as exemplified by the role of functional behavioral assessment in the development of behavior support plans.

Clarify the Relation of EBP to Other "Best Practices"

Notwithstanding the emphasis in recent laws on EBP (e.g., No Child Left Behind, Individuals with Disabilities Education Improvement Act), educators must also clearly recognize and respond to the "best practices" defined by specific state and federal laws. These laws define critical elements and drive individualized education assessment, planning, and implementation. In most cases, research-based best practices complement those based in federal laws, because the latter tend to emphasize the broad implementation of education and leave most specific recommendations regarding the teaching methods and curricula in the hands of state and local educators. One exception is the ruling that schools are not obligated to provide the best education, only one that is adequate to ensure reasonable progress. It is therefore conceivable that two practices may be equivalent within the legal standard insofar as both ensure "appropriate" progress, even though one may have stronger empirical support.

EBPs also coexist – and sometime collide – with other "best practices" defined not by empirical evidence but by strongly held assumptions that are embedded in the prevailing culture of public education. For example, the full inclusion of children with ASD and other developmental disabilities is often cited as an "educational best practice", in part because it is (mis)interpreted as the only way to meet the requirement to educate in the least restrictive environment (LRE). In response to the frankly inhumane practices in the treatment of people with intellectual disabilities prior to IDEA, the passion for full inclusion has helped increase opportunities for community integration and has improved the quality of life for countless individuals and families. It is therefore not surprising that inclusion has become a prominent goal of special education in the United States, even though the assumption that all children benefit from the same level of integration with typical peers and interaction with the typical curriculum (however thoughtfully adapted) "de-individualizes" special education. Although a thorough review is beyond the scope of the present chapter, additional research is needed to clearly demonstrate that inclusion measurably improves outcomes for students with ASD, in addition to changing the attitudes of typical teachers and students towards ASD.

The use of procedures such as physical restraint and any form of aversive consequence in response to problem behavior is even more complex and controversial, and also certainly worthy of more extensive and objective review. As we argue later, there is a clear consensus that problem behaviors can be reduced by using positive and proactive interventions linked to the hypothesized function of the behavior and this represents the most immediate opportunity for EPB to improve outcomes for many students with ASD. This is especially encouraging given that the inappropriate use of consequences in response to problem behavior ranges from repeated and unnecessary suspension from school to rare but tragic instances of death resulting from physical restraint (U. S. Government Accountability Office 2009). We believe that this functional and proactive approach to problem behavior should drive a rational process of decision-making regarding behavior support, a process that may sometimes include the temporary use of negative consequences (including restraint and other safety techniques) when all proactive approaches are in place but the behavior continues to present health and safety concerns to the education team.

IDENTIFYING BROAD AND INDIVIDUALIZED EBP

Identify First-Order EBP: Broadly Effective Methods, Approaches, or Programs

As new algorithms for defining EPB have begun to be implemented by reviewers in the present volume and elsewhere, it has become clear to us and to other reviewers that there are at least two levels of EBP recommendations (National Autism Center 2009). We would characterize first-order recommendations as addressing more general educational goals and methods for a broadly defined population: that an intervention program (e.g., early intensive behavioral intervention) or a more specific intervention method (e.g., pivotal response training) improved certain broad classes of skill (e.g., social skills) for a group of individuals with ASD (e.g. preschoolers). Such recommendations would fall short, however, of identifying specific skills and targets (e.g., increasing the initiation of joint attention) for a student with a specific skill profile (e.g., with some emerging joint attention skills).

It is clear there is at least emerging evidence to support some-first-order recommendations – for example, there is considerable evidence that interventions based in ABA produce significantly improved outcomes (National Research Council 2001; New York State Department of Health 1999). Most of the 33 practices identified as "established" or "emerging" by the National Standards Project (National Autism Center 2009) would be characterized as first-order recommendations. To the extent that the method can be specified (e.g., pivotal response training) and specific training programs are available, this recommendation may help us to set broad program priorities to train educators in the method and, perhaps, provide some general guidance regarding the classes of skill and individuals to which the method might be applied.

It seems unlikely that first-order recommendations can be easily translated into specific educational goals for specific students, for several reasons. First, truly effective teaching of a classroom of children with ASD is one of the most complex and intensive activities in the field of human services because it entails the manipulation of multiple variables that are not necessarily specific to the method under consideration.

For example, early intensive behavioral intervention includes low student–teacher ratios and intense instruction (National Autism Center 2009), a fact which led reviewers of Lovaas' original findings to question the extent to which the results reflected the overall intensity of teaching (Gresham and MacMillan 1998; Schopler et al. 1987). We can raise similar questions about whether the generally increased emphasis on reinforcement, attention to prompting, reliance on a detailed curriculum, and use of data in tracking progress may play a greater role in outcomes than the specific teaching methods outlined. As we argue later, we need more research to tease apart the impact of these nonspecific educational factors before we can draw clear conclusions about the effectiveness of broad programs (Schopler 1987). Instead of drawing conclusions about a broad program (e.g., that ABA is effective for educating all children with ASD), we prefer to speak of an ABA "toolbox" or a "multicomponent behavioral intervention package" (National Autism Center 2009) that includes a range of interrelated teaching strategies.

A second challenge is that the targets for many educational methods are so broadly defined. For example, studies of PECS have considered its role in improving communication skills (e.g., requesting, sharing interests, length and complexity of utterance), social skills (e.g., supporting peer interactions) and self-management (e.g., use of visual schedules), as well as in decreasing problem behaviors (via its impact on communication). The student's readiness to learn specific skills also varies from student to student, depending on their prerequisite skills; e.g., a student's effective use of a picture schedule may depend on their overall use of pictures to communicate. To capture this range, the National Standards Project (National Autism Center 2009) broke down treatment targets into 14 broad categories of skills and behaviors, and students into 6 groups based on age and 3 groups based on diagnosis (autism, PDD-NOS. and Asperger syndrome).

Third, there is likely considerable variation in how researchers categorize interventions: they may use different terms to describe the same method, or use the same label for two methods that may in fact differ in significant ways. The National Standards Project (National Autism Center 2009) generated 38 different treatments from their review of 775 studies but struggled because of tremendous variability between treatments: some of which were specific strategies based on as few as two studies, while others represented broad programs based on more than 200 studies.

At DAP, we sought to apply the rubric developed by Reichow et al. (2008) to explore the effectiveness of PECS (Frost and Bondy 2000) in teaching communication (Doehring et al. 2007). We chose PECS because it is in widespread use across the country (including at DAP) and we wanted to know whether the available research might point to specific uses. PECS is also particularly well-suited to this approach because it tends to focus on a discrete range of skills (e.g., early expressive communication skills), in a specific population (e.g., children with little or no independent functional communication), using a manualized method and a highly structured training protocol (Frost and Bondy 2000). While this analysis is neither exhaustive nor up-to date, it illustrates the potential for applying the resulting recommendations to public school practices.

We began by conducting a PSYCHLIT and PUBMED search for PECS-related research published in peer-reviewed journals, focusing on outcome studies written in English and readily available electronically. We eliminated studies for the reasons shown in Table 13.1. After rating studies according the Reichow et al. (2008) rubric, we also eliminated studies receiving a weak rating.

This left a total of ten studies (two group and six single case studies). Overall

TABLE 13.1   Studies eliminated from consideration

Reason for elimination	Study
Was not in English	Koita and Sonoyama (2004)
	Yokoyama et al. (2006)
Included adults or people without autism	Bock et al. (2005)
	Schwartz et al. (1998)
	Simon et al. (1996)
	Chambers and Rehfeldt (2003)
	Rehfeldt and Root (2005)
	Stoner et al. (2006)
Focused on skills other than communication	Bryan and Gast (2000)
Was not easily available electronically	Bondy and Frost (1994)
	Tincani et al. (2006)
	Peterson et al. (1995)
	Bailey et al. (2006)
	Heneker and Page (2003)
Was available but not yet peer reviewed	Malandraki and Okalidou (2007)
	Cummings and Williams (2000)
	Buckley and Newchok (2005)
	Dooley et al. (2001)
	Sigafoos et al. (2007)
Weak rating	Frea et al. (2001)
	Liddle (2001)

reliability using the algorithm presented in this volume was 85%, calculated on 25% of studies.

- Adkins and Axelrod 2002
- Charlop-Christy et al. 2002
- Ganz and Simpson 2004
- Kravits et al. 2002
- Magiati and Howlin 2003
- Marckel et al. 2006
- Tincani 2004
- Yoder and Stone 2006a, b
- Howlin et al. 2007
- Carr and Felce 2007

We then sought to generate first-order recommendations regarding the overall status of PECS as an EBP. This analysis indicated that PECS was an established EBP for teaching early expressive communication skills, with three studies (one group and two SSED) meriting a Strong research report strength rating and five studies (one group and four SSED) meriting an Adequate research report strength rating. These studies were all done by different, independent teams. Note that this differs from the overall rating of Emerging by the National Standards Project (National Autism Center 2009), because the latter is based on an average score rather than the critical threshold approach used here.

The pattern of strengths and weaknesses in the research studies is interesting. Among the primary quality indicators for these studies rated High or Acceptable, participant characteristics were most likely to fall short of the high standard (see Table 13.2). Among the secondary quality indicators common to Group and SSEDs, evidence was most likely to be absent for reporting Cohen's KAPPA, for calculating interobserver agreement, the use of blind raters, and the assessment

TABLE 13.2 Summary of ratings

Study	Design (method)	Average age Chronological (mental*language)	Adequate PQI[a]	Absent SQI[b]
Howlin et al. (2007)	Group (PECS)	7 years	PART	IOA, KAP, BR, FID, ATR, ES
Yoder and Stone (2006a, b)	Group (PECS, RPMT[c])	3 years (1.5 years)		BR
Adkins and Axelrod (2002)	Single-case (PECS)	7 years	PART	IOA, KAP, BR, FID
Charlop-Christy et al. (2002)	Single-case (PECS)	(1.8 years)	PART, VIS	KAP, BR, FID
Ganz and Simpson (2004)	Single-case (PECS)	6 years (0.6 years)		KAP, BR, FID, GM
Kravits et al. (2002)	Single-case (PECS)	6 years (2.5 years)	PART	IOA, KAP, BR, FID
Marckel et al. (2006)	Single-case (PECS)	4.5 years	VIS	KAP, BR, FID
Tincani (2004)	Single-case (PECS)	7 years (1.5 years)		KAP

[a] Primary quality indicators (PQI) considered: Participant characteristics (PART); independent variable (IV); comparison condition (CC); dependent variable (DV); data analysis linked to research question (LRQ); statistical analysis (STAT); baseline (BSLN); visual analysis (VIS); experimental control (EXP)
[b] Secondary quality indicators (SQI) considered: Interobserver agreement (IOA); Kappa calculated (KAP); blind raters (BR); procedural fidelity (FID); attrition (ATR); generalization/maintenance (GM); effect size (ES); social validity (SV)
[c] Responsive education and prelinguistic milieu teaching

of fidelity of intervention (Doehring et al. 2007). Some of these indicators are relatively easy to address (e.g., calculation of Cohen's Kappa) and efforts to remedy others can have educational benefits (e.g., better participant characterization and evaluation of fidelity), as we discuss later.

Identify Second-Order EBP: Individualized Teaching

Second-order EBP support more individualized recommendations regarding the use of specific practices to target specific skills, perhaps in a child at a specific stage of skill acquisition. For example, once a specific intervention (e.g., pivotal response training) has been broadly identified as an EBP, we consider if there is evidence that it can help to improve specific skills (e.g., the initiation of social play) for a specific group of individuals with ASD (e.g., preschoolers with the prerequisite to play skills but very limited social play). Just as it is unreasonable to expect a single program to meet all of the needs of all individuals with ASD, it is also unreasonable to expect that a single method is equally effective in teaching all skills or that all children are equally ready to learn a specific skill. For example, the relevance of PECS research to an individual student may depend only on the specific target of interest.

For this chapter, we extended the analysis of PECS studies described above to generate second-order recommendations that could be translated more readily into individual educational goals. Closer examination of the basic characteristics of the PECS studies reviewed here revealed that many dimensions could be considered when seeking to target recommendations at the individual level. We quickly realized that it was unrealistic to apply the same threshold of evidence for these second-order recommendations as we

had for the first-order recommendations because of the restricted number of studies of at least adequate quality and range of dimensions considered (see Table 13.3).

We therefore relaxed the standards of evidence for second-order recommendations, in a manner similar to that of the National Standards Project (National Autism Center 2009), and chose to focus on similar outcomes obtained across at least two studies related to specific observable skills or goals. In the summary below, we designate "consistent evidence" when similar findings were obtained across all studies that examined a specific question and "some evidence" when there was a generally positive, though not perfectly consistent, trend obtained across all studies that examined a specific question. Findings considered by only one study are indicated under the general heading "emerging evidence." It is important to note that these findings were largely restricted to preschoolers and young children, most of whom had little or no speech or other communication skills at baseline. We did not seek to interpret reported decreases in scores on the Autism Diagnostic Observation Schedule (ADOS) or data related to parent or teacher behaviors (Howlin et al. 2007) because such data are not typically considered in evaluations of individual student progress.

Most of the studies focused solely on the acquisition of PECS:

- There was consistent evidence that PECS can be mastered relatively quickly – even by children with no communication skills (Charlop-Christy et al. 2002; Ganz and Simpson 2004; Kravits et al. 2002).
- There was consistent evidence that improvement in PECS was associated with improvements in the complexity of speech, such as mean length of utterance (Charlop-Christy et al. 2002) and number of words per trial (Ganz and Simpson 2004).

TABLE 13.3   Summary of outcomes associated with Increased PECS use

Study	Significant outcomes[a]
Yoder and Stone (2006a)	Compared to RPMT[b], PECS improved frequency and range of words for children with greater initial object exploration; RPMT improved frequency and range of words for children with less initial object exploration; differences disappeared at 6-month follow-up.
Yoder and Stone (2006b)	PECS and RPMT were both effective in increasing turn-taking, but RPMT was superior; both were effective in increasing requesting and IJA but PECS was superior for subjects with little or no IJA at baseline and RPMT was superior for subjects with IJA at baseline.
Carr and Felce (2007)	PECS increased child initiations, adult responses to child initiations, and child responses to adult initiations.
Magiati and Howlin (2003)	PECS was mastered quickly; an increased number of pictures were used and frequency of PECS use increased; there was increased communication (nonverbal to using single/echoed words) and decreased problem behavior.
Howlin et al. (2007)	PECS increased initiations and PECS use but relative improvement was not maintained over time (e.g., 10 months later); there was no change in speech.
Adkins and Axelrod (2002)	Compared to sign language in teaching requesting, PECS was acquired more quickly, generalized more readily, and used spontaneously more often.
Charlop-Christy et al. (2002)	PECS was fully mastered (to Phase 6) within 17 h of training; increased spontaneous and imitative speech was generalized across sessions, mean length of utterance, and other social communicative behavior (e.g., joint attention, eye contact, and free play); problem behavior decreased.
Ganz and Simpson (2004)	PECS was largely mastered (to Phase 4) within 23 sessions (346 trials); there was an increased number of words per trial.
Kravits et al. (2002)	PECS was established (to Phase 3) and generalized across settings; there was increased spontaneous communication (including intelligible verbalizations) and duration of interactions with peers across all school settings.
Marckel et al. (2006)	PECS was used to teach children to improvise using combinations of descriptors (function, color, shape) when a picture is unavailable.
Tincani (2004)	PECS was superior in teaching requesting for a child with poor imitation skills, and sign language was superior for child with good imitation skills; vocalization was increased after training in both PECS and sign language.

[a] For group designs, differences were statistically significant; for single-case designs, improvements above baseline were consistently noted for the majority of subjects
[b] Responsive education and prelinguistic milieu teaching

- There was consistent evidence that improvement in PECS was associated with decreases in problem behaviors (Charlop-Christy et al. 2002; Magiati and Howlin 2003).

- There was consistent evidence that improvement in PECS was associated with gains in other social-communicative behavior, such as joint attention, eye contact, turn-taking, and free play

(Charlop-Christy et al. 2002; Kravits et al. 2002; Yoder and Stone 2006b).

- There was some evidence that improvement in PECS was associated with improvements in the frequency of vocalization and speech, and no evidence that it was associated with a decrease in vocalization and speech. Most studies reported a positive correlation (Charlop-Christy et al. 2002; Kravits et al. 2002; Tincani 2004; Magiati and Howlin 2003; Yoder and Stone 2006a).

Other studies compared the acquisition of PECS relative to another intervention. These studies were particularly instructive for educators insofar as they may provide emerging evidence for the differentiation of instruction according to specific student characteristics.

- PECS and responsive education and prelinguistic milieu teaching (RPMT) were both effective in increasing the initiation of joint attention (Yoder and Stone 2006b). RPMT was superior for children who frequently initiated joint attention during a pre-intervention assessment whereas PECS was superior for children who rarely or never initiated joint attention prior to intervention (Yoder and Stone 2006b).
- When considering the growth in the frequency and range of single-word use immediately between pre-treatment and at 6-month follow-up, children who were relatively low in initial object exploration benefited more from RPMT and children who were relatively high in initial object exploration benefited more from PECS (Yoder and Stone 2006a).
- PECS may by superior to sign language in teaching simple requesting to children with poor imitation skills, whereas the effect may be reversed for children with good imitation skills (Tincani 2004).

The Role of Rigorous Diagnosis and Cognitive Assessment

Educators and researchers use information about diagnosis and overall functioning somewhat differently and this may lead researchers and educators to adopt different standards. In research into ASD (as other diagnosed conditions), researchers often take great care in accurate diagnosis because the hypotheses under investigation typically address the relationship of ASD to other skills, behaviors, or characteristics of the individual. The role of diagnosis is less clear in educational planning. That is, while a medical diagnosis or educational classification may help to broadly define the intensity or funding of educational services and supports available to the student, it might also be significantly augmented by the child's IEP team who may argue in support of the need for additional evaluation, staffing support, or extension of the school day or school year to ensure adequate progress. That IEPs should vary so greatly is hardly surprising, since it is now generally acknowledged that the needs of individuals with ASD are wildly diverse.

It is perhaps not surprising that the standards used by educators to establish an ASD classification are often far less rigorous than those used by researchers. Federal regulations defining autism do not reference the broader spectrum; they emphasize unusual behaviors (some of which do not clearly align with the criteria of the *Diagnostic and Statistical Manual of Mental Disorders* (DSM-IV; APA 1994)) more than the impairments in reciprocal social interaction largely recognized as lying at the core of ASD (Carter et al. 2005). Policies and practices related to diagnosis also vary greatly from state to state (Stahmer and Mandell 2007).

In Delaware, we were concerned that the misalignment between the definition of ASD accepted by researchers and that embodied by state and federal regulation would make it impossible to broadly identify the groups of students likely to benefit from more specialized interventions identified by researchers or to project the likely number of students with ASD in the state. We first revised the state regulations to align educational classification with the DSM-IV, to encompass the entire spectrum, and to rely on multimodal assessment, consistent with the consensus-based guidelines of the National Research Council (2001). We then embarked on a program of training educational assessment teams, anchored by school psychologists, in the clinical use of the Autism Diagnostic Observation Schedule (Lord et al. 2000) and Autism Diagnostic Interview – Revised (Lord et al. 1994). A total of 85 professionals across eight school districts (serving more than 90% of the students identified with ASD in Delaware) were trained (Doehring 2008).

As in the case of diagnosis, outcome researchers have also taken great care to establish an initial level of cognitive or language functioning to render two groups comparable so that treatment effects can be more confidently attributed to the intervention, or simply to accurately characterize their population relative to that identified in other studies. For educators, the results of cognitive or language assessment are again somewhat less important, except in helping to establish the student's eligibility for special education services. Results may help to establish a starting point for broadly identifying needs and goals, or support the intensity of certain specialized services (e.g., amount of speech therapy per week), but this may be superseded in the course of creating an IEP. Similarly, the results of such assessments are not the primary measure of progress (except perhaps in cases when a major lack of progress or regression is suspected): educators more often rely on progress towards individual IEP objectives to determine the need for programmatic changes.

Nevertheless, educators seeking to implement EBP must be able to use some general criteria for identifying methods and setting goals that are reasonable for the child, given that overall rates of progress and outcomes depend in part on the child's initial level of cognitive functioning (Harris and Handleman 2000; Smith et al. 1997). Educators may also find it difficult to identify which findings and methods are broadly applicable to their particular population, because the accurate diagnosis and assessment of students may be areas of weakness for some studies. Among the primary quality indicators for PECS studies reviewed above, participant characteristics (such as diagnosis and level of functioning) were most likely to fall short of a high standard. We also conducted a simple review of all studies published in the *Journal of Applied Behavior Analysis* between 2000 and 2005 that sought to demonstrate an assessment or intervention outcome for children with ASD. We found that few studies provided information about the level of functioning and still fewer provided even basic information to support the ASD diagnosis (Doehring et al. 2007).

With the intense focus on ASD, educators and researchers have often overlooked the opportunity to extend innovations to other populations. For example, many of the ABA-based techniques used in ASD are just as relevant to children with intellectual disabilities (ID), yet schools rarely dedicate as much effort to training and supporting staff working with students with ID (even though many public classrooms mix both populations). Perhaps this is because the dramatic effects noted by some researchers for children with ASD have not been replicated to the same extent with students who have intellectual disabilities (Smith et al. 1997). In this context, it is interesting to note that the Combating Autism Act (Public Law 109–416, 2006) references both children with ASD and with ID.

The increasing shift away from a categorical approach to ASD may improve the characterization of ASD symptomatology but prove challenging for researchers and educators seeking to identify EBP. The emphasis on a dimensional model (Gotham et al. 2007) that supports a broad autism phenotype (Piven and Palmer 1999) appears more consistent with emerging evidence for the involvement of a combination of rare and common genetic variants in ASD (Wang et al. 2009), and seems likely to shape the DSM-V (Wallis 2009). Educators will need help in making the transition from a categorical to a dimensional approach to assessment, especially insofar as it makes it more difficult to broadly map EBP onto the needs of students.

Implementing EBP

Create a Culture of Data-Based Decision-Making

The emerging prominence of EBP, together with the emphasis on careful analysis of progress towards specific goals in No Child Left Behind (Public Law 107–110, 2002), may help to foster an educational culture of data-based decision-making. This is important because, even after EBPs are in place across a school, the ability of IEP teams to collect and use data to identify and evaluate outcomes for individual students requires many skills and resources: educators must not only know how to set clear and measurable objectives, how much data to collect, how to analyze the data, and how to make decisions based on progress, but they must also allocate time and other resources to accomplish these tasks. Educators will always need a defensible, data-based approach to decision-making because the failure to demonstrate adequate progress – or the promise of significantly greater progress – has been

one of the most important variables when families have successfully advocated for additional educational services or a change in educational placement.

Though the IEP process provides broad guidelines for how to collect data and how to evaluate progress, we have found additional standards are needed to foster a culture of data-based decision-making, at least for more complex cases. For example, when a family or a school requests a residential program, because challenging behaviors or pervasive deficits in skills of daily life significantly impede progress at home or at school, most public schools across the nation generally seek a full-time residential placement with a private provider. Because DAP offers Extended Educational Services within its public school program, we tended to receive many such requests and sought to implement a data-based approach to making such recommendations. We developed guidelines to urge IEP teams to identify specific IEP goals for which progress was deemed inadequate, as demonstrated via daily or weekly tracking. We also sought to verify that objectives were well-formulated, data collection procedures were appropriate, and there were sufficient opportunities and staffing support needed to teach the skill. If the data supported a clear lack of progress, we worked with the family and school to identify other program changes, including increased staffing in school, parent training, in-home training and support, or consultation or coordination with other community-based professionals (e.g., respite providers and prescribing physicians). If the data continued to show a lack of progress, we might consider increasing time in the Extended Educational Service to include overnight services.

This data-based approach was instrumental in convincing IEP teams to consider more fundamental programming changes (e.g., temporarily suspending other IEP objectives and instituting increased hours in our Extended Educational Service to teach important self-care skills, such as toileting), school districts to support creative staffing solutions (e.g., to pay for school-district staff to work intensively with an adolescent to extend behavior support programs into their home), and states to help pay for private placements when other, less expensive, options had been thoroughly tested. As a result, DAP has required full-time or private residential placement for less than 1% of the overall population of children identified with ASD in the Delaware schools (Doehring 2008). The pressure to respond to students in crisis, regardless of the evidence for a clear educational need, and the challenge of implementing the guidelines described above has made it difficult to consistently adopt this more data-based approach.

Integrate EBP in a Program of Professional Development

Even the best EBP may have a limited impact in school-based programs if they are not integrated into a cycle including a program of training derived from binding standards of practice whose implementation is closely monitored (see Fig. 13.1).

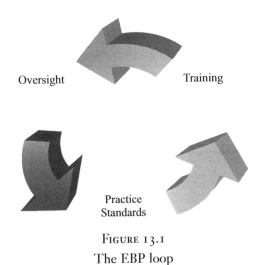

FIGURE 13.1

The EBP loop

In addition to implementing traditional training programs (e.g., traditional didactic workshops for staff and new teacher mentoring), we revised and expanded the syllabi for the required 15-credit post-graduate certification for teachers and, in some sites, added dedicated staff positions or brought in external experts to provide extensive, in-class coaching. By identifying specific practice standards and specifying training requirements, we could begin to monitor overall progress in implementation of EBP. For example, we set and then met goals to train the majority of the 400 DAP professional and paraprofessional staff statewide in key elements related to student safety, general ABA-based educational strategies, and PECS (Doehring 2008).

In the short term, we found that the most significant barrier to the completion of the EBP cycle (aside from perennial shortages of funding and training time) was the lack of specific training manuals, curricula, and associated assessments of treatment fidelity for most methods and programs. Some commonly used procedures help to set the standard. For example, the Autism Diagnostic Observation Schedule includes elements common to most tests (e.g., a comprehensive manual, detailed scoring forms, and complete test kit) as well as others that are less common but important to training (e.g., a structured workshop delivered by certified trainers and additional training to attain reliability for research purposes). PECS includes a detailed manual, an accompanying workshop, and a process for receiving coaching from a certified trainer or becoming a trainer oneself. These elements should be considered a minimum for those seeking to implement EBP system-wide.

Another significant and immediate barrier to the completion of the EBP cycle is the failure to quantify or control for "nonspecific variables" (Schopler et al. 1987). These may include intensity of support (e.g., amount of one-to-one or small group instruction, staff–student ratios, or hours of instruction per week) or the use of general teaching strategies embedded in a given approach (e.g., the increased use of reinforcement, the conscious use of prompting, the definition of clear objectives, or the more frequent collection and use of data in decision-making that is implicit to ABA).

In the long-term, educators must also become more knowledgeable consumers of research. While we have sought to weave an emphasis on EBP into all staff and parent training and provided more detailed training to teachers and other staff in understanding research, we have introduced other strategies whenever possible, such as providing annotated bibliographies of relevant outcome research, sometimes including electronic copies of specific articles; requiring staff to review and summarize outcome literature to get full credit for participation in specific training programs; and involving staff in preparing presentations for professional conferences that involve critical analysis of elements of EBP, some at which are referenced in this chapter.

Case Study: Adopting a Proactive Approach to Behavior Support

Children with ASD demonstrate a wide range of problem behavior (e.g., aggression, destruction and self-injury) that may be extremely costly to the individual, family, or the community and that may jeopardize their home and school placements. Such problem behaviors are the most common reason for children with ASD to be referred to community mental health settings (Mandell et al. 2006). At DAP, we found that the reliance on antecedent interventions informed by functional behavioral assessment to address problem behavior was perhaps the

most immediate opportunity for a public school to benefit from EBP. We describe some of the innovative mechanisms we put in place to implement these EBP statewide, by providing training and oversight linked to clear and binding practice standards. With these supports in place, we were also able to clearly document the need for a parallel program to train and oversee staff in the appropriate use of physical restraint in response to dangerous student behaviors. This example may also illustrate how "nonspecific variables" can be as important as individualized behavior supports in decreasing problem behavior.

Identifying EBP

There is a general consensus that functional behavioral assessment is very useful in identifying possible reasons or functions for the behavior (Bregman et al. 2005). Questionnaires, interviews, and rating scales are used in a functional behavioral assessment to begin to identify explanations for student problem behavior. Though functional behavioral assessment may be difficult to formally establish as an EBP using current criteria, there is no doubt that it is otherwise accepted as a "best practice" in the field of behavior support. It should be noted, however, that functional behavioral assessment potentially encompasses a range of assessment techniques ranging from checklists to interviews to experimental analysis. Each approach requires different investments in time and training and they yield different kinds of data that may not always converge (Kwak et al. 2004).

In contrast, there is clear evidence that the use of antecedent interventions to decrease problem behavior is an EBP (National Autism Center 2009). Antecedent strategies are designed to prevent the initial occurrence of the behavior, as opposed to strategies that are responses to or consequences of the problem behavior.

In the case of a student who hits a peer who is playing on the computer, antecedent strategies could include teaching an alternative skill to achieve the same likely end (e.g., teaching the student to ask for a turn), adapting the task (e.g., initially shorten the wait time and then gradually increase it), or reinforcing the student for coping (e.g., reinforce him for waiting patiently for his turn), in contrast to reprimanding or punishing the student (e.g., removing access to the computer).

Some of the advantages of initially focusing on problem behaviors are associated with the reliance on SSEDs in much of the supporting research. First, the reliance on careful observation, experimental control, individualized programming, and hypothesis testing in SSEDs is itself a model for a data-based approach for teaching students with ASD. We have found that the inclusion of SSEDs in graduate courses for teachers not only improves their acceptance of and facility with behavior support plans but also makes them more methodical and empirical in their approach to teaching more broadly. Second, educators are more likely to find very detailed descriptions of the interventions used because this is expected of articles published in behavioral journals. These descriptions fall short of a treatment manual and are not always tested by measures of fidelity but are readily understood by teachers with a basic understanding of behavior analysis. Effectively translating findings based on SSEDs presumes, however, that teachers can evaluate the fit of the child and behavior described in the article with the student who they are seeking to help.

There are other advantages to beginning a program to implement EBP by focusing on problem behavior, rather than skill deficits:

- Schools, teachers, and parents may be more highly motivated to address problem behavior. For parents, problem behaviors may stand out more dramatically than skill deficits because they may be more difficult to control. For teachers, the problem behaviors of a single child can disrupt the entire classroom. For schools, problem behaviors that result in suspension, expulsion, or injury are potentially very expensive if they lead to legal action or a private placement.

- Functional behavioral assessment and positive behavior support also provide some of the best opportunities to build partnerships between home and school and across various service agencies. Various programs have demonstrated how functional behavioral assessment can bring together families, schools, and other providers to develop a common understanding and coordinated plan (Becker-Cottrill et al. 2003; Boettcher et al. 2003).

- There are a variety of programs of schoolwide positive behavior supports that may serve as models for a system change, including a broad training program that includes all members of the school community and outcome measures of variables from suspensions to school climate. Some caution is warranted however. While the data for schoolwide interventions is promising, the outcomes for students with the most complex needs are less clear given the lack of data demonstrating individual outcomes, program fidelity, and the resources needed to achieve success.

Implementing EBP

Just as it began to emphasize proactive strategies in preventing problem behaviors among DAP students, the Peer Review Committee (PRC) recognized that clear and binding practice standards, improved data collection and analysis, and targeted staff training could be more effective than negative feedback to DAP professionals in improving behavior support plans. Broad standards for independent peer review in Delaware State Law and regulations outline the role of DAP's PRC in reviewing more restrictive procedures and we drafted binding memoranda of agreement that required participating school districts to support PRC recommendations. We extended these standards in our internal guidelines to require reviews (at frequencies of up to monthly) of behavior support plans that address behaviors that are dangerous or potentially dangerous, that necessitate intrusive procedures (e.g., all forms of time out), or that result in a relatively restrictive placement (e.g., suspension from school or change in placement to a less inclusive setting).

Other standards were added to improve the reliance on data. We required that data on behaviors and the use of key procedures are collected daily, graphed weekly or monthly (including information on key changes such as staffing, curriculum, medications, etc.), and submitted for independent review monthly or quarterly depending on the intensity of the behavior (Doehring 2006). With pilot funding from the state of Delaware, we also drafted specific standards linking the amount and quality of data needed to support a functional behavioral assessment, depending upon the intensity and complexity of the behavior, in a hypothesis-driven process. For example, when an experienced teacher and psychologist generated a hypothesis regarding a simple, frequently occurring, and nondangerous behavior that could be tested by a simple, positive, and proactive intervention (e.g., teaching an alternative skill or implementing a simple schedule of differential reinforcement), no additional assessment would be needed other than monitoring the response to intervention. Additional data collection may become necessary for behaviors that were more infrequent, dangerous, or complex (e.g., behavior that may vary according to antecedent conditions),

up to and including (in rare cases) more experimental functional analysis.

The recommendations arising from PRC's review of individual cases also informed a broad range of efforts at training and oversight. We initiated a 4-day program of training in behavior support for all psychologists and behavior analysts statewide, with an emphasis on pro-active approaches, functional behavioral assessment, and crisis response. Given the applicability of many techniques to students with intellectual disabilities, we extended an invitation to psychologists working with this population. We also recognized the limits of didactic workshops and so coupled PRC review with an option for individualized coaching and consultation. Finally, we also integrated these same principles of behavior support into the postgraduate certification in autism required of teachers.

We realized that even the best efforts cannot prevent all behaviors that are dangerous to staff and students and so we also used a train-the-trainer approach to ensure that all staff statewide could safely respond to students in a behavioral crisis, including physical restraint if clearly indicated. This was coupled with a multilevel program of oversight to ensure that each instance of physical restraint was documented, communicated to parents and appropriate staff members, and reviewed for its appropriateness according to program guidelines (Doehring 2008). We believe that this training program has been instrumental in limiting injuries and private residential placements resulting from problem behavior.

We also came to recognize that problem behaviors sometimes function as the "canary in the coalmine" because they signal poor teaching practices. When most of the students in a classroom engage in behavior that functions to gain the teacher's attention or to escape from difficult tasks, for example, this may reflect that the teacher cannot juggle individual student needs or that the curriculum is not matched to the students' ability levels. While there is no harm if the resulting multiple behavior plans all help the teacher or other staff to direct attention to successes and not failures ("catch them being good") or to adjust the curriculum, they may distract from the need for fundamental, system-wide changes (e.g., decreased staffing ratios, increased training, or curriculum modifications). Many of our recommendations also addressed general teaching practices; weaving reinforcement implicitly and explicitly throughout the school day; prioritizing the teaching of fundamental communication, adaptive, and leisure skills; ensuring a rich, stimulating schedule of activities and integration opportunities that respected students' needs, interests, and independence; individualizing the curriculum and teaching strategies as needed; and carefully monitoring students' overall health and well-being.

Conclusion

Develop a Research Network

It is wholly unrealistic for public education agencies or university-based programs to assume sole responsibility for developing and demonstrating the implementation of EBPs, though each can play a critical role in a partnership. Given the perennial budgetary pressures and the complexity and intensity involved in educating children with ASD, public education agencies cannot dedicate the resources needed to identify EBP but there are certainly increased opportunities to support their implementation: local school districts can allocate professional development days to support training in new practices and can allocate staffing resources creatively to provide on-site coaching to consolidate skills gained via training. State education agencies can spearhead efforts to develop statewide EBP

standards, gather data to demonstrate how decreased reliance on private placement for students with more complex needs might free up resources to support training and oversight statewide, and use state and federal funds to support pilot projects.

Individual researchers can also play a key role. They can shift their research focus from the effectiveness of a broad program on broad outcomes to evaluating interactions between rate of skill acquisition and current stage of development (Yoder and Stone 2006a, b) or other related skills (Tincani 2004). They can also partner with schools to validate EBPs outside of the controlled context of the laboratory or laboratory school, in the course of which they may spur the development of intervention manuals and begin to document the impact of non-specific variables. Researchers can begin by helping educators to present data and practices at professional conferences, such as those conducted at DAP and referenced in this chapter.

Collaboration among researchers, and between researches and educators, will be required to effectively address these complex questions. Multidisciplinary, community-focused, university-based programs, such as those represented by the Association of University Centers on Disabilities, are well-placed to foster such partnerships and disseminate innovative practices nationwide. Training programs funded via maternal child health (e.g., Leadership Education in Neurodevelopmental Disorders) and education (e.g., the National Professional Development Center on Autism) can also help to disseminate practices via public schools and universities.

Consider Big and Little Outcomes

Research that precisely focuses on specific questions about methodology and intervention targets in the search for EBP relevant to public schools can help educators to understand the potential application to specific students and researchers to test underlying theories. As the focus on specific EBPs narrows, we may miss other important outcomes broadly related to EBP or factors broadly contributing to EBP in schools. Fundamental gaps in services may render the best EBP less relevant – for example, there are data to suggest that there are significant variations in rates of identification between different states (Shattuck et al. 2009) and school districts (Palmer et al. 2005) and that children who are poor or from traditionally underserved populations tend to be identified later than other populations (Mandell et al. 2002, 2007). Other broad outcomes are difficult to quantify but are nonetheless important goals for educators. For example, schools should look beyond graduation to quality-of-life outcomes when planning the transition to adulthood: Can the student live independently, work at a job they enjoy, lead a healthy lifestyle, and have meaningful relationships with peers? Finally, schools need to sometimes look beyond the school day and the school's walls to other factors that might mediate outcomes, such as the need for family training and support. Research into these questions will help educators to take the final step in translating research into practice via evidence-based policy.

References

Adkins, T., & Axelrod, S. (2002). Topography- versus selection-based responding: comparison of mand acquisition in each modality. *The Behavior Analyst Today, 2,* 259–266.

APA. (1994). *Diagnostic and statistical manual of mental disorders* (4th ed.). Washington, DC: American Psychiatric Association.

Battaglini, K., & Bondy, A. (2006). Application of the Pyramid approach to education model in a public school setting. In J. S. Handleman & S. L. Harris (Eds.), *School-age education programs for children with autism* (pp. 163–194). Austin, TX: Pro-Ed.

Becker-Cottrill, B., McFarland, J., & Anderson, V. (2003). A model of positive behavioral support for individuals with autism and their families: the family focus process. *Focus on Autism and Other Developmental Disabilities, 18,* 113–123.

Boettcher, M., Koegel, R. L., McNerney, E. K., & Koegel, L. K. (2003). A family-centered prevention approach to PBS in a time of crisis. *Journal of Positive Behavior Interventions, 5,* 55–59.

Bondy, A. S., & Frost, L. A. (2001). The Picture Exchange Communication System. *Behavior Modification, 25*(5), 725–744.

Bondy, A. S., & Sulzer-Azaroff, B. (2000). *The pyramid approach to education.* Cherry Hill, NJ: PECS.

Bregman, J. D., Zager, D., & Gerdtz, J. (2005). Behavioral interventions. In F. R. Volkmar, R. Paul, A. Klin, & D. J. Cohen (Eds.), *Handbook of autism and pervasive developmental disorders* (3rd ed., pp. 897–924). Hoboken, NJ: Wiley.

Carr, D., & Felce, J. (2007). The effects of PECS teaching to Phase III on the communicative interactions between children with autism and their teachers. *J Autism Dev Disord, 37*(4), 724–737.

Carter, A. S., Davis, N. O., Klin, A., & Volkmar, F. R. (2005). Social development in autism. In F. R. Volkmar, R. Paul, A. Klin, & D. J. Cohen (Eds.), *Handbook of autism and pervasive developmental disorders* (3rd ed., pp. 312–334). Hoboken, NJ: Wiley.

Charlop-Christy, M. H., Carpenter, M., Le, L., LeBlanc, L. A., & Kellet, K. (2002). Using the Picture Exchange Communication System (PECS) with children with autism: assessment of PECS acquisition, speech, social-communicative behavior, and problem behavior. *Journal of Applied Behavior Analysis, 35*(3), 213–231.

Doehring, P. (2006). *Independent Peer Review of Behavior Plans for Students with Autism in a Specialized Public School Program.* Poster presented at the Association for Behavior Analysis Autism Conference, Atlanta, GA.

Doehring, P. (2008). *A Model for Regional Training and Service Delivery for Children with Autism.* Presentation at the International Meeting for Autism Research, London.

Doehring, P., Donnelly, L., Wagner, B., and Myers, K. (2007). *How Are Diagnosis and Cognitive Status Reported in Autism Intervention Studies Published in JABA?* Poster presentation at the Association for Behavior Analysis Conference, Boston.

Doehring, P., Reichow, B., and Volkmar, F. R. (2007). *Is it evidenced-based? How to evaluate claims of effectiveness for autism.* Paper presented at the International Association for Positive Behavior Support Conference, March, Boston, MA.

Frost, L. A., & Bondy, A. S. (2000). *The Picture Exchange Communication System training manual.* Cherry Hill, NJ: Pyramid Educational Consultants.

Ganz, J. B., & Simpson, R. L. (2004). Effects on communicative requesting and speech development of the Picture Exchange Communication System in children with characteristics of autism. *Journal of Autism and Developmental Disorders, 34*(4), 395–409.

Gotham, K., Risi, S., Pickles, A., & Lord, C. (2007). The Autism Diagnostic Observation Schedule: revised algorithms for improved diagnostic validity. *Journal of Autism and Developmental Disorders, 37*, 613–627.

Gresham, F. M., & MacMillan, D. L. (1998). Early intervention project: can its claims be substantiated and its effects replicated? *Journal of Autism and Developmental Disorders, 28*, 5–13.

Harris, S. L. (2000). Age and IQ at intake as predictors of placement for young children with autism: A four- to six-year follow-up. Journal of Autism & *Developmental Disorders, 30*(2), 137-142.

Harris, S. L., & Handleman, J. S. (2000). Age and IQ at intake as predictors of placement for young children with autism: a four- to six-year follow-up. *Journal of Autism and Developmental Disabilities, 30*, 137–141.

Howlin, P., Gordon, R., Pasco, G., Wade, A., & Charman, T. (2007). The effectiveness of Picture Exchange Communication System (PECS) training for teachers of children with autism: a pragmatic, group randomized controlled trial. *Journal of Child Psychology and Psychiatry, 48*, 473–481.

Kaufman, B. N. (1982). *A miracle to believe in*. New York, NY: Fawcett-Crest.

Kaufman, B. N. (1994). *Son-rise: the miracle continues*. Tiburon, CA: Kramer.

Kravits, T. R., Kamps, D. M., Kemmerer, K., & Potucek, J. (2002). Brief report: increasing communication skills for an elementary-aged student with autism using the Picture Exchange Communication System. *Journal of Autism and Developmental Disorders, 32*(3), 225–230.

Kwak, M. M., Ervin, R. A., Anderson, M. Z., & Austin, J. (2004). Agreement of function across methods used in school-based functional assessment with preadolescent and adolescent students. *Behavior Modification, 28*, 375–401.

Lord, C., Risi, S., Lambrecht, L., Cook, E., & Leventhal, B. L. (2000). The Autism Diagnostic Observation Schedule–Generic: a standard measure of social and communication deficits associated with the spectrum of autism. *Journal of Autism and Developmental Disorders, 30*, 205–223.

Lord, C., Rutter, M., & Le Couteur, A. (1994). Autism Diagnostic Interview – revised: a revised version of a diagnostic interview for caregivers of individuals with possible pervasive developmental disorders. *Journal of Autism and Developmental Disorders, 24*(5), 659–685.

Magiati, I., & Howlin, P. (2003). A pilot evaluation study of the Picture Exchange Communication System for children with autistic spectrum disorders. *Autism, 7*, 297–320.

Mandell, D.S. (2009). *A randomized trial of the STAR program for children with autism spectrum disorder*. [Funded] National Institute of Mental Health. 5R01MH083717-02.

Mandell, D. S., Cao, J., Ittenbach, R., & Pinto-Martin, J. (2006). Medicaid expenditures for children with autistic spectrum disorders: 1994 to 1999. *Journal of Autism and Developmental Disorders, 36*, 475–485.

Mandell, D. S., Ittenbach, R. F., Levy, S. E., & Pinto-Martin, J. A. (2007). Disparities in diagnoses received prior to a diagnosis of autism spectrum disorder. *Journal of Autism and Developmental Disorders, 37*, 1795–1802.

Mandell, D. S., Listerud, J., Levy, S. E., & Pinto-Martin, J. A. (2002). Race differences in the age at diagnosis among medicaid-eligible children with autism. *Journal of the American Academy of Child and Adolescent Psychiatry, 41*, 1447–1453.

Marckel, J. M., Neef, N. A., & Ferreri, S. J. (2006). A preliminary analysis of teaching improvisation with the picture exchange communication system to children with autism. *Journal of Applied Behavior Analysis, 39*, 109–115.

National Autism Center. (2009). *The National Standards Project: addressing the need for evidence based practice guidelines for autism spectrum disorders*. Randolph, MA: National Autism Center.

National Center for Education Evaluation and Regional Assistance (2003) *Identifying and implementing educational practices supported by rigorous evidence: A user friendly guide*. U.S. Department of Education, Institute of Education Sciences.

National Research Council. (2001). *Educating children with autism*. Washington, DC: National Academy Press.

New York State Department of Health (1999) *Clinical practice guideline: Report of the recommendations. Autism/pervasive developmental disorders, assessment and intervention for young children (0–3 years)*. Albany, NY.

Palmer, R. F., Blanchard, S., Jean, C. R., & Mandell, D. S. (2005). School district resources and identification of children with autistic disorder. *American Journal of Public Health, 95*, 125–130.

Piven, J., & Palmer, P. (1999). Psychiatric disorder and the broad autism phenotype: evidence from a family study of multiple-incidence autism families. *The American Journal of Psychiatry, 156*, 557–563.

Public Law 107–110, § 115 Stat. 1425 (2002) No Child Left Behind Act of 2001.

Public Law 109–416 (2006) Combating Autism Act.

Reichow, B., Volkmar, F. R., & Cicchetti, D. V. (2008). Development of an evaluative method for determining the strength of research evidence in autism. *Journal of Autism and Developmental Disorders, 38*, 1311–1319.

Schopler, E. (1987). Specific and nonspecific factors in the effectiveness of a treatment system. *The American Psychologist, 42*, 376–383.

Schopler, E., Short, A., & Mesibov, G. (1987). Relation of behavioral treatment to "normal function": comment on Lovaas. *Journal of Consulting and Clinical Psychology, 57*, 162–164.

Shattuck, P. T., Durkin, M., Maenner, M., Newschaffer, C., Mandell, D. S., et al. (2009). Timing of identification among children with an autism spectrum disorder: findings from a population-based surveillance study. *Journal of the American Academy of Child and Adolescent Psychiatry, 48*, 474–483.

Smith, T., Eikeseth, S., Klevstrand, M., & Lovaas, O. I. (1997). Intensive behavioral treatment for preschoolers with severe mental retardation and pervasive developmental disorder. *American Journal of Mental Retardation, 102*, 238–249.

Stahmer, A. C., & Mandell, D. S. (2007). State infant/toddler program policies for eligibility and services provision for young children with autism. *Administration and Policy in Mental Health and Mental Health Services Research, 34*, 29–37.

Tincani, M. (2004). Comparing the Picture Exchange Communication System and sign language training for children with autism. *Focus on Autism and Other Developmental Disabilities, 19*(3), 152–163.

U. S. Government Accountability Office (2009). *Seclusions and Restraints: Selected cases of death and abuse at public and private schools and treatment centers.* Rep. No. GAO-09-719T.

Wallis, C. (2009). A powerful identity, a vanishing diagnosis. *New York Times*, November 3.

Wang, K., Zhang, H. T., Ma, D. Q., Bucan, M., Glessner, J. T., et al. (2009). Common genetic variants on 5p14.1 associate with autism spectrum disorders. *Nature, 459*, 528–533.

Yoder, P., & Stone, W. (2006a). A randomized comparison of the effect of two prelinguistic communication interventions on the acquisition of spoken communication in preschoolers with ASD. *Journal of Speech, Language, and Hearing Research, 49*, 698–711.

Yoder, P., & Stone, W. (2006b). Randomized comparison of two communication interventions for preschoolers with autism spectrum disorders. *Journal of Consulting and Clinical Psychology, 74*(3), 426–435.

Evidence-Based Practices in Autism: Where We Are Now and Where We Need to Go

Fred R. Volkmar, Brian Reichow, and Peter Doehring

ABBREVIATIONS

ABA	Applied behavior analysis
ADI-R	Autism diagnostic interview – revised
ADOS	Autism diagnostic observation schedule
ADOS-T	Autism diagnostic observation schedule – Toddler
ASDs	Autism spectrum disorders
CARS	Childhood Autism Rating Scale
d	Cohen's d
DSM-IV	Diagnostic and Statistical Manual of Mental Disorders 4th edition
EBM	Evidence-based medicine
EBP	Evidence-based practice
EBT	Evidence-based treatment
EIBI	Early intensive behavioral intervention
FDA	Food and Drug Administration
fMRI	Functional magnetic resonance image
ICD-10	International Classification of Diseases and Related Health Problems *10th edition*
IDEA	Individuals with Disabilities Education Act
IEP	Individualized Education Program
N of 1	Individual trial
OCD	Obsessive–compulsive disorder
OT	Occupational therapy
PDD	Pervasive developmental disorder
PECS	Picture Exchange Communication System
PRT	Pivotal response treatment
PT	Physical therapy
RCT	Randomized control trial
RUPP	Research Units on Pediatric Psychopharmacology
SCERTS	Social communication emotional regulation, transactional support
SSED	Single Subject Experimental Design
SSRI	Selective serotonin reuptake inhibitor

B. Reichow et al. (eds.), *Evidence-Based Practices and Treatments for Children with Autism*,
DOI 10.1007/978-1-4419-6975-0_14, © Springer Science+Business Media, LLC 2011

TEACCH   Treatment and Education of
         Autistic and Related Com-
         munication Handicapped
         Children

WHERE WE ARE NOW

As shown in Chap. 1 (see Fig. 14.1 and Volkmar in press), publication on autism has increased significantly in recent years. We undertook additional analyses to determine whether this increase reflected greater interest in autism more generally or included a specific interest in autism treatments. We conducted a literature search of the terms "autism" and "autism and treatment" for the years 1990–2008. Unlike the search described in Chap. 1, which relied on the Medline database, the search described here relied on the Ovid PsycINFO database, which we felt would capture the full range of publications related to treatment. Differences and recommendations for using different databases are discussed in an appendix to this chapter. When conducting the searches, two filters were used; the "all journals" filter limited results to articles published in journals and the "year" filter limited returns to each specific year. The number of articles about "autism" and those specifically about "autism treatments" published in a journal between 1990 and 2008 (the most recent year with complete data) is shown in Fig. 14.1.

These analyses reveal a relatively flat trend in the number of publications in journals between 1990 and 1997 – about 200 per year, followed by a dramatic increase in publications from 1998 (357) to nearly 1,300 in 2008. The increase in the rate of publication has been greater than three-fold since 1998 and fivefold since 1990. These increases likely reflect the increased awareness and interest in autism. With the increasing number of journals devoted to

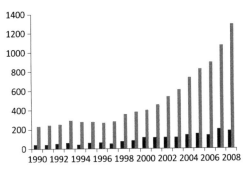

FIGURE 14.1

Articles on treatment in autism (black bars) and all articles on autism (gray bars) in the Ovid PsycINFO database, by year

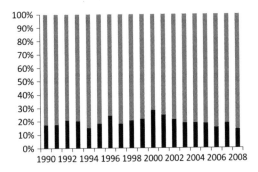

FIGURE 14.2

Proportion of autism treatment articles (dark region) to the total number of articles on autism on the Ovid PsycINFO database, by year

autism, the increasing trend in the absolute number of publications on autism is likely to continue, if not accelerate further.

A similar, albeit smaller, increase is also seen in the number of publications on autism treatments (see Fig. 14.2). Examination of the proportion of treatment studies to total studies reveals two trends over the last 2 decades. From 1990 to 2000, the proportion of articles addressing treatment increased, reaching a peak of 28% in the year 2000. The proportion of articles addressing treatment then decreased from 2000 to 2008. Fewer than 14% of articles published in 2008 focused on treatment research, which represents a reduction of over 50%. This decreasing trend is somewhat perplexing in the light of the increasing interest in early intervention since the publication of the National Research Council (2001). Regardless of the cause, the increasing number of individuals being diagnosed with autism merits greater attention on how to best serve these individuals so that they can live meaningful lives, which will best be accomplished by increasing, not decreasing, treatment research.

TREATMENT RESEARCH AND EVALUATION

Comprehensive Programs

Comprehensive Behavioral Programs. The results emerging from comprehensive programs based on the technologies of ABA (Lovaas 1987) sparked a revolution in the focus and number of early intervention programs and a new interest in the potential of outcome research to shape practice and policy. Of the ten comprehensive early intervention models outlined by the National Research Council (2001), the majority had a behavioral orientation, including many that constitute a class of interventions commonly referred to as "early intensive behavioral intervention" (EIBI). Traditionally, EIBI has involved upwards of 40 h/week of therapy, much of which is delivered in a 1:1 discrete trial format, especially during the first stages of intervention. Recent meta-analyses (Eldevik et al. 2009; Reichow and Wolery 2009) suggest EIBI can be a very effective treatment option for many children with autism. Although EIBI and other behavioral intervention approaches are often presented as if each is a distinct program, there is in fact considerable overlap in the methods, curricula, and mechanisms of program delivery. Capturing the differences that exist will require better measures

of treatment and procedural fidelity for comprehensive behavioral programs, especially measuring the relative usage and dosage of component parts. Until the active components (i.e., aspects of treatment responsible for positive outcomes) can be specified, we cannot determine whether the slight differences in program orientation have a meaningful impact.

Comprehensive Developmental and Eclectic Programs. In addition to the more strictly behaviorally focused programs, several other programs are based more explicitly on developmental theory or are more eclectic – they draw from a range of methods and procedures. As with the more behaviorally oriented approaches, the research basis for these more developmentally oriented treatments is highly variable and these programs have focused on younger children. As noted by the National Research Council (2001) and in this book (Chap. 13), regardless of theoretical orientation, there are a number of non-specific intervention variables that are common to many programs (e.g., the need for planned, structured intervention, careful attention to issues of support and generalization of skills, need for trained staff) that might in fact contribute significantly to outcomes. It is exciting, however, to speculate regarding the potential match between the orientation and methods of a given program and the child's learning style. As with the behaviorally oriented programs, the developmentally based and eclectic programs have also undergone a number of changes over the years and have evolved from more segregated and center-based service programs to more inclusive settings. It is also interesting to note how many of the more behaviorally focused programs have increasingly sought to include a more developmental perspective.

One example of a developmental approach is the Denver Model, begun in 1981 by Sally Rogers (Rogers and Lewis 1988; Rogers et al. 2000; Rogers and Dawson 2010). The program addresses core difficulties in the areas of social interaction (imitation, perception of affect, and so forth) within a strongly developmental framework, using a range of developmentally appropriate activities to foster and build communication and social skills. The program has evolved over time with an increasing focus on treating children in inclusive settings. A body of work on this approach has now appeared, which is nicely summarized in the recently published manual of the early start Denver Model (Rogers and Dawson 2010).

Two other developmentally oriented programs have been described and are widely used in practice, although though these have little or no empirical support to date. The developmental, individual-difference, relationship-based (DIR) model (Floortime) model emphasizes building relationships and seeks to improve overall social engagement, reciprocal interaction, self-regulation, and attention (Greenspan and Wieder 2009). Some supportive research is available but, to our knowledge, no controlled studies exist. The social communication, emotional regulation, transactional support (SCERTS) approach (Prizant et al. 2004) has emerged more recently and focuses on fostering social–communication skills while also addressing behaviors that may interfere with learning and social interaction. Despite considerable interest in this program, it has yet to establish a base of empirical support.

Of the various eclectic programs, the Treatment and Education of Autistic and related Communication Handicapped Children (TEACCH) Program at the University of North Carolina (Mesibov et al. 2005; Schopler 1997) has probably received the most recognition. Begun in 1972 under the leadership of Eric Schopler, this program includes various centers around North Carolina as well as special classrooms within public schools. TEACCH also provides consultation across North Carolina and training across the United States, Canada, and Europe. There is much emphasis on supporting learning, fostering communication, and increasing independence. Although studies on aspects of the TEACCH model are beginning to emerge, there is, to our knowledge, no well-controlled experimental study of outcomes associated with the TEACCH model.

Future Directions for Comprehensive Programs. Outside of EIBI, few large-scale trials have been conducted on the other approaches in the National Research Council (2001). Although many of these programs have rich empirical histories using different methodologies, validation in larger trials will help advance the field and are needed before comparisons of treatments can be made. The National Research Council (2001) concluded, "There [was] no outcome study published in a peer-reviewed journal that supports comparative statements of the superiority of one model or approach or another" (National Research Council 2001, p. 166). Ten years later, a similar conclusion would likely be reached.

The comparison of comprehensive programs with manualized treatment protocols (e.g., EIBI) to broadly defined eclectic models is particularly problematic. While an eclectic model might be considered a proxy for treatment as usual, it may be impossible to control for diffusion of treatment components (i.e., inclusion of some parts of the manualized treatment). With the lack of standardization in the eclectic model, it may also be impossible to determine if effects favoring the manualized treatment procedure might reflect improved consistency across treatment providers rather than effects more specific to the intervention. Until better measures of treatment fidelity are developed, eclectic classrooms (programs) should not be used as comparison groups in research studies.

One major problem facing schools and parents is the question of matching treatment models to the specific child and circumstance, and the choice of which approach or curricula to use (Arick et al. 2005; Olley 2005). The dearth of comparative treatment studies also complicates the issue of treatment assignment: typically, comparisons are made before and after treatment in one intervention or between "treated" and "untreated" groups. Particularly for the more complex treatment models, disentangling which aspects of the treatment/curriculum are most important will remain very challenging. After studies demonstrating the efficacy of specific models have been conducted, work on a priori predictions about treatment effects (e.g., for a given child, does one treatment work better than another) should proceed. Work on exploring child characteristics that might predict treatment response has already begun for focal interventions. The work of Yoder and Stone (2006a, b) has produced insights into the potential to tailor treatment to individuals with specific characteristics; for example, children who have high levels of initiations might do better in a milieu intervention than with an intervention based on the Picture Exchange Communication System (PECS). Work such as this with larger treatment packages would be highly beneficial and could help ensure children begin receiving the most appropriate and effective treatments as early as possible.

Social–Communication Interventions

EBPs for social–communicative dysfunction remain, in many respects, one of the most interesting and challenging areas of intervention in autism and related disorders. Since Kanner's original definition (Kanner 1943), social difficulties have been identified repeatedly (Siegel et al. 1989; Volkmar et al. 1994) as the single most robust predictor of autism and are, accordingly, more heavily weighted in the diagnostic

algorithms of the current *Diagnostic and Statistical Manual of Mental Disorders* (DSM-IV; APA 1994) and the *International Classification of Diseases and Related Health Problems* (ICD-10; World Health Organization 1992). Over the last several decades, a number of different interventions have been proposed and research has proceeded, albeit somewhat inconsistently, on these approaches with a notable upsurge of research in the last decade (Matson et al. 2007; Reichow and Volkmar 2010a).

The review of social skills interventions presented in Chap. 6 reveals that social interventions vary in many important ways including the age and developmental level of the target population, the focus of the intervention (narrow or broad), and the agent of change. Although earlier efforts in the field involved adult-directed teaching, with demonstrated effectiveness, researchers have begun to pay more careful attention to the ecology of children's social interactions in natural settings, resulting in an increased emphasis on social interactions with peers, where indeed the bulk of research has been conducted (National Research Council 2001). This emphasis on peers is consistent with a broader, ecologically organized approach focused on generalization of skills to natural and "real-world" situations (Rogers and Ozonoff 2005b) and is notably lacking in many of the adult-led, social intervention programs.

Probably the largest body of work on more general approaches to teaching social skills has emerged from the work on peer-mediated interaction (Rogers and Ozonoff 2005b). A variety of methods have been used, such as relying on children with typical development with some (minimal) training to support social interaction in children with autism and related disorders (Goldstein et al. 1992; Strain and Schwartz 2001); using role play and explicit teaching of play scripts (Goldstein et al. 1988); peer tutoring (Dugan et al. 1995); and teaching peers a pivotal response approach (Pierce and Schreibman 1997). Peer preparation can take the form of adult instruction or role play prior to exposure to the child with an ASD and peers are specifically reinforced by adults for their efforts. Several important areas of research remain to be fully addressed, including issues of exposure, consistency, and generalization, as well as the broader implications for mainstreaming (Handleman et al. 2005; Strain and Hoyson 2000).

Despite the tremendous need for more effective treatments to help adolescents with ASD (Paul 2003; Saulnier and Klin 2007), there is much less research than is available regarding younger children (Reichow and Volkmar 2010a). With the tremendous pace of social development among typical adolescents, the social impairments of adolescents and adults with autism become increasingly apparent (Klin et al. 2007) and can easily lead to social isolation, teasing, bullying, and diverse unfortunate situations (Montes and Halterman 2007). The range of approaches utilized has become increasingly sophisticated in terms of teaching strategies and materials (Volkmar and Wiesner 2009). Whereas more traditional, direct instruction disrupts the natural flow of social interaction, supports such as visual cues, visual schedules, and other minimally obtrusive strategies can be embedded more naturally and promote greater independence (Rogers and Ozonoff 2005b).

Social skills groups remain one of the most common formats for social teaching, especially among adolescents and adults. These groups make use of a range of techniques including explicit teaching, role playing, and review of social interactions (e.g., through videotape), and may include homework assigned outside the group itself (Krasny et al. 2003; Paul 2003). Unfortunately, controlled studies have been relatively uncommon and most research has relied on weaker pre/post designs. In

general, it appears that while some gains are made, these are relatively minimal (Reichow and Volkmar 2010b), especially in light of the large gap between the skill levels of the typically developing school-aged child and that of the child with autism (Rogers and Ozonoff 2005b).

In sum, much progress has been made in the area of social skills intervention and such interventions remain extremely popular among educators and parents alike. However, the effects observed tend to be relatively modest and much of the available research suffers from serious shortcomings. We recommend that future research encompass better methodological controls, include better measures of outcome (including both short- and long-term outcomes), and begin to address the needs of adolescents and adults. Social skills clearly remain a critically important "target area" for early intervention given their relevance to later learning and self-organization and generalization but better metrics and more precise measures of general social orientation will be needed to advance our understanding of the changes that occur during social skills interventions (Saulnier and Klin 2007).

Communication Interventions

Kanner (1943) noted a broad range of communication impairments in his original sample; some children did not talk at all, while others talked but in very odd ways, with echoed language, unusual pitch or prosody, pronoun reversal, idiosyncratic language, and specific impairments in the use (pragmatics) of language. Since Kanner's report, research has sought to better characterize and remediate these language-communication problems, as described in Chap. 5.

For younger children, the majority of intervention studies have employed a behavioral approach to teaching and enhancing communication skills. As with social skills interventions, various methods have been employed with the aim of encouraging specific behaviors and developing new (communicative) behaviors and a very considerable body of research has demonstrated the clear utility and effectiveness of behavioral approaches in improving communication in preverbal children with autism. Work in this area has also become more sophisticated in the use of various techniques to shape desired behaviors and build on skills in a systematic way. It appears that with earlier and focused interventions, more children with autism are now able to acquire speech, and that a host of social language functions can also be explicitly taught (Roger and Ozonoff 2005b).

For children who are nonverbal, the use of several other communication systems has also been evaluated, including PECS (Bondy and Frost 2001) and the verbal behavior approach (Sundberg and Michael 2001). Both of these behaviorally-based approaches seek to capitalize on the sources of reinforcement in which successful communication results: the former uses pictures to exploit the often intact visual recognition skills and relies on behavioral teaching strategies to shape the "exchange" implicit to all successful communication, while the latter emphasizes the use or words or sign language to teach the full range of communicative functions across a variety of contexts. Both have some support in the literature. More developmentally based approaches to teaching communication skills, such as the SCERTS model (Wetherby et al. 2000), emphasize the centrality and integration of social-communicative and social-affective behaviors (Prizant et al. 2004). Outcome research using this developmental approach has, unfortunately, been somewhat limited, despite the rich research literature documenting the specific social-communicative deficits targeted by the developmental approach.

A persistent concern on the part of parents is that augmentative approaches might actually delay the development of spoken language. Several studies suggest that children using augmentative systems can and do acquire speech (Charlop-Christy et al. 2002). However, more research in this area is clearly needed particularly since one of the better studies in the area (Yoder and Layton 1988) did not show a clear advantage in speech acquisition when a sign language system was used. This debate highlights differences in the fundamental assumptions between clinicians adopting a developmental versus a behavioral approach: the former assumes that basic social-communication skills such as imitation, eye contact, and joint attention must be prerequisites for language development and the latter assumes that communication skills can be taught as long as the environmental contingencies and sources of reinforcement are well understood.

Focal Behavioral Treatments

In addition to the growing body of evidence on EIBI for young children with autism, there is a long tradition of using focal behavioral techniques in the education and treatment of individuals with autism (see Chap. 4 and the work of Odom et al. [2003]). This tradition has yielded considerable research and many such treatments can now be considered evidence-based, following rubrics for evaluating the quality of outcome research that recognize the values of SSEDs (such as the rubric described in Chap. 2). An advantage of the reliance on SSEDs is that many of these treatments have been studied in real-world settings being delivered by "everyday" practitioners. Hundreds of SSED studies have been published on focal interventions for addressing a wide range of behaviors, from increasing existing skills (or teaching new ones) to decreasing problematic, harmful, or undesirable behaviors. Behavioral interventions have been and remain the most evidence-based treatment options for individuals with autism.

While it is gratifying that so many applications of ABA have been shown to be effective, at the same time it can be a bit overwhelming and it might not always be clear to practitioners when to use a specific technique. The vigorous debate around comprehensive behavioral programs such as EIBI, has at times overshadowed discussion of the merits of focal behavioral techniques, for which there is often a much more convincing empirical basis. Developing a concise, user-friendly system that assists service providers in making these choices would be very helpful.

Psychopharmacology

As described in Chap. 8, there have been important developments in the pharmacological treatment of the pervasive developmental disorders (PDDs). A range of medications have now been evaluated, although the research literature remains, at best, spotty, with the evaluation of apparently ineffective agents (e.g., secretin) having received much more attention than others (Levy and Hyman 2005). Unfortunately, pharmacological trials have, with a few notable exceptions, suffered from various weaknesses including small sample sizes (with attendant power issues), problems in research design, and a dearth of good dependent measures for assessment of change. As noted elsewhere in this book, some of the problems generic to autism (e.g., the tremendous range in severity of associated intellectual disability, social–communication handicap, and behavior) all pose significant obstacles for studies of pharmacological intervention. The complex problem of comorbidity with other psychiatric conditions (problems with attention, anxiety, and mood, among others) poses other, albeit potentially

intertwined, challenges. Despite these problems, a body of evidence has emerged relative to some agents, e.g., risperidone, some of the selective serotonin reuptake inhibitors (SSRIs) (fluoxetine and citalopram, in particular), and, to a lesser extent, methylphenidate (Mandell et al. 2008).

Of these various agents, the SSRIs are almost certainly the most frequently used (Oswald and Sonenklar 2007; Mandell et al. 2008). As reviewed in Chap. 8, a major rationale for the extensive use of these agents is the apparent behavior overlap, in part, of the rigidity frequently exhibited by children with pervasive developmental disorders (PDDs) and similar appearing phenomena in obsessive–compulsive disorder (OCD). Several of these agents have been approved for the treatment of the latter condition in children. The first studies of these agents in individuals with autism and related conditions suggested some age-related differences in response as well as frequent adverse reactions. Subsequent work has, unfortunately, been disappointing, with several large trials using different agents failing to show benefit (King et al. 2009). Although various issues (sample size, issues of design and measures use) always complicate the interpretation of negative results, as a group the studies have not supported the effectiveness of SSRIs for treatment of repetitive behavior in children with PDDs and, indeed, raise a question about whether the apparently similarly repetitive behaviors may, in fact, result from different processes.

In contrast, the results of studies of the newer atypical antipsychotic risperidone have been much more positive, resulting in significant decreases in a range of maladaptive behaviors (RUPP 2002). This work is built on the large body of research conducted at New York University in the 1970s and 1980s on the effects of the first-generation neuroleptics (Campbell et al. 1982). The positive results of this study led to its formal approval by the FDA for use in children with autism and subsequent work has focused on combinations of this agent with a manualized parent training (Aman et al. 2009; Scahill et al. 2009). While underscoring the importance of examining behavior and pharmacological treatments in combination, the benefit of adding a parent-training component also highlights the importance of having a plan for the development of desired behaviors that can be implemented as maladaptive behaviors decrease.

Pharmacological treatment studies have faced other challenges. Some of the most influential studies have been multi-site collaborations developed through innovative federal grant initiatives. Notwithstanding the difficulties that all treatment studies – and particularly drug treatment studies – face in funding, it is important that this model be continued. Issues of comorbidity and best approaches to conceptualizing it continue to pose general problems. Work with SSRIs has shown that superficially similar behavioral features do not always represent similar underlying phenomena. Greater understanding of basic aspects of pathophysiology, e.g., through genetic mechanisms, may significantly advance drug development (Volkmar et al. 2009) and research in this area may be increasingly important in years to come. The marriage of behavioral and pharmacological treatments is just beginning to emerge as an area of work in its own right and constitutes a critically important area for future research endeavors given the demonstrated effectiveness of behavioral methods in reducing many problem behaviors.

The Gap Between Research and Practice

Although research and our knowledge of effective treatments for autism are increasing, a significant gap remains between what is known from research studies and what is done in real-life settings (Chorpita 2003; Kazdin 2001). To help close the gap between research and practice, information coming from the research end must be made more relevant to practitioners and consumers (Hawley and Weisz 2002). Practitioners must also increase their knowledge of current methods of EBP; recent surveys suggest that the use (Nelson and Steele 2007) and knowledge (Pagoto et al. 2007) of EBP by common practitioners is low. Moreover, practitioners often feel that implementing EBP might not fit into the day-to-day reality of practice (Kratochwill and Stoiber 2002). Without a link between research and practice, defining EBP does little good since there is no exchange of information from the people in possession of the knowledge (i.e., the researchers) and the individuals who are on the front line treating the patients, clients, or students (i.e., the practitioners) (Barkham and Mellor-Clark 2003; Chorpita 2003). In order to close the research–practice gap, we must learn why traditional methods have been ineffective in transferring knowledge from research to practice and discover new and innovative methods that work (Hamilton 2007; Kennedy et al. 2004).

The limited access to research information – the second step in the model of EBM described in Chap. 1 – clearly contributes to the research–practice gap. Practitioners must be able to obtain the research if they are to evaluate the quality of research reports, learn about innovative EBPs, and participate in the EBP process. However, it is likely that many practitioners rely on antiquated and less than optimal methods for obtaining evidence regarding established treatment techniques (e.g., asking colleagues or referring to outdated textbooks) (Hatcher et al. 2005; Upton and Upton 2006). Practitioners must shift from a reliance on these antiquated methods to newer and more effective methods, such as searches of electronic databases accessed via the Internet (see the appendix).

Complicating this situation in the case of autism is the fact that many professionals working with children who have ASD do not complete courses or certificates specific to ASDs, nor does their training always include the depth of understanding in research design needed to recognize EBP. Because children with autism present such a variety of symptoms and behaviors, practitioners must be trained in a wide variety of methods and theoretical backgrounds (Chap. 12; Lerman et al. 2004; National Research Council 2001). Thus, most professionals lack training in even the most basic and most common intervention techniques (Cascella and Colella 2004; National Research Council 2001) and many believe that they are using treatments that are evidence-based when, in fact, they are not (Stahmer et al. 2005). The lack of knowledge of standard intervention techniques makes dissemination of EBP difficult and is likely one cause of the continued use of a large number of treatments used in schools and other community-based settings that are not evidence-based (Hess et al. 2008; Stahmer et al. 2005). This clearly illustrates research is not fully informing practice. To the extent that implementation of EBM in health care is a guide, several factors may help facilitate the process (Hamilton 2007). These include ready access of key personnel to development of guidelines and procedures, participation of individuals at all levels of the organization, and having "buy in" from all relevant staff. Participation of key staff and respect for the various disciplinary perspectives is critical (Ferlie 2005), as is an active program of education and training. Finally, various methods may be used to encourage participation in the implementation process.

The wide range of methods for delivering services poses other problems to outcome researchers. For example, much autism treatment – and, to a lesser extent,

research – is interdisciplinary, potentially involving psychologists, speech-language pathologists, occupational and physical therapists, physicians, general education teachers, special education teachers, and others. These disciplines speak different languages, have different research traditions, and bring their own unique perspectives to this population. The efficacy–effectiveness gap so commonly found in studies of psychotherapeutic interventions (Weisz and Jensen 1999) is further widened in autism because interventions can take place in a wide range of settings, from the clinic to the school and the home.

The extent to which intervention must be individualized will also make it hard to close the research–practice gap. Scheuermann et al. (2003) emphasized the importance of considering the unique learning style of each individual when deciding what treatment to begin with a child. Interventions addressing the behavioral characteristics of one child might not work for a different child; in research studies, it has not been uncommon for at least one participant to make no progress or even to regress on at least one outcome variable even when receiving a high-quality treatment delivered with good fidelity. With a broad, specialized training in autism techniques, practitioners who work with individuals with autism will be more able to individualize instruction for each child by considering the array of specific techniques as a toolkit from which they can draw according the needs of a particular child. To help close the research–practice gap, once treatments are identified as EBP, it is important that practitioner training programs include information on these techniques. Additionally, this training needs to emphasize the uses and limitations of EBP, especially with respect to balancing the needs of an individual child relative to proven treatments and his or her profile of strengths and weakness.

WHERE WE NEED TO GO

Future Considerations and Challenges

Over the past decade, various streams of evidence-based practice (e.g., EBT, EBM) have begun to converge in the development of more rigorously empirically based treatments. Many of the advances reviewed in previous chapters of this book have begun to enter mainstream practice and to affect the lives of children and adolescents in school programs. Although many advances have been made, much remains to be done and the question of why progress has been slow is a very legitimate one.

The slow pace of progress can be attributed to several unique challenges related to the nature of ASD and the nature of EBP. For example, the expression of ASD is highly variable across age and development – e.g., treatments developed for a verbal 5-year-old may not be at all appropriate for a nonverbal 10-year-old. Review of the treatment literature readily confirms the variability in coverage, e.g., much of the work on social skills interventions using peers has been published using preschool samples while research on teaching adults social skills is much more limited. For some populations (e.g., infants at risk of autism), treatments are only now beginning to be developed. Moving past the relatively broad confines of autism, an entirely new set of issues arise for individuals with Asperger syndrome, where the combination of better verbal ability with limited social skills raises new problems (Klin et al. in press). The following sections highlight key areas of concern that need to be addressed to advance our knowledge of reducing the symptoms and improving the lives of individuals with autism.

Addressing deficits in generalization. An important and early realization was the critical need to generalize skills, which increased the interest in home and nonspecialist treatment settings, and in parents and non-professionals as interventionists. A series of studies have now supported this move while simultaneously noting some limitations of the approach. For example, parents and others can be taught to be effective teachers as long as some ongoing training and support is provided. It also appears that outcomes are highly correlated with initial language levels (e.g., children with at least some spoken language are more likely to respond). Gains also tend to be greatest early on and the rate of gain may decrease over time (Rogers and Ozonoff 2005b). Although Lovaas (1987) noted the importance of high, intensive levels of treatment for young children in the eventual attainment of useful expressive and receptive language skills, subsequent work has tempered this view (Smith et al. 2000).

A parallel shift has been the incorporation of more developmentally oriented and naturalistic principles into interventions that retain a strong behavioral focus. For example, some of the earliest work on pivotal response training (PRT) addressed issues of naturalistic approaches to fostering speech-communication development (Schreibman and Pierce 1993; Koegel and Koegel 1995, 2006), while other work has focused on the use of incidental teaching strategies (McGee et al. 1983) and the generalization of treatment to more naturalistic settings (Goldstein 2000; Koegel 2000). While originally developed in SSED studies, group approaches using these methods have also now appeared (McBride and Schwartz 2003). The issue of the relative merits of naturalistic techniques (i.e., relative to more traditional didactic teaching) has been more controversial (Rogers and Ozonoff 2005b) though, clearly, both approaches share many similarities.

Overall, as has been shown in this book, great strides have been made in intervention research. While some studies have employed methods to elicit and teach generalization of skills across settings and behaviors, this does not always occur (Reichow and Volkmar 2010a). To create more meaningful and beneficial interventions, research must continue to explore ways to get and maintain generalization.

Differences in treatment magnitude and clinical psychopathology. Another challenge for the field will be the continued refinement and development of more powerful and efficient treatments that result in more meaningful outcomes. As outlined previously, there are now many evidence-based treatments for children with autism. A treatment can be evidence-based, however, without yielding clinically significant results. Perhaps, relatively little emphasis is placed on clinical significance or the treatment might make relatively minor differences in the lives of those receiving it.

The potential difference between those outcomes that are statistically significant versus those that are truly meaningful becomes more evident when comparing the magnitude of the social deficit in autism to the magnitude of effect from one of the most common social skills interventions for individuals with autism – social skills groups. Work by Klin et al. (2002a, b) has shown that individuals with autism have major differences in social perception (see Fig. 14.3) when compared to individuals with typical development and individuals with developmental delays.

When the differences between individuals with autism and typical development are converted to an effect size, very large differences are seen (e.g., $d = 3.81$). In comparison, a review of social skills group interventions by Reichow and Volkmar (2010b) suggested the magnitude of gains in social competence after completing a social

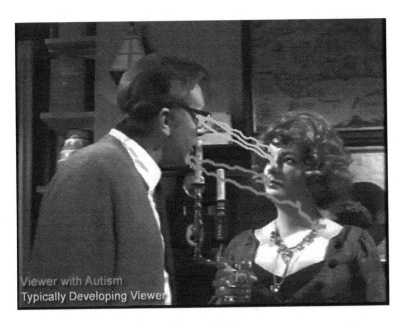

FIGURE 14.3

Visual focus of people shown a film clip of a conversation. The person with typical development (top line) focuses on the eyes in a social scene; a person with high-functioning autism focuses on the mouths of the speakers (Reprinted from Klin et al. 2002a. With permission)

skills group for individuals with autism was much smaller, with standardized mean change effect size estimates often being small (e.g., $d < .50$). Thus, the magnitude of effect for one of the most common (and thought to be one of the most effective) social interventions does not approach the magnitude of the deficits shown by individuals with autism. Clearly, interventions that are more powerful are needed.

Interventions for Infants and Toddlers

The age at which children are identified as having, or being at risk of having, autism continues to decrease, which may require adjustments to the design and the focus of outcome research. In some settings, it is now common for children under 1 year of age to be assessed (even though most of the standard screeners only become applicable no earlier than 16 months!). The ability of screening tools to help in the effective identification of young children, together with the strong endorsement of such measures by the American Academy of Pediatrics, will likely increase the number of infants and toddlers identified as at risk of ASD and the pressure to develop effective EBPs for this population. Much of the early work in this area has, understandably, focused on training parents to deliver therapies (Rogers and Dawson 2010); less work has been completed on center-based models. Although much work has been done on peer interventions for preschool-aged children with autism, infants and toddlers have very different social milieus and interact with peers in vastly different ways. Thus, novel techniques for utilizing peers in therapeutic settings for infants and toddlers with, or at risk of developing, autism are also needed. Continued research that refines these techniques and determines the most important target areas will be helpful.

Sensory Interventions

As summarized in Chap. 9 and in other reviews (Baranek et al. 2005; Rogers and Ozonoff 2005a), it is clear that the sensory dysfunction faced by many with autism is not being adequately treated and needs more sophisticated, effective, evidence-based approaches. Scholarly work on sensory dysfunction issues in autism has tended to focus on two, apparently contradictory, hypotheses – over arousal or under arousal (Rogers and Ozonoff 2005a). Although both theoretical views have been used in designing interventions, actual empirical support is, unfortunately, limited. Several different, but interrelated, issues are critical for advancing work in this area.

Obtaining a larger evidence pool for sensory interventions might require, at least in the short term, less attention to theories and interventions based upon broad and sweeping generalizations regarding sensory integration, which, to date, have lacked convincing empirical support. Research into the interrelationships of behaviors and relations of symptom clusters or patterns to key child variables (Baranek et al. 2006; Kern et al. 2007; Rogers and Ozonoff 2005a) could help facilitate treatment if shared approaches could be fostered, e.g., to facilitate interpretation of results, comparability of samples, and so forth. Clearly, for some more focused activities, good assessment instruments are presently available, e.g., for evaluation of visual–motor integration abilities (Baranek et al. 2005). Assessment of sensory-motor dysfunction is, however, much more limited. Few assessment instruments specific to the sensory-motor dysfunction in ASD have been developed and results obtained thus far using standard assessment instruments have been inconsistent (see Baranek et al. 2005). Although some attempts have been made to relate different patterns of sensory-motor dysfunction to the core social deficits in autism (Baranek et al. 1997a, b; Wing and

Gould 1979), these relations remain unclear. The methodological challenges associated with the assessment of other skills – e.g., the potential (if complex) role of age and developmental level, and the validity of parent report, observational data and self-report – are also evident in the assessment of sensory-motor skills. In order to assess accurately the effects of sensory interventions, better measures are greatly needed. Research involving very young infants at risk of autism may help clarify some aspects of the developmental course of these behaviors and suggest potential areas for future research, e.g., in relation to other areas of development or specific brain mechanisms.

Future research on sensory integrative therapies should also seek to identify the active components of the sensory therapy and to disentangle them from other behavioral or developmental therapies often delivered concurrently. As described in Chap. 9, sensory integration therapies seem to share much in common with other well-established treatment techniques (e.g., milieu teaching and incidental teaching): both techniques often involve preferred materials and play activities for children in a motivating, contextually relevant activity that together create high-quality learning opportunities. To move the field forward, research demonstrating the benefits of sensory integration above and beyond the therapies with which it is being delivered will be needed.

Research Methods

Because a majority of published intervention studies in autism utilize SSEDs (Reichow et al. 2007), the advantages of using SSEDs are worth further exploration. First, SSEDs typically involve the repeated measurement of baseline performance of an individual followed by measurement of the same variable during one or more interventions.

The repeated measurement may result in a more stable – and therefore more reliable and valid – estimate of performance and help to nullify the notorious variability in performance often seen in individuals with autism. Second, SSEDs (e.g., withdrawal design, alternating treatment design) that entail the measurement of multiple conditions (e.g., baseline and intervention) within the same individual allows the individual to serve as their own control, thus creating an experimental design that can be conducted using a very small sample (e.g., one child). Third, the documentation of improvements in skills or behaviors in an individual using such designs is much more transparent and compelling to parents and teachers than interpretations based on the statistical significance of group effects. Finally, the unit of measurement in an SSED is typically the behavior of the client (e.g., child with autism). Having the behavior in which the intervention is thought to change as the direct outcome measure helps ensure that the result of the EBP process is improvement that is clinically, and not just experimentally, significant.

The potential strength of SSEDs are recognized by some evidence hierarchies now assigning the highest rating to N of 1 randomized control trials (i.e., the performance of one individual in which sessions of intervention and placebo or control are randomized) (Guyatt et al. 2000). Two recent studies on the effects of weighted vests on the engagement of children with autism used an alternating treatment design in an N of 1 randomized control trial arrangement and failed to demonstrate any benefit of weighted vests over placebo or control conditions (Cox et al. 2009; Reichow et al. 2010). Although the results of these trials were somewhat noteworthy (see Chap. 9), the rigorous application of the N of 1 randomized design can serve as a model that researchers and practitioners should strive to use whenever possible.

Although SSEDs have advantages that need to be recognized, it should not be the only research methodology employed (Smith et al. (2007) discuss various research designs and their appropriateness for differing stages of research). Multisite trials, similar to those described in Chap. 8, should continue in psychopharmacology and can serve as a model for conducting such trials in other areas. Large-scale group design studies with adequate sample size and statistical power of common and established intervention models (e.g., EIBI, PRT, TEACCH) should be conducted. In comparing intervention models, efforts to uncover participant characteristics that predict successful outcomes should be a priority.

Regardless of the design chosen, other aspects of the nature of ASD pose important challenges when evaluating outcomes. The difficulties associated with studying highly selected samples becomes very problematic given the high potential for children with autism to exhibit other conditions, e.g., attention, mood, anxiety, or other problems. The apparent change, over time, in outcome emphasizes not only the importance of early intervention but also the need to consider previous treatments in selecting samples and interpreting results. Gender and minority issues in sample selection can be problematic, e.g., given how much less frequent autism is in girls, some studies have simply excluded such cases. Somewhat paradoxically, the large series of negative RCTs of secretin also emphasize the great potential contribution of nonspecific (placebo) effects in treatment studies (Hyman and Levy 2005; Sandler 2005; Shapiro 2000). Yet another issue arises relative to the frequent, but usually understudied and under reported, use of alternative treatments by parents (Green et al. 2006; Hanson et al. 2007).

Difficulties in evaluating the efficacy of an intervention are further complicated when multiple techniques are combined (e.g., video modeling and Social Stories or eclectic classrooms). While some combinations are methodologically complementary (e.g., video modeling and Social Stories) and theoretically compatible (because the hypothesized mechanisms of action are shared), other combinations involve interventions that unintentionally compete against or counteract one another. In either case, determining which intervention is producing the desired changes can be nearly impossible.

Although the research literature does not reflect widespread evaluations of combined treatments (i.e., few studies of combined techniques have been published), it is likely that combined techniques are much more common in real-life settings, where adherence to treatment protocol is generally lower than laboratory settings. As stated, parents often use multiple treatments simultaneously, including many treatments with little or no empirical support (Green et al. 2006; Hanson et al. 2007). In the studies that have evaluated combined treatments, some have produced favorable, although at times inconsistent, results (Sansosti and Powell-Smith 2008; Scattone 2008; Thiemann and Goldstein 2004). However, statements about the efficacy of the treatment components or parts cannot be made; i.e., conclusions can only be drawn about the relative effects of the combined approach.

Although advanced statistical techniques may help to factor out possible contributions of multiple treatments in group research studies, large samples, which have to this point been relatively uncommon in autism research, would be needed. To learn the true effects of the intervention parts (i.e., video modeling or Social Stories), component analyses using SSEDs may be a cost-effective method of evaluation. Properly designed and conducted SSEDs can help to establish the relative efficiency of each procedure alone and in combination, thus guiding the allocation of resources to individualized treatment.

Outcome Measures

The focus on infants and toddlers at risk of ASD will also increase the interest in changes in diagnostic status or overall symptom severity as outcomes. If, as expected, intervening at such a young age might slow or even reverse the "effects" of autism and shift their developmental trajectory to more closely resemble that of a child with typical development, then such "optimal" outcomes might be expected. In order to determine this, better outcome measures are needed. Diagnostic tools such as the Autism Diagnostic Observation Schedule (ADOS; Lord et al. 1999), the Autism Diagnostic Interview – Revised (ADI-R; Rutter et al. 2005), and the Childhood Autism Rating Scale (CARS; Schopler et al. 1986) were not designed as outcome measures and it is not clear how they perform as such. Additionally, downward extensions of these measures are necessary to diagnose participants for inclusion (e.g., ADOS-Toddler; Lord et al. 2008) and measures of unquestioned validity will be needed if claims of the amelioration of autistic symptomatology are to be made, which in the past has been shown to create quite a furor (Lovaas 1987). It will be challenging to obtain accurate estimates of the effect of such interventions on specific skills because children with autism are difficult to accurately assess with standardized testing procedures (Wolery and Garfinkle 2002) and this difficulty will be increased in studies of infants and toddlers. When measuring an outcome of recovery or amelioration of autism symptomatology, assessors who are blind to study inclusion, study purpose, and treatment group should be used and confirmed by observation of the child interacting with their environment in a typical manner by another equally blind observer (e.g., having an assessor observe a child's classroom without knowing the child's identity and select which child in the classroom has autism).

The development of better dependent measures in studies of psychopharmacological interventions is another high priority. Although some improvements have been made in ratings scales and checklists, it is possible, for example, that measures that tap more directly into aspects of social-communicative dysfunction may provide greater opportunities for intervention research focused on processes that underlie these areas of difficulty. The ability to identify meaningful change is limited when researchers rely upon change measures that are perhaps too broadly based (e.g., use of diagnostic instruments such as the CARS or the Clinical Global Improvement Scale) or so stringent in their criteria that the ability to identify meaningful change is limited.

The benefits of creating or refining these and other measures of outcome should not be limited to the study of very young children. Measures with reduced likelihood of bias (e.g., measures that can be administered by assessors blind to treatment status) are needed; it is time for the field to move away from studies utilizing measures with known reporter biases, such as parent report. Exploration of outcome measures incorporating state-of-the-art technology and innovations are also needed. Biological measures (e.g., galvanic skin response, eye tracking, event-related potentials, and fMRI data), which hypothetically have less bias, may supplement traditional approaches by focusing on discrete outcomes. Another measurement area that is likely to benefit from technological advances is data collection. Paper and pencil data collection, while appropriate in some instances, is becoming obsolete. Digital collection (e.g., by computer, handheld device, video recording, or web camera) should help reduce error and allow a more valid assessment of behavior across a greater number of variables. The transportability of these devices should also allow data collection and studies to evolve less obtrusively into natural settings (e.g., dinner time in a family's home without a researcher present). Smart phones (e.g., iPhone and Blackberry) also offer new possibilities because data collection applications can be readily purchased and installed. One advancement that would help tremendously would be development of a method of automated data collection, such that a parent or teacher is able to download a stream of video and receive an output on the occurrence of pre-defined behaviors. Creation of such a tool would be a bonus to both parents and researchers alike – i.e., the parents would gain access to data that could be used to monitor changes in their child while researchers would have the potential to gain large amounts of data collected in natural settings. It will be interesting to see which, if any, of these technologies make an impact on our knowledge of the condition.

Treatment Dosage

With the exception of medication studies that have compared different dosages, relatively little attention has been paid to the effects of treatment dose or intensity. For example, a child may be getting a relatively intensive ABA program with or without additional speech–communication, occupational therapy (OT) and physical therapy (PT) interventions of varying durations, which frequently go unreported in research publications. Even when the duration is known, simple metrics for approaching intensity are lacking. Is half an hour of high-quality individual work with a well-trained speech-language pathologist to be equated with 1 h of triadic (two students and one clinician) work or 1 h of individual work with a less-trained paraprofessional? As a result, the field has yet to establish the dosages of treatment recommended for optimal results. Given limited resource allocation, research evaluating (i.e., comparing) different dosages of

treatments and ways in which to increase intervention efficiency should be a priority in the coming decade.

EBP in Schools

Moving a school system into a focus on EBP presents many challenges. There is already a significant gap between what is known and shown to be effective in more structured and controlled settings (clinics or research-based interventions) and what can be readily implemented in other, often more complex, settings such as schools. Complexities in schools arise for many reasons (e.g., different disciplinary traditions and language, the variable research base of interventions, the need to develop truly individualized programs). Specific interventions may be implemented by members of diverse disciplines with varying degrees of training, knowledge, and commitment to approaches adopted by the IEP team. The individual often most intimately involved with the child, e.g., the paraprofessional or aide, may have the least formal training of all those involved. In addition, there can be, and often are, legitimate debates about the degree to which an approach can be regarded as evidence-based. All these issues can make it difficult to find common ground for discussion and program development.

With the increased emphasis on integration of EBPs into both schools and professional practice, several aspects of current treatment trends will continue to present challenges. No single intervention meets all of the needs of children with ASD at all points in their development and so most programs rely upon multiple, and sometimes overlapping, intervention modalities and targets. As noted previously, it is not unusual for children with autism to exhibit a range of problems, some of which present more pressing needs for intervention than others; for example, prioritizing self-injurious behavior, high levels of off-task behavior, or bolting may make considerable sense in real-world settings even as teachers and other professionals also consider what behaviors are desired. For more cognitively able individuals, additional considerations may arise, e.g., when a child or adolescent complains of feelings of anxiety or depression or has major attentional difficulties. Typically, educational programming will continue even when new behavioral, pharmacological, or other strategies are put into place. Finally, many parents employ alternative treatments or treatments with minimal empirical evidence without notifying school personnel. As a result of these issues, it is very common for multiple treatments to be used at one time, thus greatly complicating the task of disentangling cause–effect relationships.

The increased awareness of new methods for intervention and the documentation of approaches shown to be effective (at least for some individuals in some circumstances and in some situations) have led to a marked increase in knowledge of intervention approaches. As a result, some school districts have often adopted one model program over others as "their" program for children with autism, e.g., ABA, TEACCH, or developmental models. On the one hand, this can help to target training and increase consistency and treatment fidelity. On the other hand, the reliance on a single approach discourages the flexibility needed to truly individualize an educational intervention program, as federal law mandates. Considerable variation also exists between, and sometimes even within, states. In states such as Delaware (see Chap. 13), there are comprehensive statewide programs and considerable support from state departments of education to local districts. In most other states, services and support may vary considerably between (and even within) small towns, because of the high degree of independence

that local school districts traditionally enjoy in setting policy, adjusting curricula, and allocating resources, despite the umbrella offered by IDEA (Public Law 108–446). Though this variability may appear to offer a natural experiment, this potential has yet to be exploited.

The explicit emphasis on individualized programming under IDEA (Public Law 108–446) should not be perceived as an obstacle to applying EBP and treatment principles. Indeed, discussions regarding the strength and relevance of specific EBP approaches should guide the discussion of possible risks, benefits and costs. As discussed in Chap. 13, this level of individualization presumes the existence of second-order EBP, with evidence for the effectiveness of specific methods targeting specific skills or behaviors in individuals with specific characteristics. As in implementing EBP in mental-health settings, precise individualization requires that the team consider all relevant factors in the child, e.g., comorbid conditions that may particularly inform treatment choice. Careful diagnostic assessment (Klin et al. 2005) should be the starting point for treatment planning, with an identification of areas of strength and weakness relevant to intervention planning. Including family members in the planning process and on a continuous, ongoing basis is important for many reasons, including facilitating generalization (one of the main obstacles for children with problems on the autism spectrum). The use of EBP may also clarify when treatments (e.g., expensive alternative approaches) are not justified (Wong and Smith 2006).

FINAL THOUGHTS

Regardless of whether the increased prevalence of autism reflects an increased awareness of broader spectrum or changes to diagnostic criteria (Fombonne 2005), the impact of this increase is unmistakable: More children are being diagnosed, more families are requesting services, and more professionals are seeking guidance and training in the best available methodologies. With the estimated lifetime cost for the care of an individual with autism estimated to be between $1,700,000 (Landrigan et al. 2002) and $4,000,000 (Järbrink and Knapp 2001), the economic impact of this increase is also unmistakable. A recent analysis by Mandell et al. (2006) underscored this impact, demonstrating that children with ASD had Medicaid-reimbursed expenditures 9 times higher than other Medicaid-eligible children and 3.5 times greater than individuals receiving Medicaid who had a different developmental delay. In this light, the potential benefits of early intervention become even more striking. Children may become more likely to move into independent and semi-independent, even tax-generating, occupations and living situations as adults (Howlin 2005). Use of proven, effective EBPs can help to minimize the impact and to ensure that resources are being maximized. Unfortunately, translating EBP from research to community settings, such as homes and schools, is much easier said than done, especially given the challenges unique to autism, and so perhaps, the paucity of data on effectiveness in such contexts is not surprising.

However, evidence-based practices often confront a number of objections (see the work of Hamilton (2007) for a discussion). These include a wide range of design issues as discussed in this book: the limited data base of well-controlled treatment studies, the tendency to focus on highly selected samples, the difficulties of applying methods developed from research studies in "real-world" settings (the efficacy–effectiveness debate), potential bias in areas where research is conducted or how it is conducted, and failure to include appropriate numbers of some

groups in controlled trials (e.g., based on minority or gender status). Given some of the design challenges associated with RCTs (i.e., ethical difficulties, higher costs, etc.), we are encouraged by the increasing recognition that EBP is not demonstrated solely by RCTs but can be achieved by combining evidence across RCTs, SSEDs, and quasi-experimental group designs. The problem of positive publication bias (i.e., that it is easier for a positive outcome to be published while negative outcome studies have a much harder time surviving the rigorous peer review process) also cannot be ignored (Borenstein et al. 2009). When negative outcome studies are published, which is more the exception than the rule, the generally higher standards set for the publication of negative outcomes may lead to over-estimates of the true benefits of treatment and the increasing number of pay-to-publish journals will add to the confusion. For psychopharmacology trials, a host of ethical issues present serious challenges as well. Finally, we must combat the many misconceptions surrounding EBP: While they may appear initially to limit treatment options, they should, when informed by other aspects of the clinical process, broaden treatment perspectives and improve outcomes (Sackett et al. 1996).

In this book, we have sought to interpret and summarize important findings arising from outcome research involving individuals with autism. Notwithstanding the many challenges outlined above, this book is a testament to the considerable progress made in the last decade in helping to establish an increasingly strong basis for evidence-based treatments in autism. It is clear that the emphasis on early intervention and use of more effective practices has been associated with better overall outcomes. This in turn has presented new challenges, e.g., in supporting more able children as they move into adolescence and then adulthood. Although the pace of treatment studies has not, for many reasons, kept pace with the more general expansion of research into autism, the growing number and sophistication of studies provides good reason to hope that the coming decade will witness a major expansion in our knowledge of the best ways to intervene in autism.

REFERENCES

Aman, M. G., McDougle, C. J., Scahill, L., Handen, B., Arnold, L. E., Johnson, C., et al. (2009). Medication and parent training in children with pervasive developmental disorders and serious behavioral problems: Results from a randomized clinical trial. *Journal of the American Academy of Child and Adolescent Psychiatry*, 48(12), 1143–1154.

APA. (1994). *Diagnostic and statistical manual of mental disorders* (4th ed.). Washington: American Psychiatric Association.

Arick, J. R., Krug, D. A., Loos, L., & Falco, R. (2005). School-based programs. In F. R. Volkmar, R. Paul, A. Klin, & D. J. Cohen (Eds.), *Handbook of autism and pervasive developmental disorders* (3rd ed., pp. 1003–1028). Hoboken: Wiley.

Baranek, G. T., Foster, L. G., & Berkson, G. (1997a). Sensory defensiveness in persons with developmental disabilities. *Occupational Therapy Journal of Research*, 17, 173–185.

Baranek, G. T., Foster, L. G., & Berkson, G. (1997b). Tactile defensiveness and stereotyped behaviors. *American Journal of Occupational Therapy*, 51, 91–95.

Baranek, G. T., Parham, D., & Bodfish, J. W. (2005). Sensory and motor features in autism: Assessment and intervention. In F. R. Volkmar, R. Paul, A. Klin, & D. J. Cohen (Eds.), *Handbook of autism and pervasive developmental disorders* (3rd ed., pp. 831–857). Hoboken: Wiley.

Baranek, G. T., David, F. J., Poe, M. D., Stone, W. L., & Watson, L. R. (2006). Sensory experiences questionnaire: Discriminating sensory features in young children with autism, developmental delays, and typical development. *Journal of Child Psychology and Psychiatry, and Allied Disciplines*, 47(6), 591–601.

Barkham, M., & Mellor-Clark, J. (2003). Bridging evidence-based practice and practice-based evidence: Developing a rigorous and relevant knowledge for the psychological therapies. *Clinical Psychology and Psychotherapy*, 10, 319–327.

Bondy, A. S., & Frost, L. A. (2001). The picture exchange communication system. *Behavior Modification*, 25(5), 725–744.

Borenstein, M., Hedges, L. V., Higgins, J. P. T., & Rothstein, H. R. (2009). *Introduction to meta-analysis*. West Sussex: Wiley.

Campbell, M., Anderson, L., & Cohen, I. (1982). Haloperidol in autistic children: Effects on learning, behavior, and abnormal involuntary movements. *Psychopharmacology Bulletin*, 18(1), 110–111.

Cascella, P. W., & Colella, C. S. (2004). Knowledge of autism spectrum disorders among Connecticut school speech-language pathologists. *Focus on Autism and Other Developmental Disabilities*, 19, 245–252.

Charlop-Christy, M. H., Carpenter, M., Le, L., LeBlanc, L. A., & Kellet, K. (2002). Using the picture exchange communication system (PECS) with children with autism: Assessment of PECS acquisition, speech, social-communicative behavior, and problem behavior. *Journal of Applied Behavior Analysis*, 35(3), 213–231.

Chawarska, K., Klin, A., & Volkmar, F. R. (Eds.). (2008). *Autism spectrum disorders in infants and toddlers: Diagnosis, assessment, and treatment*. New York: Guilford.

Chorpita, B. F. (2003). The frontier of evidence-based practice. In A. E. Kazdin & J. R. Weisz (Eds.), *Evidence-based psychotherapies for children and adolescents* (pp. 42–59). New York: Guilford.

Cox, A. L., Gast, D. L., Luscre, D., & Ayres, K. M. (2009). The effects of weighted vests on appropriate in-seat behaviors of elementary-age students with autism and severe to profound intellectual disabilities. *Focus on Autism and Other Developmental Disabilities*, 24(1), 17–26.

Dugan, E., Kamps, D., et al. (1995). Effects of cooperative learning groups during social studies for students with autism and fourth-grade peers. *Journal of Applied Behavior Analysis*, 28(2), 175–188.

Eldevik, S., Hastings, R. P., Hughes, J. C., Jahr, E., Eikeseth, S., & Cross, S. (2009). Meta-analysis of early intensive behavioral intervention for children with autism. *Journal of Clinical Child and Adolescent Psychology*, 38(3), 439–450.

Ferlie, E. (2005). Conclusion: From evidence to actionable knowledge? In S. Dopson & L. Fitzgerald (Eds.), *Knowledge to action? Evidence-based health care in context* (pp. 182–197). Oxford: Oxford University Press.

Fombonne, E. (2005). Epidemiological studies of pervasive developmental disorders. In F. R. Volkmar, R. Paul, A. Klin, & D. J. Cohen (Eds.), *Handbook of autism and pervasive developmental disorders* (3rd ed., pp. 42–69). Hoboken: Wiley.

Gilbody, S. M., Song, F., Eastwood, A. J., & Sutton, A. (2000). The causes, consequences and detection of publication bias in psychiatry. *Acta Psychiatry Scandinavica, 102,* 241–249.

Goldstein, H. (2000). Commentary: Interventions to facilitate auditory, visual, and motor integration: "Show me the data". *Journal of Autism and Developmental Disorders, 30*(5), 423–425.

Goldstein, H., Kaczmarek, L., Pennington, R., & Shafer, K. (1992). Peer-mediated intervention: Attending to, commenting on, and acknowledging the behavior of preschoolers with autism. *Journal of Applied Behavior Analysis, 25,* 289–305.

Goldstein, H., Wickstrom, S., et al. (1988). Effects of sociodramatic play training on social and communication intervention. *Education and Treatment of Children, 11,* 97–117.

Green, V. A., Pitusch, K. A., Itchon, J., Choi, A., O'Reilly, M., & Sigafoos, J. (2006). Internet survey of treatments used by parents of children with autism. *Research in Developmental Disabilities, 27,* 70–84.

Greenspan, S., & Wieder, S. (2009). *Engaging autism: Using the Floortime approach to help children relate, communicate, and think.* Cambridge: Da Capo Lifelong Books.

Guyatt, G.H., Haynes, R. B., Jaeschke, R. Z., Cook, D. J., Green, L., Naylor, C. D., Wilson, M. C., & Richardson, W. S. (2000). Users guides to the medical literature XXV. Evidence-based medicine: Principle for applying the users guides to patient care. *Journal of the American Medical Association, 284,* 1290–1296.

Hamilton, J. (2007). Evidence-based practice as a conceptual framework. In A. Martin & F. R. Volkmar (Eds.), *Lewis' child and adolescent psychiatry: A comprehensive approach* (4th ed., pp. 124–140). Philadelphia: Wolters Kluwer.

Handleman, J. S., Harris, S. L., & Martins, M. P. (2005). Helping children with autism enter the mainstream. In D. J. Cohen & F. R. Volkmar (Eds.), *Handbook of autism and pervasive developmental disorders* (2nd ed., pp. 1029–1042). New York: Wiley.

Hanson, E., Kalish, L. A., Bunce, E., Curtis, C., McDaniel, S., et al. (2007). Use of complementary and alternative medicine among children diagnosed with autism spectrum disorder. *Journal of Autism and Developmental Disorders, 37*(4), 628–636.

Hatcher, S., Butler, R., & Oakley-Browne, M. (2005). *Evidence-based mental health care.* Edinburgh: Elsevier Churchill Livingstone.

Hawley, K. M., & Weisz, J. R. (2002). Increasing the relevance of evidence-based treatment review to practitioners and consumers. *Clinical Psychology: Science and Practice, 9,* 225–230.

Hess, K. L., Morrier, M. J., Heflin, L. J., & Ivey, M. L. (2008). Autism treatment survey: Services received by children with autism spectrum disorders in public school classrooms. *Journal of Autism and Developmental Disorders, 38,* 961–971.

Howlin, P. (2005). Outcome in autism spectrum disorders. In F. R. Volkmar, R. Paul, A. Klin, & D. J. Cohen (Eds.), *Handbook of autism and pervasive developmental disorders* (3rd ed., pp. 201–222). Hoboken: Wiley.

Hyman, S. L., & Levy, S. E. (2005). Novel therapies in developmental disabilities: Hope, reason, and evidence. *Mental Retardation and Developmental Disabilities Research Reviews, 11*(2), 107–109.

Järbrink, K., & Knapp, M. (2001). The economic impact of autism in Britain. *Autism, 5,* 7–22.

Kanner, L. (1943). Autistic disturbances of affective contact. *Nervous Child, 2,* 217–250.

Kazdin, A. E. (2001). Bridging the enormous gaps of theory with therapy research and practice. *Journal of Clinical Child Psychology, 30,* 59–66.

Kennedy, T., Regehr, G., Rosenfield, J., Robers, S. W., & Lingard, L. (2004). Exploring the gap between knowledge and behavior: A qualitative study of clinician action following an educational intervention. *Academic Medicine, 79,* 386–393.

Kern, J. K., Trivedi, M. H., Grannemann, B. D., Garver, C. R., Johnson, D. G., et al. (2007). Sensory correlations in autism. *Autism, 11*(2), 123–134.

King, B. H., Hollander, E., Sikich, L., McCracken, J. T., Scahill, L., et al. (2009). Lack of efficacy of citalopram in children with autism spectrum disorders and high levels of repetitive behavior: Citalopram ineffective in children with autism. *Archives of General Psychiatry, 66*(6), 583–590.

Klin, A., Jones, W., Schultz, R., Volkmar, F., & Cohen, D. (2002a). Defining and quantifying the social phenotype in autism. *American Journal of Psychiatry, 159,* 895–908.

Klin, A., Jones, W., Schultz, R., Volkmar, F., & Cohen, D. (2002b). Visual fixation patterns during viewing of naturalistic social situations as predictors of social competence in individuals with autism. *Archives of General Psychiatry, 59,* 809–816.

Klin, A., McPartland, J., and Volkmar, F.R. (in press). *Asperger syndrome* (2nd ed.). New York: Guilford.

Klin, A., Saulnier, C., Tsatsanis, K., & Volkmar, F. R. (2005). Clinical evaluation in autism spectrum disorders: Psychological assessment within a transdisciplinary framework. In F. R. Volkmar, R. Paul, A. Klin, & D. J. Cohen (Eds.), *Handbook of autism and pervasive developmental disorders* (3rd ed., pp. 772–798). Hoboken: Wiley.

Klin, A., Saulnier, C. A., Sparrow, S. S., Cicchetti, D. V., Volkmar, F. R., et al. (2007). Social and communication abilities and disabilities in higher functioning individuals with autism spectrum disorders: The Vineland and the ADOS. *Journal of Autism and Developmental Disorders*, *37*(4), 748–759.

Koegel, L. (2000). Interventions to facilitate communication in autism. *Journal of Autism and Developmental Disorders*, *30*, 383–391.

Koegel, L. K., & Koegel, R. L. (1995). Motivating communication in children with autism. In E. Schopler & G. B. Mesibov (Eds.), *Learning and cognition in autism* (pp. 73–87). New York: Plenum.

Koegel, R. L., & Koegel, L. K. (Eds.). (2006). *Pivotal response treatments for autism: Communication, social, and academic development*. Baltimore: Brookes.

Krasny, L., Williams, B. J., Provencal, S., & Ozonoff, S. (2003). Social skills interventions for the autism spectrum: Essential ingredients and a model curriculum. *Child and Adolescent Psychiatric Clinics of North America*, *12*(1), 107–122.

Kratochwill, T. R., & Stoiber, K. C. (2002). Evidence-based interventions in school psychology: Conceptual foundations of the procedural and coding manual of division 16 and the society for the study of school psychology task force. *School Psychology Quarterly*, *17*, 341–389.

Landrigan, P. J., Schechter, C. B., Lipton, J. M., Fahs, M. C., & Schwartz, J. (2002). Environmental pollutants and disease in American children: Estimates of morbidity, mortality, and costs for lead poisoning, asthma, cancer, and developmental disabilities. *Environmental Health Perspectives*, *110*, 721–728.

Lerman, D. C., Vorndran, C. M., Addison, L., & Kuhn, S. C. (2004). Preparing teachers in evidence-based practices for young children with autism. *School Psychology Review*, *33*, 510–526.

Levy, S., & Hyman, S. (2005). Novel treatments for autistic spectrum disorders. *Mental Retardation and Developmental Disabilities Research Reviews*, *11*, 131–142.

Lord, C., Rutter, M., DiLavore, P. C., & Lisi, S. (1999). *Autism diagnostic observation schedule*. Los Angeles: Western Psychological Services.

Lord, C., Rutter, M., DiLavore, P. C., & Lisi, S. (2008). *Autism diagnostic observation schedule: Toddler module*. Los Angeles: Western Psychological Services.

Lovaas, O. I. (1987). Behavioral treatment and normal educational and intellectual functioning in young autistic children. *Journal of Consulting and Clinical Psychology*, *55*(1), 3–9.

Mandell, D. S., Cao, J., Ittenbach, R., & Pinto-Martin, J. (2006). Medicaid expenditures for children with autistic spectrum disorders: 1994 to 1999. *Journal of Autism and Developmental Disorders*, *36*, 475–485.

Mandell, D. S., Morales, K. H., Marcus, S. C., Stahmer, A. C., Doshi, J., & Polsky, D. E. (2008). Psychotropic medication use among Medicaid-enrolled children with autism spectrum disorders. *Pediatrics*, *121*(3), e441–e448.

Matson, J. L., Matson, M. L., & Rivet, T. T. (2007). Social-skills treatments for children with autism spectrum disorders. *Behavior Modification*, *31*, 682–707.

McBride, B. J., & Schwartz, I. S. (2003). Effects of teaching early interventions to use discrete trial during ongoing classroom activities. *Topics in Early Childhood Special Education*, *23*, 5–17.

McGee, G. G., Krantz, P. J., Mason, D., & McClannahan, L. E. (1983). A modified incidental-teaching procedure for autistic youth: Acquisition and generalization of receptive object labels. *Journal of Applied Behavior Analysis*, *16*(3), 329–338.

Mesibov, G. B., Shea, V., & Schopler, E. (2005). *The TEACCH approach to autism spectrum disorders*. New York: Springer.

Montes, G., & Halterman, J. S. (2007). Bullying among children with autism and the influence of comorbidity with ADHD: A population-based study. *Ambulatory Pediatrics*, *7*(3), 253–257.

National Research Council. (2001). *Educating young children with autism*. Washington: National Academy Press.

Nelson, T. D., & Steele, R. G. (2007). Predictors of practitioner self-reported use of evidence-based practices: Practitioner training, clinical setting, and attitudes toward research. *Administration and Policy in Mental Health and Mental Health Services Research*, *34*, 319–330.

Odom, S., Brown, W., Frey, T., Karasu, N., Smith-Cantor, L., & Strain, P. (2003). Evidence-based practice for young children with autism: Contributions of single-subject research. *Focus on Autism and Other Developmental Disabilities*, *10*, 166–175.

Olley, J. G. (2005). Curriculum and classroom structure. In F. R. Volkmar, R. Paul, A. Klin, & D. J. Cohen (Eds.), *Handbook of autism and pervasive developmental disorders* (3rd ed., pp. 863–881). Hoboken: Wiley.

Oswald, D. P., & Sonenklar, N. A. (2007). Medication use among children with autism spectrum disorders. *Journal of Child and Adolescent Psychopharmacology*, *17*(3), 348–55.

Pagoto, S. L., Spring, B., Coups, E. J., Mulvaney, S., Coutu, M. F., & Ozakinci, G. (2007). Barriers and facilitators of evidence-based practice perceived by behavioral science professionals. *Journal of Clinical Psychology, 63*, 695–705.

Paul, R. (2003). Promoting social communication in high functioning individuals with autistic spectrum disorders. *Child and Adolescent Psychiatric Clinics of North America, 12*(1), 87–106. vi–vii.

Pierce, K., & Schreibman, L. (1997). Multiple peer use of pivotal response training to increase social behaviors of classmates with autism: Results from trained and untrained peers. *Journal of Applied Behavior Analysis, 30*, 157–160.

Prizant, B. M., Wetherby, A. M., Rubin, E., Laurent, A. C., & Rydall, P. (2004). *The SCERTS model: Enhancing communication and socioemotional abilities of children with autism spectrum disorder*. Baltimore: Brookes.

Public Law 108–446:§ 118 Stat. 2647. (2004). Individuals with disabilities education improvement act of 2004.

Reichow, B., & Volkmar, F. R. (2010a). Best-evidence synthesis of social skills interventions for individuals with autism spectrum disorders. *Journal of Autism and Developmental Disorders, 40*, 149–166.

Reichow, B., & Volkmar, F. R. (2010b). *State of the science for social skills group interventions*. New Haven: Presentation at Yale University.

Reichow, B., & Wolery, M. (2009). Comprehensive synthesis of early intensive behavioral interventions for young children with autism based on the UCLA young autism project model. *Journal of Autism and Developmental Disorders, 39*, 23–41.

Reichow, B., Barton, E. E., Volkmar, F. R., and Cicchetti, D. V. (2007). *The status of research on interventions for young children with autism spectrum disorders*. Poster presented at the International Meeting for Autism Research, May, Seattle, WA.

Reichow, B., Barton, E. E., Neeley, J., Good, L., & Wolery, M. (2010). Effects of wearing a weighted vest on engagement in young children with developmental disabilities. *Focus on Autism and Other Developmental Disabilities, 25*(1), 3–11.

Rogers, S. J., & Dawson, G. (2010). *Early start Denver model for young children with autism: Promoting language, learning, and engagement*. New York: Guilford.

Rogers, S. J., & Lewis, H. (1988). An effective day treatment model for young children with pervasive developmental disorders. *Journal of the American Academy of Child and Adolescent Psychiatry, 28*, 207–214.

Rogers, S. J., & Ozonoff, S. (2005a). Annotation: What do we know about sensory dysfunction in autism? A critical review of the empirical evidence. *Journal of Child Psychology and Psychiatry, and Allied Disciplines, 46*(12), 1255–1268.

Rogers, S. J., & Ozonoff, S. (2005b). Behavioral, educational, and developmental treatments for autism. In S. Moldin & J. Rubenstein (Eds.), *Understanding autism: From basic neuroscience to treatment* (pp. 443–474). Boca Raton: CRC Press.

Rogers, S. J., Hall, T., Osaki, D., Reaven, J., & Herbison, J. (2000). The Denver model: A comprehensive, integrated educational approach to young children with autism and their families. In J. S. Handleman & S. L. Harris (Eds.), *Preschool education programs for children with autism* (2nd ed., pp. 95–133). Austin: Pro-Ed.

RUPP. (2002). Risperidone in children with autism and serious behavioral problems. Research units on pediatric psychopharmacology (RUPP) autism network. *New England Journal of Medicine, 347*(5), 314–321.

Rutter, M., Le Couteur, A., & Lord, C. (2005). *Autism diagnostic interview: Revised*. Los Angeles: Western Psychological Services.

Sackett, D. L., Rosenberg, W. M. C., Gray, J. A. M., Haynes, R. B., & Richardson, W. S. (1996). Evidence-based medicine: What it is and what it isn't. *British Medical Journal, 312*, 71–72.

Sandler, A. (2005). Placebo effects in developmental disabilities: Implications for research and practice. *Mental Retardation and Developmental Disabilities Research Reviews, 11*, 164–170.

Sansosti, F. J., & Powell-Smith, K. A. (2008). Using computer-presented social stories and video models to increase the social communication skills of children with high-functioning autism spectrum disorders. *Journal of Positive Behavior Interventions, 10*(3), 162–178.

Saulnier, C. A., & Klin, A. (2007). Brief report: Social and communication abilities and disabilities in higher functioning individuals with autism and Asperger syndrome. *Journal of Autism and Developmental Disorders, 37*, 788–793.

Scahill, L., Aman, M., McDougle, C., Arnold, L., McCracken, J., & Handen, B. (2009). Trial design challenges when combining medication and parent training in children with pervasive developmental disorders. *Journal of Autism and Developmental Disorders, 39*(5), 720–729.

Scattone, D. (2008). Enhancing the conversation skills of a boy with Asperger's disorder through social stories and video modeling. *Journal of Autism and Developmental Disorders, 38*, 395–400.

Scheuermann, B., Webber, J., Boutot, E. A., & Goodwin, M. (2003). Problems with personnel preparation in autism spectrum disorders. *Focus on Autism and Developmental Disabilities, 18*, 197–206.

Schopler, E. (1997). Implementation of TEACCH philosophy. In D. J. Cohen & F. R. Volkmar (Eds.), *Handbook of autism and pervasive developmental disorders* (2nd ed., pp. 767–795). New York: Wiley.

Schopler, E., Reichler, R. J., & Renner, B. R. (1986). *The childhood autism rating scale (CARS)*. Los Angeles: Western Psychological Services.

Schreibman, L., & Pierce, K. (1993). Achieving greater generalisation of treatment effects in children with autism: Pivotal response training and self management. *The Clinical Psychologist, 46*, 184–191.

Shapiro, A. K. (2000). *The powerful placebo: From ancient priest to modern physician*. Baltimore: John Hopkins University Press.

Siegel, B., Vukicevic, J., Elliot, G. R., & Kraemer, H. C. (1989). The use of signal detection theory to assess DSM-III-R criteria for autistic disorder. *Journal of the American Academy of Child and Adolescent Psychiatry, 28*(4), 542–548.

Smith, T., Scahill, L., Dawson, G., Lord, C., Odom, S., et al. (2007). Designing research studies onpsychosocial interventions in autism. *Journal of Autism and Developmental Disorders, 37*, 354–366

Smith, T., Groen, A. D., & Wynn, J. W. (2000). Randomized trial of intensive early intervention for children with pervasive developmental disorder. *American Journal on Mental Retardation, 105*(4), 269–285.

Stahmer, A. C., Collings, N. M., & Palinkas, L. A. (2005). Early intervention practices for children with autism: Descriptions from community providers. *Focus on Autism and Other Developmental Disabilities, 20*, 66–79.

Strain, P. S., & Hoyson, M. (2000). The need for longitudinal, intensive social skill intervention: LEAP follow-up outcomes for children with autism. *Topics in Early Childhood Special Education, 20*(2), 116–122.

Strain, P. S., & Schwartz, I. (2001). ABA and the development of meaningful social relations for young children with autism. *Focus on Autism and Other Developmental Disabilities, 16*(2), 120–128.

Sundberg, M. L., & Michael, J. (2001). The benefits of Skinner's analysis of verbal behavior for children with autism. *Behavior Modification, 25*(5), 698–724.

Thiemann, K. S., & Goldstein, H. (2004). Effects of peer tutoring and written text cueing on social communication of school-age children with pervasive developmental disorder. *Journal of Speech, Language, and Hearing Research, 47*, 126–144.

Upton, D., & Upton, P. (2006). Knowledge and use of evidence-based practice by allied health and health science professionals in the United Kingdom. *Journal of Allied Health, 35*(3), 127–133.

Volkmar, F. (in press). Looking back and moving forward: A decade of research on autism. *Journal of Child Psychology and Psychiatry*.

Volkmar, F. R., & Wiesner, L. A. (2009). *A practical guide to autism*. Hoboken: Wiley.

Volkmar, F. R., State, M., & Klin, A. (2009). Autism and autism spectrum disorders: Diagnostic issues for the coming decade. *Journal of Child Psychology and Psychiatry, 50*(1–2), 108–115.

Volkmar, F., Klin, A., Siegel, B., Szatmari, P., Lord, C., et al. (1994). Field trial for autistic disorder in DSM-IV. *American Journal of Psychiatry, 151*, 1361–1367.

Weisz, J., & Jensen, P. (1999). Efficacy and effectiveness of child and adolescent psychotherapy and pharmacotherapy. *Mental Health Services Research, 1*, 125–157.

Wetherby, A. M., Prizant, B. M., & Schuler, A. L. (2000). Understanding the nature of communication and language impairments. In A. M. Wetherby & B. M. Prizant (Eds.), *Autism spectrum disorders: A transactional developmental perspective* (pp. 109–141). Baltimore: Brooks.

Wing, L., & Gould, J. (1979). Severe impairments of social interaction and associated abnormalities in children: Epidemiology and classification. *Journal of Autism and Developmental Disorders, 9*(1), 11–29.

Wolery, M., & Garfinkle, A. N. (2002). Measures in intervention research with young children who have autism. *Journal of Autism and Developmental Disorders, 32*, 463–478.

Wong, H. H., & Smith, R. G. (2006). Patterns of complementary and alternative medical therapy use in children diagnosed with autism spectrum disorders. *Journal of Autism and Developmental Disorders, 36*(7), 901–909.

World Health Organization. (1992). *International classification of diseases and related health problems* (10th ed.). Geneva: Switzerland.

Yoder, P., & Layton, T. L. (1988). Speech following sign language training in autistic children with minimal verbal language. *Journal of Autism and Developmental Disorders, 18*(2), 217–229.

Yoder, P. J., & Stone, W. L. (2006a). Randomized comparison of two communication interventions for preschoolers with autism spectrum disorders. *Journal of Consulting and Clinical Psychology, 74*(3), 426–435.

Yoder, P., & Stone, W. L. (2006b). A randomized comparison of the effect of two prelinguistic communication interventions on the acquisition of spoken communication in preschoolers with ASD. *Journal of Speech, Language, and Hearing Research, 49,* 698–711.

APPENDIX: RESEARCH DATABASES FOR INFORMATION ON AUTISM TREATMENTS

Database	Brief description	Types of source	Advantages	Disadvantages
PsycINFO http://www.apa.org/pubs/databases/psycinfo	This database is managed by the American Psychological Association and has over 2.8 million records.	• Journal articles • Books • Book chapters • Theses • Dissertations	• Good source for information on treatments • Regularly updated	• Need subscription to see search results • Some sources not readily available (e.g., theses and dissertations) • Might not cover all psychopharmacologic treatments
Education Resources Information Center (ERIC) http://www.eric.ed.gov	This database is managed by the Institute for Education Sciences (IES) of the US Department of Education and contains over 1.3 million bibliographic records.	• Journal articles • Books • Research syntheses, including reports from the What Works Clearinghouse • Conference papers • Technical reports • Policy papers • Theses • Dissertations	• Links to many full-text documents • Regularly updated • Contains unpublished material (i.e., gray literature)	• Focus on education is narrow – most journal articles and books are found in PsycINFO • Gray literature might not be of same quality as published materials
PubMed http://www.ncbi.nlm.nih.gov/pubmed	This database is maintained by the National Center for Biotechnology Information at the US National Library of Medicine, located at the National Institutes of Health (NIH), and comprises more than 19 million citations.	• Journal articles	• Uses MeSH classification system, which can provide greater specificity • Provides list of related articles • Links to some full-text articles from PubMed Central or publisher	• MeSH classification system might not be familiar to users • Limited to journal articles • Many social science journals are not indexed, thus, it will miss many relevant articles, especially concerning psycho-educational treatments

| Cochrane Library http://www.thecochranelibrary.com | The Cochrane Database of Systematic Reviews contains the systematic reviews conducted for the Cochrane Collaboration and other review organizations. Note, most resources that can be located using the Cochrane Library are reviews. | • Cochrane reviews
• Database of abstracts of reviews of effects
• Cochrane central register of controlled trials
• Cochrane methodology register
• Health technology assessment database
• NHS economic evaluation
• Database | • No subscription needed to perform search and the summaries and abstracts are provided without fee
• Reviews undergo rigorous process and typically have good methods | • Subscription required to view full reviews – some countries, states, or provinces have agreements to provide access
• Few reviews regarding autism, mostly limited to studies using RCTs |

INDEX

A

AAC. *See* Augmentative alternative communication
ABA. *See* Applied behavior analysis
Aberrant Behavior Checklist (ABC) rating scale, 233, 234, 238, 240–241
Accardo, P.J., 11
Acquisto, J., 70
Adams, C., 97, 106
Adams, J.B., 282
Adams, L.A., 81, 84, 149
Adaptive behavior
  definition, ASD, 297–299
  measurement, 303
  treatment, 300–303
  Vineland-II, 307–308
Adaptive daily living skills (ADLs), 300
Addison, L.R., 75, 130
Adelinis, J., 134
ADHD. *See* Attention deficit hyperactivity disorder
ADI-R. *See* Autism diagnostic interview-revised
Adkins, T., 349, 350, 352
Adler, T., 186, 187
ADLs. *See* Adaptive daily living skills
ADOS. *See* Autism diagnostic observation schedule
ADOS-T. *See* Autism diagnostic observation schedule-Toddler
Ahlsen, E., 139
Aimonovitch, M.C., 283
Akullian, J., 175, 177
Alazetta, L., 119
Alberto, P.A., 66
Aldred, C., 97, 106
Allen, E.M., 93
Allen, S., 285, 286
Alter, P., 135
Aman, M.G., 241, 284
Amerine-Dickens, M., 103
Amminger, G.P., 278, 283
Andersen, I.M., 283
Anderson, A., 121
Anderson, S.R., 98
Andrews, S.M., 183, 185
Angermeier, K., 139
Anxiety and mood disturbance. *See* Mental health comorbidities, ASD
Apple, A.L., 155
Applied behavior analysis (ABA)
  antecedent interventions, usage, 357–358

applications, 372
behavioral momentum
  aggressive, disruptive and self-injurious, 76
  practice parameters, 77
  reinforcer quality, 75–76
  stimulus fading effect, evaluation, 75
  task avoidance, 75
  use and effectiveness, 74–75
behavioral programs, 367
data-driven instruction, 318
differential reinforcement of alternative (DRA) behavior, 68
DTI method
  communication skills, 97–105
  Young Autism Program, 96
early intensive behavioral intervention (EIBI), 304, 367–371
evidence-based assessment, 219–221
experimental analysis, behavior, 57–58
functional behavior assessment, 59–67
functional communication training (FCT), 68–71
methodology, intensive training, 317, 375
modules, 318
noncontingent reinforcement (NRC), 70–73
program comparison, 346
SD, 246–247
techniques, 354
verbal behavior, 125–132
Aripiprazole, 237–238
Arnold, L., 241
ASDs. *See* Autism spectrum disorders
ASHA, 11
Ashwal, S., 11
Asperger syndrome (AS)
  ASD sample, 298
  disorder comparison, 299
Aspy, R., 324
Attention deficit hyperactivity disorder (ADHD). *See also* Mental health comorbidities, ASD
  children with PDD, 69, 232
  comorbid diagnosis, 201
  symptoms, 234
  treatment, 216, 232–234
Atwood, K.D., 267, 268
Auditory integration training (AIT)
Auditory interventions, 264–267
Augmentative alternative communication (AAC), 132–141

393

B. Reichow et al. (eds.), *Evidence-Based Practices and Treatments for Children with Autism*,
DOI 10.1007/978-1-4419-6975-0, © Springer Science+Business Media, LLC 2011

The Research Units on Pediatric Psychopharmacology
  (RUPP) autism network
  guanfacine, 234
  risperidone, 238, 240
  trial phases, 232
Richardson, W.S., 11, 13
Richdale, A., 72, 80, 133
Richman, D., 133
Richmond, J.A., 282
Rickert, V.I., 81, 83, 84
Rietveld, W.J., 283
Rimland, B., 280
Risley, T.R., 58, 80
Risperidone
  ABC irritability subscale score, 238, 241
  approval, risperidone, 240
  atypical antipsychotics, 237
  average weight gain, 239
  CARS results, 241
  CGI-I, 241
  conservative dose scheme, 242
  dosing strategy, 240
  drawbacks, haloperidol, 238
  drooling, 239
  HSQ score, 241
  mean dose, risperidone, 238–239
  "negative" symptoms, schizophrenia, 238
  "placebo non-responders," 239
  relapse rate, 239–240
Roberson-Nay, R., 204
Roberts, H., 9
Rocha, M.L., 109, 173
Roche, M., 282
Rodgers, J., 280
Rodriguez-Catter, V., 72
Roeyers, H., 179, 180
Rogers, S.J., 7, 8, 13, 367
Rosenberg, W., 11, 13
Ross, D.E., 128, 134
Rossignol, D.A., 278, 285
Rossignol, L.W., 278, 285
Royer, J., 180, 182
RUPP. *See* Research Units on Pediatric
  Psychopharmacology
Rush, K.S., 69

S
Sackett, D.L., 11, 13
Sahl, R., 234
Sahoo, T., 283
Salets, M., 241
Sallows, G., 102
Sandberg, A., 139
Sandler, A.D., 277
Sandler, R.H., 284
Sansosti, F.J., 150, 151, 157, 183, 184

Sarokoff, R., 145
Sasso, G.M., 64–66, 133, 181
Saulnier, C.A., 298–299
Sautter, R., 130
Savery, D., 280
Scahill, L., 231, 234, 241
Scattone, D., 150, 183, 184
SCERTS. *See* Social Communication, Emotional
  Regulation, Transactional Support
Schaaf, R.C., 245, 247, 249–251
Schaefer, K., 283
Schafer, M.R., 278, 283
Schaller, J.L., 180
Schalock, M., 273, 274
Schepis, M., 136
Scherer, M., 84
Schertz, H.H., 109
Scheuermann, B., 374
Schilling, D.L., 267, 268
Schindler, H., 134
Schizophrenia, 4
Schlosser, R., 139, 140
Schmeidler, J., 284
Schneider, C.K., 278, 284, 285
Schopler, E., 5
Schreck, K.A., 78
Schreibman, L., 106, 109, 130, 172–175, 179, 267,
  268, 300
Schultz, J.R., 175, 178
Schultz, R.T., 234, 376
Schulz, M., 240
Schwartz, I.S., 117, 155, 174–176, 267, 268, 349
Schwenk, H.A., 247
Scotese-Wojtila, L., 282
Scottish Intercollegiate Guidelines Network, 16–17
Scripting and fading
  design studies, 145–146
  event structure, 144
  evidence-based techniques, 144
  social goals, 143
Seeely-York, S., 138
Selective serotonin reuptake inhibitors (SSRIs)
  behavioral features, 373
  repetitive behavior, treatment, 372
  treatments
    benefits, 237
    dose strength, 237
    repetitive behavior, 235
Sensory dysfunction (SD)
  class activities, 246
  interventions, 247–249
Sensory-integrative approach
  Ayres sensory integration approach, 255
  occupational therapy, 250–252
  self-stimulating behaviors, 253
Sensory treatments
  auditory training interventions, 264–266

37971619R10239

Made in the USA
San Bernardino, CA
29 August 2016